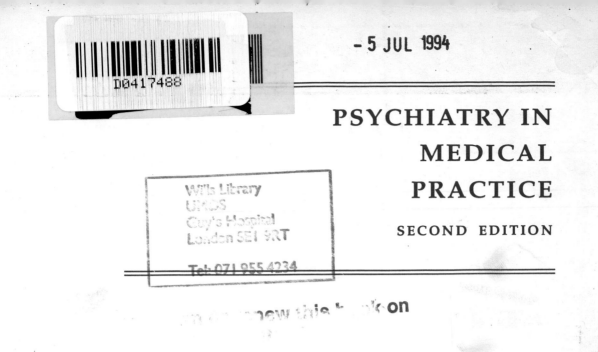

PSYCHIATRY IN MEDICAL PRACTICE

SECOND EDITION

Psychiatry in Medical Practice is an essential textbook for medical students and young doctors in training. This fully updated and revised second edition provides a reliable framework within which to understand the psychiatric illnesses they are likely to encounter in general medical settings. It also gives clear guidelines for good practice.

Important features of the book are:

- a detailed treatment of the medical interview, showing how the doctor's manner influences the patient
- use of the ICD-10 classification throughout, helping the reader become familiar with the new international classification of disease
- a full account of the psychological aspects of AIDS
- a discussion of post-traumatic stress disorders
- clear models and diagnostic criteria for each psychiatric syndrome
- an up-to-date account of the neurochemistry of mental disorders
- an extended description of abnormal illness behaviour
- a chapter specially written for house officers
- an invaluable 'pocket card' summarizing essential information

Written in straightforward and practical language, *Psychiatry in Medical Practice* provides an excellent introduction to the subject for all medical students, and particularly for those who intend to enter psychiatry or general practice.

David Goldberg is Professor of Psychiatry and Director of Research and Development, Institute of Psychiatry, London. **Sidney Benjamin** is Senior Lecturer in Psychiatry at the University of Manchester. **Francis Creed** is Head of the School of Psychiatry and Behavioural Science at the University of Manchester.

PSYCHIATRY IN MEDICAL PRACTICE

SECOND EDITION

David Goldberg

Sidney Benjamin

Francis Creed

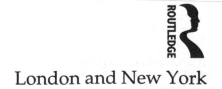

London and New York

First published in 1987 by Tavistock Publications
Reprinted 1989 (twice), 1991 by Routledge
Second edition published in 1994 by Routledge,
11 New Fetter Lane, London EC4P 4EE

Simultaneously published in the USA and Canada by Routledge,
29 West 35th Street, New York, NY 10001

© 1987, 1994 David Goldberg, Sidney Benjamin and Francis Creed

Typeset in Times by LaserScript, Mitcham, Surrey
Printed and bound in Great Britain by Clays Ltd, St. Ives PLC

British Library Cataloguing in Publication Data
A catalogue record for this book is available from the British Library.

Library of Congress Cataloging in Publication Data
Goldberg, David P.
  Psychiatry in medical practice/David Goldberg, Sidney Benjamin,
  and Francis Creed. – 2nd ed.
  p. cm.
  Includes bibliographical references and index.
  1. Psychiatry. I. Benjamin, Sidney. II. Creed, Francis.
  III. Title.
  [DNLM: 1. Mental Disorders. WM 100 G6168p 1994]
  RC454.G588   1994
  616.89 – dc20
  DNLM/DLC   93-32987
                                                       CIP

ISBN 0–415–10611–7 (hbk)
ISBN 0–415–10612–5 (pbk)

CONTENTS

PART 1: THE CLINICAL APPROACH TO THE PATIENT

vi / Contents

PART 3: DISORDERS RELATED TO STAGES OF THE LIFE CYCLE

ILLUSTRATIONS

FIGURES

TABLES

PREFACE TO THE SECOND EDITION

The success of the first edition of what has become known as the 'Red Book' has exceeded our most optimistic expectations: it is read widely in the United Kingdom and Eire, and it has been translated into Bulgarian, Italian, and Chinese. We are indebted to our students, our consultant colleagues, and reviewers of the first edition for many helpful and constructive comments which we have incorporated into this new edition.

The book is written from the standpoint of a medical student setting foot for the first time in a Department of Psychiatry, but we have anticipated needs that a young doctor will have after qualifying, in both primary care and general hospital settings. We have focused on somatic aspects of psychological ill-health, since these are the commonest syndromes that will be encountered in these settings. We give major emphasis to the medical interview, and include a special chapter called 'Psychiatry for the Houseman' which covers important aspects of a doctor's work which are often neglected, since they are not examined in Finals.

Our book is unusual in giving a simple and clear framework in which to understand psychological illness, and showing how it relates to major classifications like ICD-10 and DSM-4. We distinguish between syndromes which are not age-related, and those which are peculiar to stages in the life cycle – since in our view much unnecessary confusion occurs in students' minds unless this distinction is grasped. Our classification does not use either the term 'neurosis' or the term 'hysteria', although we explain what these terms have meant in the past. However, in this edition we have reverted to the older terms 'delirium' and 'dementia' for what we called acute and chronic brain syndromes in our earlier edition.

The sciences that underpin clinical psychiatry are neurochemistry, epidemiology, and psychology: our book gives an up-dated account of all three, as well as emphasizing the relationships which exist between psychological and physical ill-health. Finally, we continue to provide students with a card small enough to fit into pocket or handbag, which will serve to remind them of questions that are useful to ask in everyday clinical work in accident room and general ward.

There have been many changes in the six years since our first edition: the International Classification of Disease has come out in its tenth edition (ICD-10), two new groups of anti-depressants have appeared, a new use has been found for clozapine, and changes have been made to the classification of epilepsy. We have brought our definitions of illnesses into line with ICD-10 guidelines, and given the ICD-10 codes for the various disorders. We now include a thorough treatment of AIDS, and also discuss post-traumatic stress disorders – both of which have achieved greater salience since we wrote our first edition. We also now include a brief treatment of preventive psychiatry in Chapter 1.

In response to a reviewer we have greatly expanded and rethought our treatment of abnormal illness behaviour and somatization (Chapter 15), and we believe that we have made this confusing area much clearer to students – as well as to ourselves! – by so doing.

The arrival in Manchester of Richard Harrington, Alastair Burns, and Nick Tarrier has allowed us to make extensive revisions to the sections on child and adolescent psychiatry, old age psychiatry, and cognitive and behavioural treatments. Neill Simpson has kindly rewritten the chapter on mental retardation. Bill Deakin, Ian Anderson, Danitza Jadresic, Brian Hore, Angus Campbell, Nick Seivewright, and Lynne Webster have all made amendments to parts of the text on our behalf. Substantial sections of text originally written by Elemir Szabadi on psychopharmacology still survive from the first edition, as well as those sections written by David Jolley, Peter Maguire, Frank Margison, Chris Bradshaw, and Michael Wang.

We are grateful to all our colleagues who have helped us in this way, but responsibility for any errors must rest with us as authors.

David Goldberg
Sidney Benjamin
Francis Creed
Manchester, 1993

1 / INTRODUCTION

This book sets out the knowledge you will need to enable you to understand and manage the common psychiatric disorders and psychological problems that you will encounter among your patients in your pre-specialist years. It contains everything you are likely to need for your Finals examination, and then some more. It does not pretend to be a textbook for psychiatrists, but it should provide a useful introduction to the subject even for those students who intend to enter psychiatry or general practice.

THE CLINICAL APPROACH TO THE PATIENT

We start by giving an account of those **interview techniques** that are necessary in order to evaluate the importance of psychological factors in the individual case. We follow with a chapter on the **mental state examination**. Next come chapters dealing with the **classification, aetiology, assessment and treatment** of purely psychiatric disorders, and this section concludes with a chapter explaining how you should set about the **formulation** of an individual patient's problems.

   The chapters in this first part are fundamental to understanding what goes on in a department of psychiatry and are also relevant to work in the general wards. They will help you to elicit data relevant to a proper understanding of a patient's psychological problems, and then go on to make appropriate plans for treatment and management.

SYNDROMES OF PSYCHIATRIC DISORDER

The second part of the book gives a general account of the commoner syndromes of psychiatric disorder. We start with psychological disorders which commonly accompany physical diseases, and include sections on epilepsy and pain. We then start at the top of a *hierarchy* of psychiatric disorders: starting with **organic brain syndromes**, going on to **schizophrenia** and then considering **affective disorders** (disorders of mood). We next consider **maladaptive behaviours** such as alcohol and drug dependence, eating disorders, and obsessional states. We end with a consideration of **abnormal illness behaviour** such as somatization, hypochondriasis, dissociative disorder, and malingering.

The disorders described in this part are defined in terms of **syndromes** or collections of symptoms that commonly occur together, and in this respect they are therefore fairly similar to illnesses you will already have come across in general medicine, such as migraine or asthma.

DISORDERS RELATED TO STAGES OF THE LIFE CYCLE

In the third section we will consider disorders which either take their onset at a particular stage of human development, or are peculiar to a stage of the life cycle. We start with **mental handicap** since this group of disorders reflects problems arising at conception, during intra-uterine development, or from events during or shortly after birth. We then work our way through the life cycle with chapters on **disorders of childhood and adolescence** followed by **sexual and reproductive disorders**, and finally **disorders of old age.**

PSYCHIATRY IN THE GENERAL HOSPITAL AND LEGAL ASPECTS

In the final part we return to the general wards of the hospital with a section on psychiatry for the houseman and legal aspects of the subject.

We will give a **short form of clinical assessment** suitable for use in other parts of the hospital where time for such assessments may be short – we give special emphasis to the detection of three problems: affective illnesses, alcohol-related problems, and the detection of organic cerebral damage. However, we hope that those who have mastered the longer techniques described in Part 1 will readily be able to use these principles in order to make fuller assessments.

EPIDEMIOLOGY

We will be giving you figures for each illness in later chapters: here we will consider overall rates for *any psychiatric diagnosis* in various populations. In a random sample of Londoners one can expect about 6 per cent of men, and 12 per cent of women, to receive a psychiatric diagnosis at any point in time.

The prevalence of such illnesses is considerably higher in populations seeking medical help: general practitioners themselves consider that approximately 14 per cent of the population registered with them will consult them and be considered psychiatrically ill in the course of a year, with just over 5 per cent of these illnesses being new illnesses. If we consider consecutive attenders at general practitioners' surgeries, then somewhere between 25 and 35 per cent of them will meet research criteria for psychiatric illness.

Figures for those admitted to medical wards of general hospitals are approximately similar: recent estimates range between 20 and 40 per cent. Most of these illnesses are states of anxiety or depression, and such disorders are usually an integral part of the various physical disorders for which help is being sought (see Chapters 10 and 11 for a fuller discussion). It is for this reason that an understanding of the assessment and management of psychiatric illness is an essential part of your medical training. Nor should it be thought that most people do not experience such illnesses: one well-conducted study in Sweden showed that a man who survived to the age of 65 had just over a 40 per cent chance of having an episode of a mental illness at some point in his lifetime, while the corresponding figure for a woman was just over 70 per cent!

SKILLS TO BE ACQUIRED

With the help of this book and the opportunity to interview patients, you should aim to acquire the following skills between now and the time that you qualify:

1. To **take a history** from a patient in such a way that you are able to assess the importance of psychological factors.
2. To **make a short assessment of a patient's personality** and to distinguish it from illness.
3. To **carry out a mental state examination** of a patient with a psychiatric illness, and to assess dementia.
4. To **adapt your interview techniques** to special types of clinical interview, for example interviews with children, with old people, with immigrants and those with communication problems.
5. To **write a formulation** of a patient's illness.
6. To **assess an episode of self-poisoning**.
7. To **assess suicidal risk**.
8. To **take a history from a relative**.

KNOWLEDGE OF MANAGEMENT PROCEDURES

By the time that you qualify you should aim to acquire knowledge of the following management procedures. You should aim to cover most of them during your time in the department of psychiatry. It helps a great deal if you have actually seen them carried out, but there is no need for you to have done them yourself.

Medical procedures

1. The management of **delirium tremens.**
2. The management of an **acutely psychotic** patient.
3. **Electroconvulsive treatment.**

Psychological procedures

1. (On the general wards)
   - How to break bad news.
   - Dealing with malignant disease.
   - Helping patients who have had mutilating surgery.
   - Helping the dying patient.
2. (In the paediatric department)
   - How to interview a child.
3. The management of violent behaviour in hospital settings.
4. Emergency procedures under the Mental Health Act.

PREVENTION OF MENTAL DISORDERS

Prevention in medicine is conventionally divided into three types: primary prevention, which aims to prevent the disorder occurring; secondary prevention, which aims to abort the course of a disorder by early detection; and tertiary prevention, which is aimed at treating established cases of illness, and thus reducing prevalence.

Primary prevention includes measures to reduce psychosyndromes associated with head injury by seat belts and safer cars; health education to prevent AIDS by reducing promiscuous sexual contact or by use of appropriate contraceptive techniques; health education to provide clear guidance about safe levels of alcohol ingestion; measures to reduce sexual and physical abuse of children and to reinforce the desirability of providing children with a secure, caring environment and so reducing vulnerability to later anxiety and depression.

Secondary prevention is best directed at high-risk groups: those who have experienced mutilating surgery, young widows, and women who have experienced previous episodes of puerperal depression are all examples of such groups. A broader group of people at high risk of depressive illness would be working-class women with young children at home and no intimate confidante.

Tertiary prevention can best be directed at those with mental disorders that will otherwise be long-term and will be associated with great disability: examples would be those with chronic psychosis and young adults with head injury.

HOW TO READ THIS BOOK

We have written the book in the order you should read it: Part 1 deals with fundamental aspects of the psychological approach to clinical problems. Try and read Chapters 2, 3, and 4 right away: although you can skip the remaining chapters in Part 1 until you have clerked your first patient. In particular, there is more information than you need to pass Finals in the chapter on 'Treatment': however, you will need this information to manage common psychological disorders adequately – so we make no apologies for the surplus!

As soon as you have interviewed a patient with a particular problem read up the appropriate chapter in Part 2, as well as relevant bits of the chapters on investigation and treatment. Aim to read the whole of the first two parts in the first week of your time in the department of psychiatry.

Parts 3 and 4 can safely be left until the earlier parts have been absorbed, although all parts are equally important.

THE CARD NOT INCLUDED

We have included a card with this book which you may wish to carry about with you until you have got used to carrying out clinical assessments. On one side we have shown you, in note form, the main headings to be used in taking a *history* and carrying out a *mental state examination* with especial attention to assessments for organic damage. You will most often need this side of the card in the department of psychiatry, although you will find it useful on the general wards as well from time to time.

On the other side we give you the abbreviated 'Newcastle scales' for the assessment of cerebral impairment in elderly patients. We remind you of some of the common manifestations of *mood disorders* that accompany physical disorders in the rest of the hospital. We also provide you with useful screening questions for the detection of alcoholism in patients with medical problems. A further section reminds you of the questions that need answering when you make an assessment of *suicidal risk* in the accident room. Get into the habit of using all these questions in your routine clinical work. You will not be sorry.

In case you lose the card, we have reproduced its content at the end of the book.

PART 1
THE CLINICAL
APPROACH TO THE
PATIENT

2 / INTERVIEW TECHNIQUES AND HISTORY-TAKING

A medical interview should allow you to obtain the most accurate possible account of the patient's illness, and the events in the patient's life that are relevant to it, within a reasonably short time. If time is not to be wasted, you must create conditions from the outset so that the patient finds it easy to talk to you. To start with, you must look like a member of the medical staff. On the general wards this is quite easy since you will be wearing a white coat, but in settings like the department of psychiatry or in general practice it is important that you dress in such a way that patients who may be much older than you nevertheless see you as someone from whom help may be sought.

Start by saying who you are, and explaining the purpose of the interview. Show consideration by asking whether it is a convenient time for the patient: it usually will be, but people like to feel that they have been consulted. Let us suppose that you have been asked to see a forty-four-year-old woman called Mrs Woods, who has been referred to hospital with a severe central chest pain. You are working for a consultant called Dr Johnson:

> *Good morning Mrs Woods. My name is Brian Matthews . . . (shake hands) . . . I'm a student doctor working with Dr Johnson. He has asked me to see you to ask you about the illness that has brought you to hospital. Is this a convenient time to talk to me?*

In the medical wards the next step is to establish some privacy by drawing the curtains so that others in the ward will not be able to eavesdrop on what the patient tells you. If you can do anything to make the patient more comfortable – for example, helping an orthopnoeic patient to sit up on his pillows – this also shows consideration, and you will be rewarded by a better history. In places where interview rooms are available you should now lead the way to the room, resisting the temptation to start the interview until you are both seated and the patient is comfortable.

You should be aware that communication between yourself and the patient will be

Figure 2.1 *Poor communication*

Figure 2.1 (*cont.*) *Good communication*

affected by the distance between you, and your relative positions. For example, a doctor who stands at the foot of a patient's bed while taking a history is making three mistakes at once: he is too far away, he is face to face, and he is looking down on the patient. You should be sitting about a metre from the patient, on the same level, and sitting in such a way that you can always look at the patient, but he can look away from you without difficulty. In out-patient work this is usually achieved by having the patient sit beside the doctor's desk, while on the wards one draws up a chair beside the bed (see *Figure 2.1*).

Start by explaining what you are going to do, and then tell the patientwhat you need to hear about first. Remember to ask permission to take notes. Patients may be reluctant to give full details about their illness to medical students if they think your notes may be left around on the bus, or in the students' union.

> *Mrs Woods, I'm going to have to ask you quite a lot of questions about yourself, but I'd like to **start** by asking you to tell me about the illness that has brought you into hospital. I'll need to jot down a few notes while you are talking, but the notes I make are confidential, and will be kept with your other medical notes.*

In fact, don't dream of writing down anything yet. Look at your patient and, as you listen to the first few sentences, notice as much as you can about the sick person who is seeking help. There is a great deal to take in, and eventually it will become as automatic as the complex series of actions taken by a driver as he starts a car and drives off into a busy city street. However, at first you will have to break it down into its component parts. We will concentrate on those aspects of the patient's non-verbal behaviour that should alert you to the possibility that he or she is psychologically unwell. These are called **non-verbal cues**.

The **posture** may be dejected, with the patient slumped in his chair; or it may indicate anxiety, with the patient being so tense that either the back of his chair does not take the weight of his body, or as he lies in bed the weight of his head is unsupported by his pillow. Valuable cues are also in the **handshake**: the warm dry feeling of health contrasting with the cold, clammy feeling of anxious over-arousal. The **voice** also contains valuable information quite apart from what is being said: the monotonous, uninflected sound of depression; the strained, distressed sound of pain and anxiety; the altered pitch of anger; and the whining note of someone who feels he is always left with the dirty end of the stick. The patient may **avoid eye-contact** with you, sometimes because he is distressed and perhaps ambivalent about confiding emotional problems, but sometimes just because he is feeling ill. There may be motor activities which suggest inner tension: either **tremor** or **restlessness**.

In addition to these non-verbal cues, the patient may mention things that suggest that they have been worried or depressed, or have had unusual experiences: these are of course **verbal cues**.

THE HISTORY OF THE PRESENT CONDITION

This is a clear account of the development of the patient's symptoms starting from the time the patient last felt well until she was admitted to hospital. It is up to you to leave out things that are clearly irrelevant, and to arrange symptoms and events into chrono-logical order. All times are given relative to the date of admission to hospital: thus, *'Mrs Woods began to feel a pain in her chest three weeks before her admission'*, rather than ' . . . on 3rd January' or '. . . on the day of the Cup Final'.

'Probe' questions like 'And what happened after that?' help to emphasize to the patient your interest in a sequential account of her problems.

It encourages the patient to speak in the early minutes of the interview if you utter **facilitations** – these may take the form of noises like *'uh-huh'*, words like *'yes, I see'*, or repeating what the patient has just said with a different inflection: *'you fell down the stairs?'* Sometimes patients start by telling us the most dramatic events, and only gradually tell us about what actually happened to them first. If you think that this is happening, say something like:

> *I need to know the order in which these things happened to you. What was the first thing you noticed that was wrong?*

After each incident is described, remind her of the same need by saying:

> *And what happened after that?*

Sometimes patients start by pouring out an account of their current social problems without really mentioning medical symptoms at all. If this happens you will need to interrupt quite soon, saying something like:

> *What effect did (that) have on your health?* or

> *I'd like to come back to that in a minute. Could you start by telling me about your health (or about how you have been feeling in yourself)?*

During the course of giving the history patients will often mention key symptoms about which you will need to know many details. **Pain** is the most obvious example: you will need to know its site, quality, intensity, radiation, things that make it worse, and things that ease it. Sleep disorders, depression, and bowel disorders are other examples where there are many questions that need to be answered before you can pass on to the next topic. In your anxiety to leave nothing out, you have perhaps already got into the habit of asking patients many probe questions about each of these areas, but this is not the right way of going about things. It takes too long, and patients who are suggestible often agree to things that they have not actually experienced. Get into the habit of asking **directive questions** about such important topic areas:

> *You say you developed a pain in your chest. Could you describe it to me?*

> *How have you been sleeping?*

The student has indicated to the patient that this is an important area, but phrases his question in such a way that the patient must use her own words to convey her experience, rather than having words put into her mouth. It is often necessary to ask several directive questions.

Patients often use vague phrases to describe their symptoms – such as 'these heads of mine', or 'my dizzy turns' – and when this happens you must try to find out exactly what the patient is experiencing:

> Please describe your dizzy turns to me exactly

and follow this up with any probe questions that are necessary, like 'do they come on at any particular time?', 'how do they start?', 'can you do anything to influence them?', and so on. This technique is called **clarification**, and you must get into the habit of doing it carefully. Occasionally you will ask **closed questions** which the patient can answer with a simple '*yes*' or '*no*', but generally only when the patient has told you what he can, but has left out some detail that is potentially important.

Sometimes you will notice that the patient looks emotionally unwell as she describes her physical symptoms, a **non-verbal cue** suggesting psychological illness. The thing you notice could be any of the cues already mentioned, but in the case of Mrs Woods her eyes are red and swollen.

As she mentions her mother's death, she dabs her eyes with her handkerchief. Instead of politely ignoring this, the student deals with it by drawing attention to it. This in effect gives the patient permission to talk about her feelings:

> Mrs Woods, I can see you're still very upset about your mother's death. Have you found yourself crying a lot?

This procedure is called a **reflection** of the patient's feeling, and it can be used for other feelings as well, such as anger or tension.

Sometimes patients mention their feelings at the same time as they give you important information about a physical symptom. An insensitive interviewer simply picks up the physical symptom and asks further questions about that, never returning to the abnormal mood. Remember to prick up your ears when you hear these **verbal cues** relating to psychological illness. You may well want to finish hearing about the pain first, but remember to come back to the abnormal mood, and ask a **directive question** about it:

> You mentioned a moment ago that you've been feeling depressed. Could you tell me more about that?

It has been known for some time that some doctors are very good at detecting psychological disorders, while others miss most of these illnesses. The way that you interview the patient will affect the number of both verbal and non-verbal cues that they show you: doctors who hurry the patient, or tend to interrupt the patient, who ask many questions derived from theory, or who ask many closed questions will inhibit the release of these cues; while those who ask questions that follow on from what the patient has just said, who make sympathetic comments when they are appropriate, and who make a habit of asking directive questions will find that patients are prepared to allow their distress to show.

Your questioning therefore proceeds in a systematic way moving gradually forward in time, so that eventually you arrive at the day of admission. This should remind you to carry out a brief **systems review**. In the department of psychiatry some parts of this are particularly important, so be sure you remember to ask for:

1. Changes in **appetite**.
2. Changes in **weight**.
3. Changes in **sleep**.
4. Changes in **sexual feelings**.
5. Changes in **bladder and bowel habit**.
6. Decreased ability to **enjoy oneself**, including **loss of usual interests**.

Sometimes students feel embarrassed asking older people about their sexual feelings. You need not be. The patients aren't embarrassed, if you aren't. Everyone knows what sexual feelings are, whether or not they are currently having a sexual relationship with someone. If the patient isn't consulting for a sexual problem, it is usually sufficient just to ask whether there has been any *change* in their sexual feelings recently, at the same part of the interview as you are asking about other functions such as appetite and sleep.

Anyway, when you have completed the 'systems review' questions you should be thoroughly up-to-date. This should remind you to **recapitulate** the history to the patient. This only takes a few moments, and it is an excellent habit to get into. Patients frequently correct things which (often through no fault of your own) you have got wrong, and they are often reminded to put in something important that they forgot to tell you the first time:

> *Well, Mrs Woods, you seem to have been well until your mother died unexpectedly three weeks ago. You cried quite a bit on the day she died and since then you've gradually become sure that she wouldn't have died if only you had done more for her when she stayed with you six months ago. On the day of the funeral you developed a severe pain in your chest which you have had, off and on, ever since. It is just below your left breast, and feels like a dull ache. It seems to get worse when you cry a lot, but doesn't seem to be helped by resting, or by aspirin. You have been eating very little since she died as you have lost your appetite, and have lost twelve pounds in weight. You have great difficulty falling asleep, and in the past week you have been waking three hours earlier than usual. You have been feeling unlike your usual self: you said it was as though a black cloud had fallen over you.*

THE FAMILY HISTORY

Now that you have heard the nature of the present illness, you are in a far better position to know how much detail to take about the family history. Not everything is equally important. In Mrs Woods' case, for example, we certainly want to know about the illness that caused her mother's death, and to know something about the relationship between mother and daughter. Did her mother have a chest pain in her last illness? Had there been bad feelings between mother and daughter to help us to understand the guilt the patient now reports? Is there a tendency for depression to run in the family? These are questions in our minds, but we do not ask them right away. However, they will influence us in the amount of detail that we collect. The family history is a voyage of discovery.

However, before we embark we utter a sentence to let the patient know that we have finished one area, and are about to go on to another. These statements are called **transition**

statements – think of them as a form of professional good manners – and go straight on with your first question:

> *Now that I've heard about your present problems I'd like to go on to ask you a few questions about your family. Could we start with your father? Is he still alive?*

We are aiming to get answers to the following questions about each parent:

Age, or age at death and year of death (so that you can work out how old the patient was at the time); occupation; health; whether parent suffered with 'nerves' (if so, details: were they seen by a psychiatrist; did they have any treatment?); what the parent was like; how the patient got on with them.

Go on to siblings. List them in order, showing where the patient comes in the family. If the patient uses first names, use these both in your notes and in questioning the patient, otherwise use the patient's terminology: *'so your older sister was always your mother's favourite, and you found that you never really could please her?'* You are interested in the health of all first-degree relatives, but not of relatives by marriage. The family history should tell us whether any of Mrs Woods' first-degree relatives have had mental illnesses, as well as giving us some idea of the sort of family she comes from. Do not ask about the patient's spouse or children yet: they come later.

We started our family history with some hunches about the patient: we should by now have begun to confirm or refute them, and often we now have some new insights: the voyage of discovery can continue. . . .

THE PERSONAL HISTORY

At first you will take very full and detailed personal histories, because you won't really know what is relevant and what is not. Don't worry about that, you need the practice, and you will discover some very interesting things about your patients in the process. However, once more, not everything is equally relevant. How a girl received her sex education will have great relevance if the patient is asking for help because she has not been able to consummate her marriage, but it will probably matter very little in a spinster of seventy-five who is complaining of loss of memory.

Childhood

It is helpful to take the personal history in chronological order, starting from childhood. A patient's mother may be able to tell you what her health was like in the pregnancy that produced your patient, and to give you details of the delivery and age on reaching 'milestones': however, information on the same points from the patient is likely to be unreliable. Students often begin their account of the personal histories of their patients with an air of spurious accuracy: 'Mrs Woods was born in Bermondsey as a full-term, normal delivery. Her milestones were normal, and there were no neurotic traits in childhood . . . .'

Don't do this unless you can obtain information which seems to be reliable. It doesn't matter whether she was born in Bermondsey or Hoxton, and she probably doesn't really know whether her delivery was normal or not. Nor does she have much idea whether her motor milestones were normal, and it doesn't matter two pins whether or not an adult patient reports 'neurotic traits' in childhood! Although birth injury and delayed motor milestones are of great medical interest, it is better to say that you have no information than to say that things were normal when they in fact were not. However, if the patient has been told that her birth or early years were abnormal this is certainly worth recording; otherwise confine yourself to things which the patient can actually remember, and which are of interest in understanding disorders in adult life.

So, start the personal history with a transition statement:

> *Now you've told me a bit about your family I'd like to ask a few questions about your early life. Were you ever told anything about your birth?*

Go on to ask:

> *Do you remember your childhood as happy or unhappy?*

Happy childhoods can be passed over quickly, but get details about unhappiness. What was wrong, and how did it affect her? Was she separated from her parents? (If so, for how long, and how did she manage?) In patients with mixtures of physical and psychological symptoms, ask about physical health in childhood, and the attitudes of care-givers to them when physically ill. It is helpful to ask routinely whether or not there were serious physical illnesses in childhood.

School

If you are taking a detailed history start with primary school – how did they get on? What were they good at? Did they make friends? (If not, were they teased; what about?) How did they get on with teachers? Then, pass on to secondary school. The briefest school history will record age of entering and leaving full-time education, and the highest level of education achieved. Make a note of any public examination passed, since this information is especially important in the assessment of possible organic cerebral damage.

Sexual history

Move on to the sexual history by asking female patients about their age at the menarche, and go on to a menstrual history. Ask whether their mother prepared them for their menarche, and whether sexual matters could be discussed at home. Go on from there to ask about boyfriends. You are interested in their capacity to form loving relationships, as well as obtaining a detailed account of any problems encountered in the physical side of sexual relationships.

Ask male patients at what age they learned the facts of life, whether sexual matters could be freely discussed at home, and so through a similar sequence of questions. Once more, do not confine yourself to an account of the purely physical problems which the patient may describe, but try to assess the patient's capacity to form loving relationships.

Do not ask about homosexual activities unless the patient volunteers information, or unless there is some reason to suspect it and it is relevant to the patient's present problems. If you need to discuss such problems, do so without embarrassment. If anal intercourse has occurred, has the patient been worried about the possibility of AIDS?

If the patient presents with a sexual problem you will of course need to get fuller details than this brief outline suggests: these are given in Chapter 18.

Marital history

The marital history follows naturally on: once more, happy marriages can be recorded briefly. If the patient has been married more than once obtain a description of the first marriage and how that marriage ended. At what age did they meet their spouse, and get married? What is the age, health, and occupation of the spouse? Can they confide in their spouse? Have there been problems? (An example of a problem would be separations, or threatened separations.) If there have been no problems, record this briefly; otherwise obtain a description of the problems.

Is the sexual side satisfactory? Ask about children, recording separate notes about each child: age, health, any problems?

Occupational history

The occupational history gives valuable information about the patient's personality, as well as the range of his abilities. What is the patient's current occupation: if none, how long has the unemployment lasted? How many jobs have there been, and how long did the longest one last? Why do changes occur? Promotions and changes forced by circumstance require no explanation, but get someone who is constantly changing jobs to tell you what goes wrong. A list giving exact names of employers and dates is of little value: but this part of the history and the marital history give you some idea of the patient's capacity to form enduring relationships and stick at things, as well as allowing you to judge his strengths.

Present social circumstances

Finish this part of the history by trying to assess the patient's present living circumstances. Who is there at home? How do they get on? In what sort of accommodation do they live?

Forensic history

Whether or not you take such a history depends largely on the patient's presenting problem. They should routinely be taken in patients with drug or alcohol problems.

Start with truancy and problems at school, both with teachers and with other students. Go on to ask if they have ever been in trouble with the police. If they have, be sure to start with the first time, not the most recent! Have they appeared before a court, either juvenile or adult? if so, what was the charge, were they convicted, and what was the sentence?

Previous medical history

If there are important medical, surgical, or psychiatric illnesses in the **past history** these should be recorded in the usual way.

Life charts

If there appear to be relationships between life events, physical illnesses, and psychiatric illnesses it is very helpful if these are brought together as a **life chart**. An example of Mrs Woods' life chart is shown as *Figure 2.2*.

THE PRE-MORBID PERSONALITY

Some personality types are at greater risk than others of developing psychiatric illnesses: for example, people with cyclothymic traits are more likely to develop manic-depressive illness, or those with obsessional traits are more likely to experience obsessional symptoms when depressed. This is discussed more fully in Chapter 5 (see also p. 200).

However, there are two major problems in relying upon information from the patient. Unless you're very careful, patients tell you what they're like now, rather than what they used to be like. Also, people cannot tell you things that they don't know themselves, and if they are depressed they will tend to see themselves in a bad light. Always see a relative if you want accurate information. Nonetheless, there are some things that the patient can tell you about himself, and you should start, as usual, with a transition statement:

> *Mrs Woods, I want to ask you some questions now about the sort of person that you were before you became ill. Could you remember how you were a year or so ago? Could you start by telling me about your interests?*

Aim to collect information under headings: interests, mood, friendships, habits – including alcohol and drugs.

INTERVIEWS WITH SPECIAL GROUPS

Children and old people

Special points that should be borne in mind with patients at either end of the life cycle are discussed in Part 3: interviews with children on pp. 261–2 and interviews with old people on p. 306.

Figure 2.2 *Example of a life chart for Mrs Vera Woods*

age	year	life events	psychical illness	mental illness
	1940	Born 10.9.40		
1	1			
2	2			
3	3			
4	4			
5	5	Started school		
6	6			
7	7			
8	8	F. died		
		M. → Dep'd	Investigated for abdo. pain	
9	9			
10	1950		Appendicectomy	
11	1			
12	2			
13	3			
14	4			
15	5	Left school; clerical job		
16	6			
17	7			
18	8			
19	9			
20	1960	1st engagement		
21	1	Broken off		Anxiety; No Rx
22	2	2nd engagement		
23	3	Marriage		
24	4			
25	5	Stopped work; daughter born		
26	6			
27	7		Hysterectomy: 'menorrhagia'	
28	8			
29	9	Husband unfaithful; leaves		
30	1970			
31	1			
32	2	Divorces husband		
33	3	Second marriage		
34	4			
35	5			
36	6			
37	7			
38	8			
39	9			
40	1980			
41	1			
42	2			
43	3	Daughter to univ.		Dep'd; Rx GP
44	4			
45	5	M.'s illness discovered Aug.		
46	6	M. died 18.2.86		Onset present illness

Deaf people

Don't shout at them. Make sure that they can see your mouth, and speak slowly and clearly. Ask them to let you know if they cannot hear any of your questions, as you will be pleased to repeat them. If a particular question is really important, and you are unsure whether the patient really understood it, write it down.

People who do not speak English very well

Often you can manage just by speaking slowly and clearly, and *avoiding long words*. If this does not work, you will need an interpreter: these are usually available, so make proper enquiries! When the interpreter appears and you have introduced yourself, put the patient in the usual chair and address your questions to him or her, not to the interpreter. Watch the patient's face as they reply to each question: even if you do not understand a word of their language, you will learn a great deal.

INTERVIEWING A RELATIVE

Use the same headings when you see a relative, but be sure to include your impression of your informant. Include any anecdotes that are mentioned. You should learn about the patient's capacity to form friendships, as well as patterns of relationship within the family. Look now at the following example:

Mrs Vera WOODS
Ward M4
13 March 1994

Informant: husband
Mr John Woods
s/a as patient

Impression of informant

Mr Woods is a heavily built man who seems very concerned about his wife's illness. He thought carefully about some of his answers, pausing for emphasis on things he thought important. He asked particularly to be told if there was anything else that he might do to help, but appeared to have difficulty seeing how his wife's depression could have much to do with her chest pain.

Present illness

Little to add to patient's account except that she told him her mother wouldn't have died if she'd been a better daughter, and that she felt wicked.

Early life

Always trying to please her mother, but mother found fault with her. Wanted to have mother live with them last year, but informant wasn't keen as there were always arguments.

Marital history

Informant met her aged thirty-two, a few months after she had divorced her first husband for desertion and mental cruelty. They married after about six months and were initially quite happy, although she was possessive. Intercourse satisfactory for both of them and occurred regularly until her mother's death. There was some tension in the early years because he did not get on with her mother, but in the past two years the old lady had been to stay for several long visits.

Children: Dorothy, aged 21: tends to be nervous and tearful. Pt. was rather over-protective, wouldn't let her play with other children.

Previous psychiatric history

Nil.

Pre-morbid personality

Usually cheerful, but tends to be gloomy for weeks if things go wrong. During such times she is irritable, sleeps poorly, and seems listless.

Always very houseproud. 'You could eat your breakfast off her kitchen floor.' Tends to check gas-taps and switches at the best of times. Very sensitive, thought people at her work were criticizing the way they brought up their daughter: couldn't see this wasn't so.

Likes making clothes for herself and their daughter, also interested in country dancing and Help the Aged. Works tirelessly for other people: tremendous energy. Has many friends and leads an active social life. Drinks only socially; non-smoker; no recreational drugs. Tranquillizers from GP only once, about three years ago, he thinks.

Brian Matthews
Medical Student

3 / EXAMINATION OF THE MENTAL STATE

The examination of the mental state is an orderly and systematic procedure like that of the physical examination. It is carried out routinely for each new patient and is repeated, either in whole or in part, on every subsequent occasion that the patient is seen. A summary of the main aspects of the mental state follows this introduction. Each of these aspects is then considered in turn, with a description of the observations that are to be made and the tests that will be carried out, the interpretation of these observations, and their relevance to diagnosis. The division of the mental state into these parts is convenient, but to some extent arbitrary, because they tend to overlap.

The emphasis in this chapter is on the accurate evaluation of the most important symptoms and signs of mental illness. The student is advised to start by learning how to carry out well the tests presented here and how to evaluate the significance of the results. Many other symptoms, particularly those seen in schizophrenia, are described in the chapters on those disorders.

As in other branches of medicine the history of the disorder should suggest the diagnosis, and the examination should help to confirm it. Although an experienced clinician will be able to concentrate on certain aspects of the mental state, the inexperienced student will only learn to carry out the mental state examination rapidly and effectively by keeping to the routine described for each patient examined. The novice can expect to take as long as an hour to carry out the examination in some cases, but by the end of a few weeks should be able to carry out at least an initial examination in about twenty minutes. (A total of one hour is the customary time allowed for a history and clinical examination of a 'long case'.)

A full and accurate account of the mental state should always be recorded in the medical notes, for both clinical and medico-legal purposes. As with all medical records each note must be dated and signed. Observations must be noted separately from opinions. For example:

> *The patient insists that Dr Smith is his father, refers to him as 'Dad' and describes his real father as an imposter when he comes to visit. He cannot be argued out of this belief*

should be recorded, and separately the opinion:

> *(This belief appears to be a delusion.)*

The latter might not be the only interpretation of the finding. It might be an overvalued idea, or intentional play-acting. Records that contain only opinions, for example, 'The patient is suffering from delusions', are of little value. Another doctor, seeing the patient a few days later, may find no evidence of delusions and will probably decide that the recorded opinion is wrong and based on inexperience if he does not also have available the data on which the opinion was based.

Negative findings are as important as positive findings and should be recorded. For example, the note of orientation in time should specify the patient's replies to questions on the time, day of the week and date, together with the correct answers, rather than the opinion 'Well orientated in time'. Similarly 'Mood normal' is not an acceptable alternative for 'Describes his mood as "contented" and shows appropriate modulation of mood throughout the interview'.

Verbatim accounts by the patient should be recorded if they are particularly illuminating or provide an example of some morbid phenomenon and should be indicated by using inverted commas. It is especially important to record examples of speech which you consider to be abnormal: once more, a note which reads 'patient's speech grossly thought disordered' is valueless – you must record an actual example. You should also record the context in which the statement is made, or whether in response to a question.

Some of the words to be found in this chapter are also used in colloquial English, when they often have a less precise meaning. For example, 'obsession' is a term used generally only to mean a preoccupation, whereas in psychiatry it has a more specific meaning which is precisely defined and should only be used in this way. Throughout the following account we shall use technical terms, some of which may be unfamiliar to you. Rather than break up the text each time this occurs, we have gathered these together at the back of the book in a **Glossary**, and have used asterisks to indicate that a Glossary definition is available. Thus, if you come across '**akathisia** (*p. 335)' this means that a full account of that term is to be found on p. 335.

APPEARANCE AND BEHAVIOUR

General description

The mental state examination should start with a brief description of what the patient looks like, so that another person hearing the account might recognize the patient in a crowded room. Include the physique, clothes, cleanliness, hair, make-up, and whether these seem appropriate to the age, sex, cultural group, and social class of the patient.

Signs of self-neglect (poor hygiene, stubbly beard, body odour, stained clothes, or loose clothes due to weight loss) occur in many mental illnesses, particularly depressive disorders, dementia, and schizophrenia, as well as being due to poverty.

Always note any evidence of disorders of the **level of consciousness**. Is the patient fully awake and alert, responding normally to stimuli, drowsy, or unrousable? Apart from normal tiredness, an impaired state of consciousness is strongly suggestive of an organic cerebral disorder, particularly delirium, but inattention also commonly occurs in affective disorders. Tests of orientation may help to differentiate these.

Reaction to interviewer

The manner of the patient towards the interviewer should be described next. Is he friendly, cooperative, complaining, suspicious, or critical? Students tend to assume either that they themselves are at fault when occasionally a patient refuses to cooperate, or alternatively that the patient is being 'difficult'. However, this is an important part of the patient's mental state and provides some indication of how the patient relates to others at the present time. One must then consider whether such behaviour is the patient's reaction to an unfamiliar and stressful experience, is a symptom of illness, or is an indication of personality problems.

Motor activity

This is sometimes referred to as 'psychomotor activity'. Included here are the facial expression, posture, and gait. Note particularly the speed of movement, the quantity and the presence of abnormal movements. Is there any evidence of repetitive, apparently purposeless or involuntary movements?

There may be *too little* movement. Distinguish between **akinesis** (*p. 335) in which there are reduced voluntary movements especially affecting the face, and **retardation** (*p. 339) in which all movements are slowed. Loss of **volition** (*p. 340) is where the patient generally doesn't have much 'go' in him, and **stupor** (*p. 339) is when the patient does not move at all, although fully conscious.

There may be *too much* movement. Distinguish between a generally increased level called **over-activity** (*p. 338), or an anguished, driven restlessness which leads to **agitation** (*p. 335). **Akathisia** (*p. 335) is a state of restlessness and over-activity produced by neuroleptic drugs. Ask yourself whether any increased level of activity is associated with **disinhibition** (see p. 204).

There may be **involuntary movements**. Some of these are of especial interest to psychiatrists. You are probably already familiar with **tics** (*p. 340), and will have seen **choreic** movements on the neurological wards. The movements of **acute dystonia** (*p. 335) are painful spasms and **tardive dyskinesia** (*p. 339) refers to a wide variety of repetitive and distressing movements, both brought on by neuroleptic drugs.

DISORDERS OF TALKING AND THINKING

Knowledge of another person's thoughts is only available through speech or some other form of communication, such as writing or gesture. Talking and thinking are closely related, in that thought usually precedes speech; however, thoughts may remain unspoken. We therefore consider talking and thinking together.

Students often have some difficulty in understanding the essential difference between the form and the content of talk. Briefly, the **form** is how we talk, whilst the **content** is what we say. For example, we may talk quickly in a disjointed manner (the form), but this gives no indication of whether we are talking about the weather or our next meal (the content).

The speed of talk

The speed of talk varies greatly from one person to another, so that a moderately fast or slow rate of talk cannot be assumed to be morbid. Extremes of speed may be associated with changes in volume and also in the quantity of speech.

RETARDATION OF SPEECH

Retardation of speech (*p. 339) refers to a delay in starting to speak as well as in the rate of speech.

MUTISM

Mutism (*p. 337) is total absence of speech. **Elective mutism** is characterized by mutism which occurs in some settings but not in others.

Changes in the amount of speech occur in depression and mania. A reduction in talk may sometimes be seen in dementia, where patients may say very little; alternatively, they may talk a great deal but communicate little.

PRESSURE OF SPEECH

Pressure of speech (*p. 338) describes a rapid outpouring of ideas which are often difficult to interrupt.

Continuity of talk

Note whether talk is hesitant, with longer than usual interruptions for thought, and whether it is coherent and relevant to the current conversation. Remember that this should be judged more by what is relevant to the patient, who may be preoccupied with a crisis in his life, than by what is relevant to you the interviewer. Hesitancy in speech is a common feature in those who are anxious or depressed, indecisive or preoccupied with worries. Deafness, often unsuspected, is also a common impediment to the free flow of conversation.

Does the patient use words of his own making (**neologisms**: for example, 'my mind is *spired*') or strange grammatical constructions?

Does talk **follow a sequence** in which consecutive ideas follow logically, working towards an identifiable goal, or is it circumstantial, tangential, or over-inclusive? If any disorder is possibly present, record verbatim samples of speech to illustrate this, together with the question that you asked beforehand:

> *How long have you been in hospital?*

> *I came in last Wednesday: that was a fine day for mushrooms. Do you like omelettes?*

The patient may talk circumstantially, or he may wander from one subject to another, apparently with little purpose other than social contact. This must be differentiated from a breakdown of normal associations of ideas, in which talk apparently attempts, but fails, to follow a logical sequence. *ie "looseness of association"*

SCHIZOPHRENIC THOUGHT DISORDER

In **schizophrenic thought disorder** the logical sequence of ideas may break down so that consecutive sentences are unconnected; a single sentence may contain two unrelated elements:

> *I want to go home because this hospital is nearer to the shops than the last one.*

Here there is an apparent attempt to provide an explanation in the second half of the sentence for the wish expressed in the first half, yet there is no real explanation, and the two ideas appear to be disconnected. Always ask the patient to explain the association between ideas if you are unable to discern a meaningful connection. This may result in an even greater breakdown in logical thinking or a logical explanation that was not initially evident. Asked to explain the previous statement, the patient may say:

> *Shops frighten me and if I stay here I may be expected to go to the shops. I wouldn't mind going to the other hospital.*

This now begins to make sense. Alternatively, he may say:

> *I mean I want to go home because it's near the shops and the shops are near the hospital.*

This makes even less sense than previously. In extreme disorder there may be a jumble of unrelated words (**word salad**).

FLIGHT OF IDEAS

Flight of ideas describes the way in which the speech of manic patients may move rapidly from one subject to another, usually with some discernible association, which may be rather flimsy. For example:

> *I don't like this place. It's really rather boring. The patients keep snoring. It's just a great yawn: I'd rather have soft porn. Are you a softie, doc?*

Here the ideas are associated and there is a return at the end to the initial theme. Such 'flight' is usually associated with pressure of speech, unlike schizophrenic thought disorder. However, the form of the disorders of thinking and speech in schizophrenia and mania may be so similar in practice as to defy differentiation.

If the patient suddenly seems to go blank during your examination the most likely explanation is just that he is anxious, but consider the possibility of **thought block** (*p. 339) and ask him what was happening during the pause. Another possibility is **epileptic absence attacks** (see p. 145).

PERSEVERATION

Perseveration is the repetition of a response when it is no longer appropriate. For example:

> *What day is it today?*
> *Monday. (Correct)*
> *Which day did you come into hospital?*
> *Monday.*
> *What is the name of the ward?*
> *Monday.*

Verbal perseveration is often associated with motor perseveration: 'Hold up your left hand.' The patient does so. 'Hold up your right hand.' The patient again raises his left hand. Perseveration is usually an indication of organic brain disease.

DISORDERS OF MOOD

The examination of mood has four main components: subjective mood, objective observation, autonomic activity, and thought content. The last of these is considered further in the next section.

Subjective mood

Always ask first about the patient's subjective mood state with an open-ended question:

> *How have you been feeling recently?* or
> *How have you been in your spirits?*

If the response is non-committal, follow up with:

> *Have you been feeling mainly happy or sad?*

If the reply indicates sadness, ask:

> *How sad? Can you snap out of it?*

If the patient describes depressed mood, always remember to ask:

> *What do you find yourself thinking about when you feel like that?*
> *How do you feel about the future?*

Do you ever feel completely hopeless?
(If 'yes' to previous question:)
As though life isn't worth living?
(If 'yes', continue with questions about suicide, see p. 31)

Objective observation of mood

Moods of sadness, anxiety, or happiness are conveyed through facial expression, posture, and motility. 'Normal' mood modulates frequently, depending on the thoughts and experiences of the individual.

There are two separate points to note:

1. What is the predominant mood during the course of the interview?
2. To what extent does the mood fluctuate, are fluctuations appropriate, and in what direction are these fluctuations?

Occasionally patients deny unpleasant mood states, such as depression, perplexity, or suspicion, although there may be ample alternative evidence to show this is present. In particular there may be a deliberate attempt to conceal depression by refusing to answer questions, and this should alert the interviewer to the risk of suicide.

Sadness is a feature of depressed mood, but it is not of course in itself indicative of mental illness. **Weeping** is commonly associated with sadness, although it may merely be a way of releasing pent-up tension.

In less severe depressive states the mood may improve when the patient is distracted by amusing incidents, that is to say, the mood reacts to the circumstances (this is the proper meaning of **'reactive depression'**). In more severe depressive states weeping is less common, and there tends to be a more constant melancholic mood, lacking normal modulation, which may easily be mistaken for **affective blunting** (see below). The patient may describe the experience of an inability to have feelings or to care about others, such as family members or friends.

Smiles and laughter are associated with cheerfulness and **euphoria**, in which case they usually have an 'infectious' quality. However, they can also be produced in the unhappy as an indication of irony or of social expectation, when they fail to convey real enjoyment. The manic patient is not always cheerful: he will often display irritability and impatience if frustrated by those trying to limit his activities. **Irritability** is commonly seen in all affective illnesses.

The patient may display **labile mood**(*p. 337) in that he has little control of emotion. Less commonly, you may notice examples of inappropriate or **incongruous affect** (*p. 337), or he may display **blunting of affect** (*p. 336) in that the capacity to experience emotion seems to have been lost.

Autonomic activity

Affective changes are accompanied by fluctuations in autonomic activity. You may have noticed a cold, sweaty palm as you shook hands with the patient.

Increased arousal is characterized by sweating, palpitation, dry mouth, hyperventilation, frequency of micturition which may be evident during mental state examination, while raised diastolic and systolic blood pressure, tachycardia, and increased gastro-intestinal motility may be found on physical examination. High arousal commonly occurs in all psychiatric disorders associated with anxiety, including anxiety states, depressive illness, and both acute and chronic schizophrenia.

THOUGHT CONTENT

The content of thinking is evident primarily through the patient's talk, but also through aspects of behaviour. In this respect 'actions speak louder than words'. For example, the patient may deny that he is suspicious of others, but opens the office door to see if anyone is listening outside.

Preoccupations

Themes which are predominant in a patient's thought content are likely to be revealed in his spontaneous speech. Note any topics to which he may return repeatedly during the course of the interview and the difficulty which you encounter in trying to steer him from these subjects back to other aspects of the history and mental state examination. If preoccupations are not evident, ask:

> *What are your main worries?* or
> *Do you have some thoughts that you just don't seem to be able to get out of your head?*

Many people have preoccupations, but these are appropriate to the circumstances. For example, it is appropriate for a patient about to undergo major surgery to be preoccupied with the possible hazards, the likely outcome, the provision for dependants, etc., even though there may be encouragement from others to keep these thoughts to himself. However, some preoccupations are morbid, and their content may be important in understanding the diagnosis of the disorder.

Ruminations are repetitive ideas and themes, usually having an unpleasant content, on which the patient may brood for prolonged periods. They commonly occur in anxiety states and depressive illnesses when their content reflects the **affective state**: for example, they may include ideas of guilt, low self-esteem, or hypochondriasis. These should be differentiated from delusions (see below) in which the content may be the same but the form is different. Ruminations also occur in **obsessional states** (see p. 228), in which case they reflect the state of indecision.

Suicidal ideas are of special importance, because of the risk to the patient's life. A patient who has said that life is not worth living should be asked:

Have you ever thought of ending your life?
Have you planned what you will do?
Do you intend to carry it through?

Perhaps surprisingly most patients answer such questions honestly, but be particularly wary of the patient who avoids answering. Although commonest in depressive illness, suicidal ideas are by no means limited to that disorder.

Abnormal beliefs

Ideas which are shared by many people within a particular cultural or ethnic group may seem strange to others; for example, particular religious beliefs and practices. Individuals too may have ideas which seem idiosyncratic or eccentric, but are not necessarily symptomatic of mental illness.

Over-valued ideas are beliefs which are strongly held about matters which are of special importance and preoccupy the subject. They are not delusions, because they lack the quality of unshakeable conviction. For example, a patient with anorexia nervosa may develop the characteristic belief that they are fat although they know that they are grossly underweight; indeed, they would regard others of the same weight as dangerously thin. Over-valued ideas are not necessarily indicative of illness.

Delusions are mistaken beliefs which are held with conviction, which are not shared by others of the same cultural or social background and intellect, and which persist despite all the evidence to the contrary. For example, a patient insists that there are men plotting to kill him, hidden in the hospital grounds behind the shrubs and trees. The doctor takes him round the grounds and they look carefully in potential hiding places. Eventually they return to the ward, and the doctor points out that there was no one there.

'Of course not,' says the patient, 'they knew we were going to look for them and they left, but I know that they're back in the grounds now.'

Primary delusions are not secondary to other morbid processes such as abnormal moods or hallucinations. However, they may be prompted by non-morbid processes. For example, a patient may see three clouds in the sky (a normal perception) and realize that these are a personal message to him from God telling him that he is a member of the Holy Trinity. Primary delusions are generally associated with schizophrenia provided that they occur only in a setting of clear consciousness. There are several kinds of primary delusion, but of particular importance is the **delusional perception**, of which an example is presented above. Here the perception is normal, but it is given delusional significance.

Secondary delusions are secondary to some other morbid process. For example, a patient wrongly believes he is being persecuted by his neighbours. This belief may be secondary to an abnormal mood state of depression in which he believes he is guilty and worthy of punishment; or secondary to voices, which he identifies as belonging to the neighbours, saying 'Kill him'. Secondary delusions occur in many different disorders, but their content may be related to the diagnosis. For example, delusions about having disease or dying are usually associated with depressed mood whilst grandiose delusions are more likely to occur in mania.

The possible presence of delusions usually becomes evident whilst taking the history. For example, the patient with delusions of persecution may tell you about the way others are acting against him, his efforts to stop them by complaining to the police or consulting solicitors, or he may appear suspicious in the course of an interview.

Do not ask about delusions routinely: only when other aspects of the history or mental state indicate that they might be present. Then ask:

> *Do you think that others are trying to harm you?*
> *Do you ever feel guilty, or to blame?*
> *Do you think that your body has changed in any way?*
> *Do you think that you have been specially chosen, or have special powers?*

If the patient agrees to any of this, detailed questioning will be necessary to discover whether such ideas, if present, satisfy the criteria of delusions. Is there evidence supporting the patient's views? Do others share his views and encourage him in them? Are his beliefs shakeable?

Delusions occur in many different mental illnesses, in fact all those commonly labelled as **psychoses** (see p. 46). Persecutory and hypochondriacal delusions occur in many disorders and are of little help with diagnosis. Others are more suggestive of diagnosis (see above) and are described in Part 2 or in the Glossary.

PERCEPTION

Most of the time we are aware of our own thoughts, our bodies, and the world around us only to a limited degree, but we can focus our attention on each of these, and they have qualities and order which we recognize and take for granted. This sense of familiarity may be morbidly disrupted. Disturbances may occur in each of the modalities of our perception of ourselves and the outside world.

It is not necessary to ask every patient detailed questions about disorders of perception but it is useful to ask most patients a few 'screening' questions and to pursue these more vigorously if indicated by the history or mental state examination:

> *Have you noticed any changes in yourself or your surroundings that you can't account for?*
> *Have you heard voices of people that you couldn't see?*

The patient may have an unpleasant feeling that although his environment is the same, he or his body has changed – this is suggestive of **depersonalization** (*p. 336) Alternatively he may feel that although he is the same, the surrounding environment has altered in some way – this suggests **derealization**.

Depersonalization and derealization do not necessarily indicate morbidity but occur commonly in states of fatigue and high arousal, particularly in association with anxiety and depression; and less often in schizophrenia, epilepsy, and drug-induced states.

Illusions

Illusions are misinterpretations of external stimuli. They may affect each of the sensory modalities. Commonest are auditory illusions, in which the patient misinterprets what is heard, and visual illusions, in which there is a misinterpretation of visual stimuli. Illusions are not necessarily morbid, and most people are familiar with 'optical illusions' or with the tendency to 'hear' footsteps following them when walking alone in the dark. Emotional states, such as anxiety, often result in such misinterpretation.

Probably the commonest pathological cause of illusions is sensory deficit, as in partial blindness or deafness, and a similar effect may result from diminished sensory input, such as the effect of darkness. Lowering of the state of consciousness has similar effects, and illusions are particularly liable to occur in delirium. In this state it is common for the movement of shadows to be misinterpreted as, for example, the movement of dangerous animals, or the movement of bedclothes against the skin may be misinterpreted as the movement of insects. Not surprisingly, patients experiencing such illusions often appear terrified.

Hallucinations

Hallucinations are perceptions which are not based on external stimuli. For example, a voice is heard talking, but no one is there speaking, and others present hear nothing. Like illusions, hallucinations can occur in any modality of perception, but auditory hallucinations are by far the commonest.

AUDITORY HALLUCINATIONS

Ask:

> *Do you ever hear voices when there is no one there, or no one is talking?*

If 'yes':

> *Are these real voices, coming from outside your head, or your own thoughts inside your head?*
> *Do you ever hear your own thoughts, spoken aloud, outside your head?*

Also ask about the content of the voices:

> *What do the voices say?*
> *Give me an example of what you heard today, or yesterday.*

Always record verbatim accounts of the patient's experiences, including the content of the hallucinations.

Auditory hallucinations can occur in many disorders, including schizophrenia, organic brain syndromes, and manic-depressive illness, and their content tends to be related to the nature of the disorder. For example, in manic states they may be grandiose, such as a voice telling the patient that he has special powers; whereas in depressive disorders they are likely to be abusive and consistent with the state of low self-esteem. Features suggestive of schizophrenia are described on p. 175.

VISUAL HALLUCINATIONS

Visual hallucinations are uncommon and most likely to occur in acute organic states (for example, intoxication with drugs such as amphetamines, or other delirious states), although they occur occasionally in schizophrenia and in affective disorders. Disorganized visual hallucinations (lacking normal form) may result from occipital lobe disease.

OTHER HALLUCINATIONS

Olfactory and gustatory hallucinations may occur as symptoms of temporal lobe disease, for example, in complex partial seizures. **Tactile and somatic hallucinations**, that is, perceptions arising from the body surface or internally, are described, but difficult to differentiate from illusions. All of these occasionally occur in schizophrenia.

Hallucinations occur commonly during dreams, and also in the twilight state between waking and sleeping (**hypnagogic hallucinations**), in which case they have no morbid significance. Simple hallucinations – that is to say, bangs or flashes of light – may occur in conditions of extreme fatigue. You should therefore always ask about the circumstances in which hallucinations are experienced:

> *Was it during the day or at night?*
> *Were you in bed with the lights out?*
> *Were you awake or dozing?*

It is sometimes difficult to differentiate between an illusion and a hallucination. If, for example, a patient says he heard a voice saying 'You have been specially chosen', ask:

> *Where did the voice come from?*
> *Was anyone else present at the time?*
> *Were they speaking?*

Pseudohallucinations lack the qualities of vividness and reality which are possessed by normal perceptions and by hallucinations: they have an 'as if' quality, and they are experienced in inner subjective space. Thus a voice is heard inside one's head, or a vision is seen as if by an 'inner eye'. Ask:

> *Did it sound just the same as a real voice, like listening to my voice now?*

Pseudohallucinations, like illusions, have little diagnostic specificity. They may occur in any mental illness, and also in those who are not mentally ill, particularly those who are highly imaginative or of dull intellect. Failure to discriminate between pseudohallucinations and hallucinations sometimes results in a patient being wrongly regarded as psychotic.

INTELLECTUAL FUNCTIONS

These tests should be used for most patients seen in the department of psychiatry and in particular should be carried out whenever there is a possibility that a patient is suffering from an organic brain syndrome. The tests described must be presented accurately if the results are to have any value. You should start by explaining what you are going to do, and why:

Now I am going to ask you some other questions to find out how well you are keeping up with things. It's important that you try to do your best even if you find them very easy or very difficult.

Record correct and incorrect answers. Also note the patient's attitude to the tests. Is he really trying? Is he *unable to cooperate* because he is very anxious, or very depressed? Does he lose patience or refuse to attempt them, for example on the grounds that they are too trivial? When interpreting the results remember that to some extent they are affected by both intelligence and education, and the history of education and occupation should, therefore, be taken into account when trying to decide the significance of difficulties that are encountered.

Orientation

Orientation in time and place should be examined first. Ask:

What day of the week is it today?
Without looking at your watch, about what time is it now?
Can you tell me the date and the year?
What is the name of this place?

If these are inaccurate ask more detailed questions:

What sort of place is it?
What town are we in?
How would you get here from your home?
What is your name?
Who am I?

If the patient is unable to do any of these, ask:

Is it daytime or night time?
Is it nearer to 9.00 a.m. or midday?
Would you say it's Monday or Tuesday today?
The beginning or end of the month?

All patients should be able to answer the questions about identity correctly. They should also know they are in hospital and its name. They should have an accurate knowledge of the day of the week and of the time of day to within about one hour. Record verbatim replies to your questions together with the correct answers (in brackets).

Note any other observations suggesting disorientation. For example, the patient may have difficulty finding his way about a hospital ward several days after arrival or he may get into the wrong bed.

Disorientation is the cardinal sign of clouding of consciousness, which is a feature of delirium. This may be accompanied by a diminished awareness and grasp of the surroundings, and attention is also likely to be impaired. Delirious patients may be unaware of the time of day, the nature of the place, or of the function of people around them. However, inaccurate replies to questions about orientation may also be due to poor memory (in dementia), or to a narrowed range of interest in the affective disorders.

Attention and concentration

Defects in attention and concentration will usually be evident whilst the history is being taken. It may be difficult to attract the patient's attention, or once attracted it may be poorly sustained. The patient may be distracted by events in the environment which would usually be ignored during a medical consultation, such as birds singing in the garden or a book on the table, and attention may flit rapidly from one object to the next. Attention may be diverted by experiences not shared by the interviewer, such as voices to which the patient listens. Specific tests of attention are based on the ability to keep track of sequences of material which is familiar to the patient and does not, therefore, require new learning.

Allow the patient as much time as he needs to complete each test, but note unobtrusively how long the patient takes and record this:

> *Tell me the days of the week backwards, starting with Saturday.*
> *Tell me the months of the year backwards, starting with December.*

As usual record the patient's replies verbatim and the length of time taken for each task. Unimpaired subjects should be able to complete these rapidly, without mistakes:

> *Starting with one hundred, subtract seven and then continue to subtract sevens as far as you can.*

If the patient does not understand the task, ask:

> *What's seven from one hundred?*
> *And seven from ninety-three?*

Carry on like this until he's got the idea. If the patient still does not understand, or says it is too difficult, ask him to subtract threes from twenty.

Performance is more dependent on educational and intellectual attainment than the previous tests, and results must, therefore, be interpreted in the light of the history of schooling and employment. Disorders of attention are common and can occur in almost any psychiatric disorder, particularly organic states and affective disorders.

(Patients who show definite evidence of impaired attention on these tests will usually be unable to attend to the following tests of memory, in which case they will not provide any additional information and need not be carried out.)

Registration and short-term memory

DIGIT SPAN

This is a test of registration and immediate recall. Start by explaining:

> *I am going to give you some numbers to remember. When I stop I want you to repeat them to me. For example, if I say '2 4 7', you would repeat '2 4 7'.*

Give a series of three digits, at an even speed of about one per second, and avoid laying emphasis on some more than others. Ask the patient to repeat them immediately.

If he is correct, give four digits, using a new sequence, then five, and so on, until the patient makes a mistake, say at seven digits.

Finally note the maximum number of digits that can be correctly repeated in sequence. Most unimpaired adults of average intelligence can manage seven digits forwards. Five or less is strongly suggestive of impairment.

STANFORD-BINET SENTENCE

This is a test of registration and immediate recall, which makes allowance for intelligence. Explain:

> *I am going to ask you to remember a sentence. Listen carefully and then repeat the sentence as accurately as possible.*

One of the following sentences should then be read out slowly. Select the one best suited to the patient's probable intellect. Then immediately ask him to repeat it. If he makes a mistake, try an easier sentence. If his repetition is accurate, try a more difficult sentence. Only read out a sentence once, slowly and clearly. Then record the response verbatim.

Sentence to be given to adults of dull intellect (completed successfully by 50 per cent of eleven-year-olds):

> *Yesterday we went for a ride in our car along the road that crosses the bridge.*

For dull average adults (50 per cent of thirteen-year-olds):

> *The aeroplane made a careful landing in the space which had been prepared for it.*

For adults of average intellect:

> *The red-headed woodpeckers made a terrible fuss as they tried to drive the young away from the nest.*

For adults of superior intelligence:

> *At the end of the week the newspapers published a complete account of the experiences of the great explorer.*

NAME, ADDRESS, AND FLOWER

This tests registration, immediate recall, and short-term memory. Explain:

> *I am going to give you the name and address of an imaginary person, and the name of a flower that he likes. It is a routine test of your memory which we give everyone. I want you to try to remember it and repeat it back to me as soon as I have finished. The name is:*
> Mr William Thompson
> 118 Hamilton Terrace
> Chorlton
> Manchester 13.
> *The flower is a daffodil.*
> *Now please repeat that back to me.*

Record both the name and address that you give the patient and his immediate response. Note that there are nine items to be remembered, apart from 'Mr'. In selecting a name and address avoid very common names, for example, John Smith, or local addresses which are familiar to the patient. If the patient makes a mistake, read back the same name and address as before and ask him to repeat it. Continue until he is entirely accurate, noting the number of trials required. When the patient is entirely correct, say:

> *I want you to try to remember that name and address and I will ask you again later on.*

Then continue with other tests, for example remote memory. After two minutes ask the patient to repeat the name and address. This time do not correct any mistakes. After a further three minutes again ask for a repetition. Record the responses each time. Was there evidence of poor registration? Once the material has been correctly registered, is there accurate recall? If mistakes are made, are they the same on each occasion, or is performance worse after five minutes than after two?

   If the same test is used on subsequent occasions, use different names and addresses each time, of similar length and complexity to the example provided. Most people are able to repeat the name and address without mistakes immediately and after five minutes. Three mistakes or more at five minutes are strongly suggestive of a clinically significant deficit.

Longer-term memory

Recent memory can be tested by asking about personal experiences in the last few days: if possible ask questions to which the correct answers can be verified. For example, ask:

How long have you been in hospital?
Who brought you here?
Can you tell me about the television programme you watched last night?
What's in the newspaper you were reading this morning?

Test remote memory by asking about personal experiences, for example:

Can you tell me the name of your last school?
And the name of the headmaster?
What was the date when you got married?

Past general events, for example, the dates of the Second World War or the names of the last five prime ministers, are concerned with general knowledge rather than long-term memory, and answers depend on intelligence and education as well as memory. Thus, poor performance can be due to poor education as well as dull intellect or organic brain disease:

Can you tell me the names of five cities in England?
And five sorts of fruit?
What is the name of the Prime Minister?
And the one before that?

Evidence of difficulty with longer-term memory often comes to light during the process of taking the history. For example, the patient may show major contradictions in his age, the year of his retirement, or when his wife died.

Defects in short-term memory alone, as revealed by the above tests, are actually defects of new learning. Memory of events prior to the onset of brain disease remains intact, but there is a disorder in the registration and retention of new experiences.

Defects in longer-term memory may involve **retrograde amnesia**, that is, the loss of memories of events experienced before the onset of brain disease.

Patients with dementia often have difficulty with short-term memory, but appear to have remarkably good memory for the details of early life. However, beware of **confabulation** – the invention of replies to questions to hide poor memory. As dementia progresses, eventually even long-term memory deteriorates.

Intelligence

An impression of the patient's level of intelligence will be gained during the course of history-taking, from the extent of the vocabulary used, from the complexity of the concepts expressed, and from the Stanford-Binet sentence remembered correctly. If these appear to be consistent with the patient's known history of education and employment, and if there is no evidence of impairment in tests of memory, then tests of intelligence are unlikely to be helpful.

Possible **mental retardation** may be assessed by simple tests of comprehension, such as:

What is three times nine?
Sixteen divided by four?

What is the difference between a fence and a wall?
If a flag is being blown towards the west, from which direction is the wind coming?

Illiteracy may be a serious handicap, which patients often fail to mention and may not be suspected. If in doubt, ask:

Did you learn to read and write at school?
Would you mind reading to me from this newspaper?

ABSTRACTION

Tests of abstraction can be helpful in eliciting thought disorder, and should be given only if this is suspected (see p. 27). Ask the patient to explain the meaning of one or two **proverbs**. Start by giving an example:

Proverbs are sayings which have general meanings. For example, 'Too many cooks spoil the broth' means 'If too many people do the same job it is likely to go wrong'. Have you heard people say 'Make hay while the sun shines'?
(If 'yes') Could you tell me what it means?

Record the reply and if it is satisfactory ask a more difficult proverb:

Now tell me the meaning of 'People who live in glass houses shouldn't throw stones'.

Consider the extent to which the patient's answer shows thought disorder (which may indicate schizophrenia) on the one hand, or concrete thinking (suggestive of organic damage or dull intellect) on the other.

INSIGHT AND JUDGEMENT

An understanding of the presence and nature of mental illness and of its causes is never complete and is rarely totally absent, therefore avoid generalizations, such as 'good insight' or 'bad insight'. The patient's insight may be indicated at different stages through the history and examination. The following are all quite common:

There's nothing wrong with me. I'm not ill. It's my doctor who wanted me to see you.
My wife's the one who needs to see you.
I just need some stronger sleeping pills.

Sometimes a patient's statements about insight appear to contradict his non-verbal behaviour. For example, he may insist that he is not mentally ill, but agrees voluntarily to admission to a psychiatric unit and to take medication for mental illness. So, ask:

Do you think you are ill?
What sort of illness do you think you have?
Do you think it might be a nervous or mental illness?

To what extent does he correctly identify the relevance of his symptoms? For example, does he recognize that feelings of guilt and suicidal thoughts are due to depressive illness from which he may recover? Does he regard his auditory hallucinations as abnormal experiences, indicative of mental illness and requiring treatment; or as a normal experience, shared by others and not requiring medical attention?

Further questions may be needed to find out the patient's views about the cause of his illness and the appropriate treatment:

> *What do you think might have caused this illness?*
> *Has anything happened to upset you?*
> *What sort of help do you think you need now?*

How realistic are the patient's views?

The assessment of insight has important implications for management. A patient who does not recognize that his suicidal thoughts are symptomatic of a treatable illness with good prognosis is more likely to act on such thoughts and, therefore, will require closer observation, possibly as an in-patient. The patient with persecutory delusions who is unaware that his fears are due to illness is more likely to defend himself by attacking others. A patient who shares the doctor's opinion of appropriate management is more likely to be compliant, for example by either taking medication or involving himself in psychotherapy. Insight has, therefore, an important bearing on prognosis (see Chapter 8).

INTERVIEWER'S REACTION TO PATIENT

What is your own subjective response to the patient? Did you enjoy meeting the patient, or did he make you feel sad, frustrated, or angry? Was it easy or difficult to control the interview in order to obtain necessary information? Ask yourself what happened in the interview which caused you to feel this way. Your responses indicate something about you, as well as about the patient, and your relationship with each other. Is the patient a passive, dependent person, who induces in you frustration as much as sympathy; an aggressive, bombastic, or egocentric person, who took over the interview, prevented you from obtaining essential information and left you feeling inadequate and angry; or one who makes frequent statements about how others, particularly doctors, have let him down and, therefore, induces feelings of guilt?

If you found some difficulty in developing a working relationship with the patient, consider to what extent this is determined by the patient's behaviour and whether this is symptomatic of his present illness. Alternatively, have you elicited evidence of lifelong difficulties which the patient has had in his relationships with family, workmates, or others? It is likely that your own reaction to the patient is similar to the reactions of others and may tell you much about the patient's personality.

EXAMPLE OF A MENTAL STATE EXAMINATION

Appearance and behaviour

Mrs Woods is a rather plump, middle-aged lady who is not wearing any make-up. On introduction she shook hands limply and avoided eye-contact but her manner was cooperative. She walked slowly to the interview room, then sat slumped in her chair in the same posture throughout the interview with little movement except of her hands, which she clasped and rubbed together particularly when talking about her bereavement.

Speech

Talk is slow with slight delay before replying to questions and there is little spontaneous speech except about her physical health. However, her answers are coherent and to the point, and there is no evidence of formal thought disorder.

Mood

She describes her mood as 'I've got a bit low recently. I'm worrying all the time about my mother'. Says she regards life as worth living 'because of my family'. Appears sad and tense through most of the interview, weeps when talking about her mother, but smiles appropriately on several occasions.

Thought content

Describes herself as 'brooding' about her mother. On several occasions refers to her recent chest pains and asks at the end of the interview whether I think she might have had 'a heart attack'. She expresses an idea of self-blame: 'If only I had done more for my mother, I'm sure she wouldn't be dead now' . . . 'I wasn't a good daughter'. Denies that there is anything specific that she could have done but this belief is firmly held. No other abnormal beliefs. She denies suicidal thoughts.

Perception

Mrs Woods admits on direct questioning that she thought she heard the voice of her mother on three or four occasions since her death saying: 'Don't worry about me. I'm all right now'; and felt 'as if her mother was present with her in the room. 'It must have been my imagination, but it seemed real at the time.' (These seem to have been auditory hallucinations.) She also describes a feeling of 'numbness' on the day of the funeral which has gradually diminished since then. There are no other disorders of perception.

Orientation

'Thursday, about ten o'clock, November 1994; I'm not sure, is it the 26th?'

(All correct except 28th November.)
'In the Psychiatry Department, Manchester Royal Infirmary.' (Correct.)

Attention and concentration

Generally attentive during the interview except when preoccupied with the bereavement and her own health.
'Saturday, Friday, Thursday, Wednesday, Tuesday, Monday, Sunday.'
(Slow and hesitant in 25 seconds.)
'December, November, October, September . . . September, August, July, March . . . no, where was I? I'm sorry.'
(40 seconds.)
'100, 93, 86, 80, 73, 65, 60, did you say seven from a hundred? 60, 50, no 53, 45, no, I'm sorry.'
(4 mistakes; 2 minutes 10 seconds.)
'20, 17, 14, 11, 9, 7, 5 . . . no, that's not right is it?'
(25 seconds.)

Registration and short-term memory

Not tested in view of obvious problems with attention.

Long-term memory

Gives detailed and consistent account of early life.
Cities: Manchester, London, Birmingham, Liverpool, Chester.
Knows the name of the Prime Minister and the President of the USA but cannot remember their predecessors.
Dates of world wars 1914–1918, 1939–1945.

Intelligence

Probably average in view of school to age of fifteen and semi-skilled work; consistent with present use of vocabulary.

Insight

'It's the pain in my heart . . . I don't think it's a mental illness . . . do you think I need another ECG? Well perhaps I've got a bit low since my mother died.'

SUMMARY OF THE MENTAL STATE EXAMINATION

1. **Appearance and behaviour**
    Description: reaction to interviewer; motor activity

2. **Speech**
    Speed; quantity; continuity; relevance

3. **Mood**
    Subjective account; observed mood; autonomic reactivity

4. **Thought content**
    Preoccupations; morbid thoughts; abnormal beliefs

5. **Perception**
    Illusions; hallucinations; depersonalization

6. **Intellectual function**

    6.1 Orientation
    Time and place

    6.2 Attention and concentration
    Days of week and months of year backwards
    Serial sevens or threes

    6.3 Registration and short-term memory
    Recent news; your name; consultant's name
    Digit span; Stanford-Binet sentence
    Name, address, and flower

    6.4 Long-term memory
    Early life; five cities
    World leaders; world wars

    6.5 Intelligence
    Assessed from personal history

7. **Insight**
    Nature of illness; causes of illness; appropriate treatment

FURTHER READING

Fish, F. (1985) *Psychopathology*. Bristol: John Wright. (Ed. M. Hamilton.)

4 / SYNDROMES AND DIAGNOSIS

THE PURPOSE AND LIMITATIONS OF DIAGNOSIS

The purpose of a diagnosis is to bring together illnesses which have the same characteristics. Ideally, a diagnosis should identify disorders having the same underlying pathology, the same causes, and the same likely response to treatment. However, such an ideal is rarely achieved. Thus a diagnosis of **Huntington's chorea** identifies a necessary cause (an autosomal dominant gene), a pathology (cortical and extra-pyramidal degeneration), a clinical presentation (dementia and choreiform movements with onset usually between ages thirty and fifty), and a course (progressive deterioration resulting in death). Ideally the diagnosis should also indicate an expected response to treatment, which in this example is at present limited to genetic counselling and symptomatic care. Although this diagnosis identifies a disease process, there are some limitations in its value, because not all those who suffer the disease will conform to this typical pattern. For example, some will show choreiform movements with little or no evidence of dementia. The age of onset will vary, and occasionally presentation may occur in childhood or old age. This illustrates the fact that all disease processes are subject to considerable variability.

Pulmonary tuberculosis is a diagnosis which deviates further from the ideal. All patients will have a similar basic pathology in the same organ, but the clinical presentation will vary from a chance radiological finding with no clinical features to an acute fulminating disorder. The course of these will differ widely, as will the management. All cases will have a similar necessary cause (the tubercle bacillus), but this is not a sufficient cause, and many other different factors will play a part in the aetiology of different cases (for example, the state of nutrition, accommodation, and socio-economic status).

Other 'diagnoses' tell us even less and are mainly a means of identifying clinical syndromes. A common example is **congestive cardiac failure,** which identifies a set of symptoms and signs, but provides only limited information about the underlying aetiology or pathology, and little about the course or response to particular treatments. However, even such a limited clinical label may alert us to a range of possible causes.

Most psychiatric diagnoses are syndrome diagnoses. Like the example of congestive cardiac failure, they tell us the symptoms and signs that characterize the disorder, but only a little about the aetiology, which must be considered separately. A diagnosis of **delirium** will convey the clinical presentation, but does not tell us which of the many different causes of this syndrome is relevant to a particular case (see p.152), and therefore does not tell us which specific treatment will be appropriate.

However, it does direct our attention to known causes of delirium, just as the diagnosis of depression directs our attention to known causes of depressive illness. Cause and treatment must, therefore, be considered separately from diagnosis for each patient.

A further complication arises because not only may a syndrome have a different cause in different cases, but often there are multiple interacting factors all contributing to the aetiology of a single case. In the example of pulmonary tuberculosis, contact with a case of pulmonary tuberculosis exposes an individual to the risk of developing the disorder, but he will not necessarily become infected unless other factors are also involved. Similarly a woman's susceptibility to the development of a **depressive illness** will be increased by the death of her mother before the age of eleven, having no close supportive relationship, and having three children or more below the age of fourteen. However, not all women with these experiences will develop depressive illness. Just as malnutrition may predispose an individual to many different physical illnesses, the same aetiological factors may increase susceptibility to several psychiatric syndromes.

THE TRADITIONAL ORGANIZATION OF DIAGNOSTIC CATEGORIES

It has been traditional to differentiate between categories of psychiatric disorder in two ways. The first divides them according to clinical presentation, into **psychoses**, **neuroses**, and **personality disorders**. The second has regard to aetiology, and divides them into '**organic**' disorders that are secondary to known brain disease, and '**functional**' disorders whose physical basis is unknown.

Both the psychoses and the neuroses share a widely accepted criterion of illness, that is, a deterioration from a presumed previous state of health and the development of symptoms. By contrast **personality disorders** do not involve change. They are identified by the presence of personality characteristics (traits) which are relatively constant throughout life and cause the subject and/or society to suffer.

The differentiation between the psychoses and neuroses is essentially arbitrary, and based mainly on historical beliefs and practices. The **psychoses** include those disorders traditionally regarded as madness, in which strange beliefs and perceptions, often accompanied by violent and destructive behaviour, at one time resulted in incarceration in mental asylums. It has long been recognized that some of these illnesses are secondary to structural disease of the brain and these are therefore called **organic psychoses**, while others occur in brains that appear histologically normal, and are therefore called '**functional**' psychoses.

However, recent research shows that demonstrable structural or neurochemical changes also occur in the functional psychoses, so that the distinction between them and organic psychoses no longer has much substance.

The term **neurosis** was first used in 1769 by William Cullen to describe what were believed to be organic diseases of nerve tissue. Patients with these disorders presented to physicians with complaints generally thought to indicate physical illness, such as lassitude, dizziness, weakness, and poor appetite. They were considered to be suffering literally from 'weak nerves', and the terminology survives, even though there is usually no corresponding underlying physical disease of nerve tissue. During the nineteenth century there was an increasing awareness that these physical complaints could have their foundation in mental rather than physical mechanisms. The development of psychoanalysis from the 1890s, and behavioural psychology from the 1920s, led to increasing awareness of the way that mental mechanisms might operate to produce these symptoms.

By the beginning of the twentieth century psychiatrists saw those who presented with physical symptoms that were without known organic cause (dissociative disorders and hypochondriasis), and also began to see patients with wholly psychological disorders such as anxiety state, obsessional neurosis, and phobic neurosis.

In the United Kingdom psychiatrists only began to be appointed to the staff of general hospitals in any numbers in the 1930s, and departments of 'psychological medicine' arose, to which patients with somatic symptoms unaccompanied by physical disease – the 'neurotics' of the previous century – were referred. However, most psychiatrists continued to work in mental hospitals, where their clinical work was mainly concerned with 'psychotic' illnesses. Thus patients with neuroses and psychoses were seen and treated in different hospital settings and often by different groups of psychiatrists. Although these barriers have almost disappeared the separation between neuroses and psychoses lingers on as a vestigial remnant.

By the middle of this century psychiatrists were working more closely with colleagues in general hospital settings, were seeing patients referred by general practitioners, and were beginning to be asked to see increasing numbers of patients with **maladaptive behaviours** which cannot be fitted into the categories of either psychosis or neurosis. These disorders include disorders such as alcoholism, anorexia nervosa, bulimia nervosa, and drug dependency; self-damaging behaviours such as self-poisoning and self-mutilation; and certain sexual disorders.

We will now consider the distinction between each of the various categories which we have discussed so far.

Organic versus functional psychosis

The disorders at present referred to as 'organic' should more accurately be thought of as those where we have a clear idea of an aetiology, and that aetiology is a physical disease. They include conditions where the structure of the brain is abnormal such as Alzheimer's disease or psychoses secondary to cerebro-vascular disease, and conditions where the brain is structurally normal – such as delirium associated with typhoid fever, pneumococcal pneumonia, or alcohol withdrawal ('delirium tremens'). It could be argued that the latter group are in a sense 'functional', and that as knowledge of neurochemistry advances we can expect to gain a greater understanding of many – if not all – of those psychoses at present referred to as 'functional', such as schizophrenia and manic-depressive illness.

For the present, there are clear advantages in making a distinction between those conditions where the aetiology is either coarse brain disease or physical disease elsewhere in the body, and those where the disorder arises from disordered functioning of the brain itself.

Neurosis versus psychosis

Previous claims that psychoses differ from neuroses because they are more 'severe' are not valid, because many neurotic patients also suffer from chronic, severely disabling illnesses. Although psychotic patients are said to be less in touch with reality (or to show 'defects in reality testing') and to have less insight into their illness, it will be remembered from the previous chapter that insight is never completely present or absent. Psychotic patients rarely have no insight at all, and neurotic patients never have perfect insight. It is a matter of degree, so insight cannot be a basis on which two categories of disease can be separated.

The only criterion by which these groups of disorders can be separated reliably involves an arbitrary operational definition. Psychotic illnesses are characterized by the presence of 'psychotic symptoms', specifically delusions and hallucinations. Such symptoms occur only in the psychoses, whereas 'neurotic symptoms' occur in both the neuroses and the psychoses. Thus if delusions or hallucinations are found in a particular mental illness, by definition it is a psychosis; if absent, it is a neurosis. The reason for making the distinction at all is that patients experiencing psychotic phenomena are more likely to have grossly deranged neurochemistry, and are therefore more likely to respond to physical treatments such as psychotropic drugs and ECT. They are also more likely to have severely disturbed behaviour requiring in-patient treatment.

However, the word 'neurosis' applies to a kind of illness which can come and go, while the word 'neurotic' refers to long-standing attributes in a person. There are many indi- viduals who have episodes of allegedly 'neurotic' illness such as depressive illness who are not especially 'neurotic' people. The term 'neurosis' should really be abandoned, but it will probably obstinately live on, if only because it is a pithy way of saying 'non-psychotic'. However, we shall not be using it in the remainder of this book.

Non-psychotic illnesses therefore form a large residual category of disorders. Within this category the mood disorders – those related to depression and anxiety – are most like medical syndromes such as migraine, but there are also other patterns of maladaptive behaviour such as alcoholism and self-poisoning and patterns of abnormal illness behaviour which the doctor must understand, and these will be described in the chapters which follow.

THE HIERARCHICAL MODEL OF DIAGNOSIS

We have seen that the various syndromes of psychiatric disorder can be arranged in a rough hierarchy, where the top level (*'level one'*) represents those conditions which have a known 'organic' aetiology, the second (*'level two'*) those psychotic conditions where there are likely to be severe neurochemical derangements in cerebral functioning, and then there is a rather heterogeneous residual group. It is reasonable to make a distinction between disorders where concepts of treatment and recovery are appropriate (*'level three'*): affective disorders, maladaptive behaviours, and abnormal illness behaviours; and those which represent stable attributes of human functioning (*'level four'*): personality disorders and disorders of gender identity and sexual orientation.

The latter should not be thought of as illnesses, but they are often relevant to understanding the aetiology of illness, they may complicate treatment plans, and they are associated with suffering – either for the patient, or those with whom he lives. The scheme is shown in *Table 4.1*. From the student's point of view, the main advantage of such a hierarchy is to remind you that certain symptoms have more specificity than others in leading to a syndrome diagnosis.

Thus symptoms in the 'intellectual function' section of the mental state examination indicate that serious consideration must be given to the possibility that the patient can be recruited to the top of the hierarchy. If we decide to do this, we will give less attention to other symptoms from lower in the hierarchy that might be present. For example, if we decide a patient has delirium we will pay little diagnostic attention to anxious mood since we will be preoccupied with finding (and treating) the cause of the delirium.

Within the psychotic stratum, it is now usual to put clear manic symptoms 'above' schizophrenic symptoms, and to put these in turn 'above' depressive symptoms (see below). This is because many studies have shown schizophrenia-like symptoms in manic patients who have recovered completely from such illnesses and gone on to develop clear manic-depressive (or 'bipolar') illnesses. However, providing manic symptoms are absent, 'disintegrative delusions' (thought reading, thought withdrawal, or ideas of passivity) are suggestive of schizophrenia, *providing that features indicating an organic disorder are absent.* This is because certain organic illnesses can cause schizophrenia-like symptoms (see p. 179), and if these illnesses are present it is usual to diagnose them rather than schizophrenia.

In this way 'schizophrenia' becomes a name attached to disorders which have certain typical symptoms but for which no organic aetiology has been identified and which are not clearly manic: and it is in this sense that organic illnesses and mania are 'above' schizophrenia in the hierarchy. On the other hand, mood disorders such as depression and anxiety occur commonly in the setting of schizophrenia but do not alter the diagnosis of schizophrenia since they are said to be 'below' schizophrenia. Thus, a depressive illness would only be diagnosed if signs of schizophrenia and of an organic state were absent.

The third level of the hierarchy contains all possible symptoms except those pathognomonic of organic disorders or strongly suggestive of psychotic illness. These symptoms are non-specific in the sense that they can also occur at the higher levels, but if they do they will not alter the diagnosis. They only attract syndromal labels when they occur on their own. You will notice that the concept of 'depression' appears in both levels 2 and 3. This is because in its severe form depression can be accompanied by psychotic symptoms, whereas the commoner forms of depression have symptoms that are more readily

Table 4.1 *The hierarchical model of diagnosis*

level one: ORGANIC DISORDERS	**delirium** ('Acute brain syndrome') **dementia** ('Chronic brain syndrome') **Korsakow's syndrome**
level two: 'FUNCTIONAL' PSYCHOSES	**mania** **schizophrenia** **psychotic depression**
level three: NON-PSYCHOTIC DISORDERS	**depressive illness** **anxiety disorders** anxiety state specific phobias agoraphobia panic disorder post-traumatic stress disorder **maladaptive behaviours** alcoholism drug dependence anorexia nervosa and bulimia obesity obsessive compulsive disorder **abnormal illness behaviour** somatization disorder persistent somatoform pain disorder hypochondriacal disorder factitious illness malingering dissociative disorders
level four: PERSONALITY DISORDERS	**paranoid** personality **schizoid** personality **dissocial** personality **emotionally unstable** personality **histrionic** personality **obsessional** personality **dependent** personality

understandable. This alerts you to the fact that the distinction between 'functional psychoses' and less severe forms of mental disorder is but a convenient fiction.

ONE DIAGNOSIS OR TWO?

In the case of 'maladaptive behaviours' it will often be useful to diagnose these *in addition to* a diagnosis based on experienced symptoms.

For example, if a patient with schizophrenia (a *level 2 diagnosis*) also has symptoms of alcoholism (a maladaptive behaviour) we should diagnose both conditions, since the second diagnosis gives important information not contained in the first. There is no underlying assumption about their relationship: they might be coincidental, or either might be a factor contributing to the aetiology of the other. It is usual to ask ourselves whether there might be a relationship whenever we make more than one diagnosis: in this example the patient may have developed a typical form of auditory hallucinosis after many years of heavy drinking (in which case we speak of **alcoholic hallucinosis**), or he may only drink because the voices tell him to (primary diagnosis therefore **schizophrenia**), or there may be no obvious relationship, in which case we simply make two diagnoses, putting the one highest on the hierarchy first.

Further examples of related diagnoses, where the second label gives information not implicit in the first, would be

1. *Agoraphobia,*
2. *Alcoholism,* or

1. *Anorexia nervosa,*
2. *Depressive illness.*

The second diagnosis is necessary since by no means all agoraphobics develop alcohol problems, and not all anorexics are depressed. In each case, the presence of the second diagnosis is likely to influence the treatment plan proposed for the patient. Note that the maladaptive behaviour has been put first in the latter example, implying that it may be causally implicated in the depression.

Diagnosis of a personality disorder may also be complementary to other diagnosis, and either help us to understand the aetiology or influence our management of the problem, for example:

1. *Paranoid psychosis,*
2. *Paranoid personality,* or

1. *Self-poisoning,*
2. *Emotionally unstable personality.*

Having said this, it should be emphasized that two diagnoses should only be made if one will not do, so that one tries first to find a single diagnosis which will accommodate all the symptoms and signs. Only if this is not possible consider a second diagnosis.

Differential diagnosis is a quite separate process, which is concerned with alternative rather than complementary diagnoses, and is discussed in the chapter on formulation.

CLASSIFICATORY SYSTEMS

The terminology used to label the different syndromes is embodied in various systems of classification. The tenth revision of the International Classification of Disease (ICD-10) includes a classification of mental disorders in its fifth chapter. There are 458 categories of mental disorders listed in this chapter, and they are grouped in ten major groups. Most of these are rare disorders, or are subvarieties of some of the larger groupings described in this book. The fifty-one disorders described in this book are shown in *Table 4.2*, grouped according to their official codes in the ICD-10. This is the system that has been most widely used, both in the United Kingdom and abroad. It has been shown that different psychiatrists working in different hospitals, and in different countries, reach a high level of agreement in making diagnoses for the same patients when applying this classification. The World Health Organization has produced a much simpler version of this classification for use in primary care and general medical settings, called the ICD-10 PHC: each of the twenty-four conditions included in this classification is accompanied by clear advice on the management of the disorder.

The Diagnostic and Statistical Manual of the American Psychiatric Association (now in its fourth revision, thus DSM-IV) provides another classification which has recently aroused much interest. It differs from the International Classification of Disease in some important respects, notably in that it tends to give more emphasis to clear operational rules in making diagnoses.

Table 4.2 *Ten major groups of Chapter V of ICD-10 and their relationship to the main disorders described in this book*

F0	**Organic, including symptomatic, mental disorders**	
	F00	Alzheimer's disease
	F01	Vascular dementia
	F02	Other dementias
	F05	Delirium
F1	**Mental and behaviour disorders due to psychoactive substance use**	
	F10	Disorders due to alcohol
	F10.2	Alcohol dependence
	F10.6	Korsakow's syndrome
	F11–19	Disorders due to other substances
F2	**Schizophrenia and delusional disorders**	
	F20	Schizophrenia
	F22	Persistent delusional disorder ('paranoid psychosis')
	F25	Schizoaffective disorder
F3	**Mood (affective) disorders**	
	F30	Manic episode
	F31	Bipolar affective disorder
	F32.0	Depressive episode
	F32.3	Depressive episode with psychotic symptoms
	F34.0	Cyclothymia
F4	**Neurotic, stress-related, and somatoform disorders**	
	F40.0	Agoraphobia
	F40.1	Social phobias
	F40.2	Specific phobias
	F41.0	Panic disorder
	F41.1	Generalized anxiety state
	F42	Obsessive compulsive disorder

Table 4.2 *Continued*

	F43.1	Post-traumatic stress disorder
	F43.2	Adjustment disorders
	F44	Dissociative (conversion) disorders
	F45.1	Somatization disorder
	F45.2	Hypochondriacal disorder
	F45.4	Persistent somatoform pain disorder
F5	**Physiological dysfunction associated with mental factors**	
	F50	Eating disorders
	F50.0	Anorexia nervosa
	F50.2	Bulimia nervosa
	F51.0	Non-organic insomnia
	F52.0	Lack of sexual desire
	F52.11	Lack of sexual enjoyment
	F52.2	Failure of genital response
		(includes male impotence; female lack of arousal)
	F52.3	Orgasmic dysfunction
	F52.4	Premature ejaculation
	F52.5	Vaginismus
	F52.6	Dyspareunia
	F53	Puerperal mental disorder
F6	**Abnormalities of adult personality and behaviour**	
	F60.0	Paranoid ('sensitive') personality
	F60.1	Schizoid personality
	F60.2	Dissocial ('anti-social') personality
	F60.3	Emotionally unstable personality
	F60.4	Histrionic personality
	F60.5	Obsessional ('anankastic') personality
	F60.7	Dependent personality
	F64	Gender identity disorder
	F68.1	Factitious disorder
F7	**Mental retardation**	
	F70–73	Mild; moderate; severe; profound
F8	**Developmental disorders**	
	F84.0	Autism
F9	**Behavioural and emotional disorders of childhood or adolescence**	
	F90	Hyperkinetic disorders
	F91	Conduct disorders
	F93	Emotional disorders

FURTHER READING

American Psychiatric Association (1993) *Diagnostic and Statistical Manual of Mental Disorders. DSM-IV*. Washington, DC.

Kendell, R.E. (1975) *The Role of Diagnosis in Psychiatry*. Oxford: Blackwell Scientific.

World Health Organization (1992) *The ICD-10 Classification of Mental and Behavioural Disorders: Clinical Descriptions and Diagnostic Guidelines*. Geneva: World Health Organization.

5 / AETIOLOGY

In this chapter we will look at the general principles that underlie the causes of mental disorders and the way in which these can be used to form hypotheses about the aetiology of an individual patient's illness. An accurate assessment of aetiology is important but should be based on well-observed data rather than wild speculation. It then serves as a logical basis for the plan of management (Chapter 7). The particular causes of each syndrome will be considered in Part 2.

AETIOLOGICAL FACTORS

When we look for the aetiological factors of a patient's illness we are in effect trying to answer the following questions:

> *Why this disorder?*
> *Why at this particular time?*

In more chronic disorders we must also ask:

> *Why no recovery?*

Aetiological factors can contribute at different stages: first by predisposing to illness, then as precipitants and finally as maintaining factors. The first of these questions deals with predisposition, the second with precipitation, and the third with maintaining factors.

Predisposing factors

Predisposing factors are those which increase an individual's vulnerability to developing an illness at any time in the future. They address the '*Why this disorder?*' question. The predisposition may operate in a general way (for example, **personality traits** of anxiety) so that the patient is at increased risk of developing different illnesses at a later stage in his life; or it may operate in a highly specific way (for example, a **genetic predisposition** to Huntington's chorea) to increase the risk of one particular disease. Some kinds of **abnormal personality** are at higher risk of particular illnesses, and these will be described at the end of this chapter.

Precipitating factors

Precipitating factors determine when the illness starts (*'Why at this particular time?'*). Some people are vulnerable to mental illness but may go for many years without becoming ill, so we have to determine the factors that bring about this change from health to illness. Usually precipitating factors act in a non-specific way, that is, they determine when the illness starts but not the type of illness: for example, **life events** (see p. 57) which involve loss can help to precipitate almost any disorder to which the patient has a predetermined vulnerability.

Maintaining factors

In addition we have to consider whether there may be additional maintaining factors which prolong a disorder, if it continues for longer than would usually be expected (*'Why no recovery?'*). For example, the majority of affective disorders lead to recovery within weeks or months so, if the condition persists for longer, is there any evidence of causes which continue to affect the patient and prevent recovery?

A systematic approach

We should use the available data to answer these questions for each patient that we assess. *Table 5.1* provides a guide to a systematic approach and each stage needs to be considered in turn. At each stage the aetiological factors may be divided into biological, social, and psychological. Consider whether you have discovered anything about your patient which might fit into these categories, in turn, but you are likely to use only a few of these for each patient.

Aim to write a systematic account of the possible aetiological factors that you have discovered after you have taken the history and completed the examination of the mental state. This will form part of the formulation (see Chapter 9).This initial hypothesis will have to be tested, and perhaps modified, when you attempt to support it by investigations (see Chapter 6).

In the past there was some controversy about whether the origins of mental illnesses are mainly genetic or acquired: nowadays it is more appropriate to consider the extent to which each makes a contribution.

Table 5.1 *Examples of aetiological factors*

1. *predisposing*

A biological: genetic; intra-uterine disadvantage; birth trauma; or disorders of later onset resulting in cerebral disease or physical handicap. Some forms of personality disorder.

B social: physical or emotional deprivation during childhood due to family discord, bereavement, or separation. Chronic difficulties in work, marriage, housing, or finance. Lack of supportive relationships

C psychological: inappropriate parental models, e.g. agoraphobic mother or violent father: constitutional predisposition to neurotic traits (may be partly biological), low self-esteem. Some forms of personality disorder. Habitual use of particular defence mechanisms.

2. *precipitating*

A biological: recent physical disease, e.g. infections, injury resulting in disability, malignant disease with threat of disfiguring surgery or death.

B social: recent life events, particularly those involving threat and loss, such as redundancy, child leaving home, separation or divorce, loss of a supportive relationship.

C psychological: subject's responses to biological or social factors, e.g. following bereavement or mutilating surgery; feelings of loss of self-esteem; helplessness; hopelessness.

3. *maintaining*

A biological: physical handicaps; pain from physical disease; failure to take medication or unwanted effects of medication.

B social: adverse social circumstances; no intimate relationships; negative interactions at home; no support from key relative; inappropriate medical management.

C psychological: hopelessness (no expectation of recovery); marked adverse personality traits, e.g. low self-esteem, excessive dependency or anxiety traits.

THE GENETIC CONTRIBUTION

Evidence for the inheritance of a mental illness is based on the following:

1. Higher prevalence rates in first-degree relatives than the risk for the general population.
2. Higher prevalence rates in the children of probands who are adopted by healthy parents.
3. Higher concordance rates in monozygotic than dizygotic twins.
4. The persistence of this increased concordance, even when monozygotic twins have been separated in infancy and reared apart.

There is a considerable variation in the extent to which different diagnostic categories have a genetic contribution. For example, the concordance rate for first-degree relatives of schizophrenics is between 5 per cent and 15 per cent compared with a lifetime prevalence of about 1 per cent in the general population. The concordance rates for monozygotic twins is between 40 and 60 per cent and this remains almost as high in twins that are raised separately by adoptive parents. The picture for manic-depressive (bipolar affective) disorder follows a similar pattern.

From these figures there can be no doubt that there is an important genetic contribution to the aetiology of these illnesses. However, the nature of this contribution is in doubt. It cannot be determined by either a simple dominant or recessive gene because concordance rates are too low. It has therefore been suggested that inheritance is likely to be due either to poly-genetic interactions (that is, a number of different minor genes acting to complement or modify each other) or to a single gene with incomplete penetrance. The fact that the concord-ance rates in monozygotic twins are considerably less than 100 per cent demonstrates the importance of the contribution from environmental factors.

There are few mental disorders in which the genetic contribution is substantially greater than this and these are due to single gene transmission following the recognized Mendelian patterns. Examples are:

Huntington's chorea (autosomal dominant inheritance)

and some of the uncommon causes of severe mental handicap such as:

tuberose sclerosis (autosomal dominant) and
phenylketonuria (autosomal recessive).

The genetic contribution to most of the common psychiatric disorders – the non-psychotic forms of affective disorder – is probably small and based on the inheritance of a general tendency rather than a predisposition to specific diseases. It is greater for anxiety states and obsessive compulsive disorders than for depressive disorder. It has been suggested that individuals who score high on 'neuroticism' scales may readily form conditioned responses when anxious.

Some mental illnesses are **familial** in the sense that they tend to aggregate in particular families, even though the evidence for a specific genetic contribution is not very good. Depressive illness is an example of this, but it is not known in what way members of a family 'communicate' depression to each other.

ENVIRONMENTAL FACTORS

Many different factors in the environment that play a part in the aetiology of mental illness have already been mentioned. Some specific events – like bereavement in child-hood – can have a long-term effect which may not be evident until much later in life. Others are more chronic difficulties, such as physical or sexual abuse in childhood, an unhappy marriage, or an unrewarding job, which may have a cumulative effect over many years.

LIFE EVENTS

Life events refer to discrete changes in a person's environment that may cause some form of threat or stress to the individual. Some studies have been concerned with specific types of stressful event, while others have dealt with the effects of any kind of stressful event. In the former type of study, groups of subjects who have all had a similar experience – such as death of their spouse – have been followed up prospectively to find out how many develop mental illness during the following year compared with control subjects who have not been bereaved.

In the latter type of study, a group of patients suffering from the same illness – for example, depression – are studied to see whether they have experienced more stressful events than controls in the months prior to the onset of illness. Careful research has excluded those events which might have been the effect rather than the cause of the illness, and demonstrated which types of events are important in the aetiology of various psychiatric illnesses. Events which can precipitate an episode of schizophrenia are any that involve change and include such 'desirable' events as promotion, getting a new job, and moving house in addition to undesirable events. In the three weeks prior to an episode of schizophrenia there is a three-fold increase in life events of all types compared with controls. The brevity of this increased period of risk indicates that the event is merely concerned with the exact *timing* of an episode of illness – we must look elsewhere for predisposing factors.

By contrast, research into life events prior to the onset of depressive disorders shows a five-fold excess only of undesirable events, and these may occur throughout at least the six-month period preceding the onset of illness. 'Loss events' such as bereavement, divorce, severe illness in a close relative, or redundancy have been shown to be particularly important. This means that the contribution of life events to the precipitation of a particular episode of depression is relatively greater than in schizophrenia. Of course many people experience such events without developing schizophrenia, depressive disorders, or any other mental illness, and this demonstrates the essential interaction between life events and predisposition. In the case of depression a stressful life event is much more likely to be followed by an episode of depressive illness in a woman who lacks an intimate confidant (a social predisposing factor) and who has low self-esteem (a personality factor).

PSYCHOLOGICAL DEFENCE MECHANISMS

The description of psychological defence mechanisms stems from the psychoanalytic work of Sigmund Freud (1856 to 1939). These are *unconscious* processes (the subject is not aware of them) used to *protect the individual from anxiety* arising from inner impulses or environmental threat. The subject is consciously unaware of painful experiences and of the unpleasant feelings attached to them. Individuals tend to have particular mechanisms which they acquire in childhood and use habitually, although sometimes they may emerge for the first time in the face of an unusual crisis. However, if a particular mechanism is used habitually it sometimes helps us to answer the *'Why this disorder?'* question, since different mechanisms tend to be used in different illnesses.

Repression and denial

Defence mechanisms are a part of the healthy repertoire of all people, since we all need to ward off anxiety. **Repression**, for example, refers to the exclusion from our awareness of impulses or emotions which would otherwise cause us distress. It would be difficult to remain healthy if we were unable to suppress unpleasant material, but it is easy to see that the process could go too far. Sometimes the defence against anxiety may prevent the subject from being aware that there are problems in his life which require constructive action. At other times the defence mechanism used may lead the subject to act in inappropriate ways which are maladaptive.

Thus defence mechanisms play an important part in the aetiology of mental illness: sometimes helping to protect against them, at other times contributing to their predisposition or precipitation. We shall be concerned only with those mechanisms which are of particular importance to an understanding of illness.

Denial is a mechanism by which experiences or feelings that might cause anxiety are denied, or prevented from entering conscious awareness.

> *A widow may keep all her late husband's personal possessions intact, cook meals for him, and anxiously await his return: she is said to be denying his death.*

Patients who have been told by their doctors that they have malignant disease may afterwards not remember that they have been told and behave as though they are certain of recovery: they have *denied* the information.

Projection

Projection is a process by which your own feelings or impulses are attributed to others.

> *For example, a patient does not accept his doctor's reassurance, and complains that no one will be able to help him. He is projecting his own feelings of helplessness into his doctors.*

Projection is an important mechanism in paranoid psychoses, which are illnesses in which the patient is convinced that others are persecuting him: his own self-critical feelings are being attributed to others.

Introjection

Introjection is the reverse process by which aspects of another person may be incorporated into the subject's perception of himself.

> *A patient may constantly criticize himself for being a failure in life, even though objectively he has done well. His criticism of himself stems from his father's critical attitude towards him which he has now introjected: it has become part of his perception of himself.*

Idealization

Idealization is a means by which ambivalent feelings towards another person may be split, so that the bad feelings are denied, or sometimes introjected, and the other person is then regarded as perfect. It is thus a feature of being in love. However, it is also a common feature of morbid grief.

> *For example, Mrs Woods (see p. 123) had an extremely ambivalent relationship with her mother, being very dependent on her but never able to please her. Following her mother's death Mrs Woods responded by unconsciously using idealization so that she remembered only her mother's good qualities and her own feelings of affection towards her mother. Her more negative feelings of anger and resentment were introjected and took the form of ideas of guilt and self-blame: it was no longer her mother whom she regarded as at fault, but herself. (A further example of introjection was the way in which she developed chest pain similar to that suffered by her mother. This also involved 'identification', a process by which she fused – or confused – her own identity with that of her mother.)*

Somatization and conversion

The term **'somatization'** can be used in a descriptive sense to indicate a psychological disorder presenting primarily with physical symptoms (see p. 233) but can also be used to describe a defence mechanism by which the focus on physical complaints serves to divert the subject from awareness of anxiety-provoking conflicts. Closely associated with this is the concept of **conversion**. This refers to the process by which the affect caused by a conflict is replaced by (or 'converted' into) a physical symptom. Idealization is also commonly associated with conversion: in extreme cases the patient claims that he has no problem of any kind in his life other than physical illness and if this is cured his life will be perfect in all respects (a truly remarkable state).

> *An example was a man who had been severely disabled due to headache for three years. He insisted that he could not remember any distressing event that occurred in the year prior to the onset of his symptoms. The history from his wife revealed that during that year he had experienced the bereavement of his father, a brother, and his closest friend, and had been so distressed that he could not attend the funerals.*

Dissociation

Dissociation is a defence mechanism which involves the splitting of two (or more) mental processes which would otherwise be integrated, one part then becoming unconscious. The splitting of conscious awareness is thought to result in such phenomena as **dissociative amnesia** or **fugue states** in which highly organized behaviours are carried out despite gross disturbance of memory or grasp of the environment. Dissociation and conversion are the defence mechanisms thought to predominate in **dissociative disorder** (see p. 239), and the resulting symptoms are described as 'dissociative' and 'conversion' symptoms, respectively.

PERSONALITY DISORDERS

A person's personality refers to long-standing ways of behaving in a wide variety of situations. The characteristic ways of behaving are called **traits,** and particular constellations of traits are said to constitute **personality types**. Thus, normal populations may be described in terms of 'extraversion–introversion', of 'stable–neurotic', or of other dimensions of personality derived by multivariate analysis of responses to questionnaires. We shall not give a full account of normal personality here, but there is a wide range of information available in postgraduate textbooks.

We shall be concerned with those aspects of personality that are of especial importance to doctors: either because they *increase an individual's vulnerability* to a particular disease, or because they help us to understand *how an individual is likely to behave when he is ill.*

Personality disorders refer to characteristics of individuals that cause them to suffer or which cause others in society to suffer: they have been described by the International Classification of Disease as:

> *deeply ingrained maladaptive patterns of behaviour generally recognisable by the time of adolescence or earlier and continuing throughout most of adult life, although often becoming less obvious in middle or old age.*

Two points must be emphasized from the outset. First, a personality disorder is not an illness, so concepts of 'treatment' and 'recovery' are simply irrelevant. It is sometimes possible to modify habitual patterns of behaviour to some extent, although typically such modification takes a great deal of time and effort if it succeeds at all. Second, by their very nature, personality disorders are dimensional rather than categorical. That is to say, there are infinitely graded steps between normality and any of the 'disorders' described below. The distinction between having, and not having, such a disorder is arbitrary: individuals present such traits to a greater or lesser extent, and it is possible to have some traits but not others under each heading.

Possession of some of the traits can be quite adaptive: for example, mildly obsessional people make good doctors, accountants, or lawyers; mildly histrionic people are good public speakers and fun to be with; schizoid people may run a good computer system; and dependent personalities may play supportive roles in human organizations. People with cyclothymia can be very creative during upswings of mood.

It is better to get into the habit of describing which traits best describe your particular patient rather than forcing them into one of the descriptions given below.

Paranoid personality (F60.0)
(also known as 'sensitive personality')

DESCRIPTION

The patient has displayed excessive sensitivity to humiliations and rebuffs; a tendency to misconstrue neutral or friendly actions of others as hostile and contemptuous, and a combative and tenacious sense of personal rights. There may be proneness to jealousy or excessive self-importance. Such people feel easily humiliated and put-upon, and there is excessive self-reference. They bear grudges, and are unforgiving.

AETIOLOGY

Unknown. There is a high incidence of this disorder in first-degree relatives of patients with paranoid psychoses.

MEDICAL RELEVANCE

Those with pronounced sensitive traits are especially likely to develop ideas of reference when depressed; some will even progress to frank persecutory symptoms during illnesses which respond to treatment with anti-depressants.

In the general wards of the hospital such patients readily misinterpret medical advice, and may be hostile and critical about treatment given to themselves or to their relatives.

Schizoid personality (F60.1)

DESCRIPTION

A withdrawal from social and interpersonal contacts with emotional coldness and a preference for fantasy and introspection. The patient will have had few friends outside his immediate family and is often indifferent to praise or criticism from others. Prefers solitary activities – such as computing. He tends to be aloof and cold, and has little enjoyment in close personal relationships and no desire for sexual experience. Rarely experiences strong emotions such as anger or joy.

AETIOLOGY

Uncertain; probably genetically related to schizophrenia. Increased incidence of schizoid personalities in the first-degree relatives of schizophrenic probands.

MEDICAL RELEVANCE

Schizoid personalities are at somewhat greater risk for developing an episode of schizophrenia, and, having developed such an illness, the prognosis will be worse. However, it must be emphasized that only a minority of schizoid personalities develop schizophrenia; and many schizophrenics have normal personalities before they become ill.

Dissocial personality (F60.2)
(originally called 'psychopathic personality' or 'anti-social personality')

DESCRIPTION

A lifelong tendency to disregard social obligations, and lack of real feeling for other people which may show itself either in impetuous violence or by callous unconcern. The patient may be abnormally aggressive, and tends to be affectively cold and irresponsible. They tolerate frustration poorly and tend to be impulsive. They tend to blame others or offer plausible rationalizations for the behaviour which brings them in conflict with society.

The assessment is made from the personal history, which will show at least four of the following features:

1. An *inability to sustain enduring relationships* with others: most easily indicated by an *unstable work record,* with significant periods of unemployment at times when work was available, repeated episodes of absence from work, or repeated episodes of walking out of jobs without good cause; and a failure to sustain a monogamous *sexual relationship* for a prolonged period of time.

2. *Failure to conform to social norms* indicated by admitting to offences that have not been detected, a repeated failure to honour financial obligations, or a *forensic history* showing episodes of larceny, destroying property, assault, etc.

3. *Low tolerance for frustration,* with irritability and aggressiveness indicated by fights, assaults, wife-beating, or child-abuse.

4. *A callous unconcern for the feelings of others,* and a marked tendency to blame others for behaviour that brings the patient into conflict with society. Lacks remorse.

5. *Failure to plan ahead, and impulsive behaviour:* travels without clear destination; long periods with no fixed address.

6. *No regard for truth:* repeated lying, use of aliases, or 'conning' others.

7. *Disregard for own personal safety and the safety of others:* drives while drunk or disqualified; recurrent speeding offences.

8. If a parent or guardian, *neglects the child,* squanders money that should be spent on the child.

AETIOLOGY

Perhaps because of its enormous social importance, much work has been done on the aetiology of what has been called 'sociopathic personality'. Both genetic and environmental factors are undoubtedly important. There is a very much higher concordance for criminality in monozygotic than in dizygotic twins. Adoption studies show that adopted offspring of criminal parents have a much higher expectancy of sociopathic personality than adopted children whose biological parents were not offenders. In one Danish study the expectancy of criminality in adopted children whose biological parents were not known to the police was not affected by criminality in the father of the adopting family. However, since the MZ concordance rate for criminality in twins is only about 50 per cent, it is evident that environmental factors must also be important.

Criminality and social deviance in parents have repeatedly been shown in surveys of anti-social behaviour, as have conflict-ridden and 'broken' homes, lack of early training, and lack of caring supervision. Parents have repeatedly been shown to use poor disciplinary techniques: thus mothers have little control over their (delinquent) children and don't enforce obedience, while fathers are either too lax or too strict.

MEDICAL RELEVANCE

Many of the injured patients you see in an accident room on a Saturday night will either have been injured by dissocial personalities, or be dissocial personalities who have managed to injure themselves in fights. Dissocial personalities are at higher risk than others for alcoholism and drug dependence.

Emotionally unstable personality disorder (F60.3)
(includes explosive personality; borderline personality)

DESCRIPTION

A marked tendency to act impulsively without considering the consequences, combined with easily aroused symptoms of anxiety and depression. In the 'explosive' type, outbursts of intense anger often lead to violence with minimal provocation. The individual has outbursts of violence or threatening behaviour, often accompanied by feelings of tension.

In the 'borderline' type the same tendency for emotional instability is accompanied by chronic feelings of emptiness and lack of clarity about emotional preferences and long-term aims. The patient's anger is often directed against the self. Intense and unstable relationships are associated with attempts to avoid abandonment with suicidal threats and self-harm.

AETIOLOGY

Little is known.

MEDICAL RELEVANCE

'Explosive' patients often injure others, and may themselves ask for medical help in controlling their temper. They are best dealt with by teaching them 'anger management' in which they learn to recognize early signs of becoming angry, and either remove themselves from the encounter or learn to engage in displacement activities. They sometimes derive benefit from beta-blockers like propanolol.

'Borderline' patients most often come to medical notice in accident and emergency departments after they have taken overdoses or tried to harm themselves after a crisis in some interpersonal relationship. They respond poorly to most forms of medical treatment.

Histrionic personality (F60.4)
(originally, and confusingly, called 'hysterical personality')

DESCRIPTION

The patient – who is usually female – behaves in a histrionic way, tending to exaggerate and dramatize her descriptions of both symptoms and circumstances. Aspects of her own behaviour which are inconsistent with the romanticized version she relates are either ignored or denied. Displays of emotion (both weeping and angry tantrums) commonly accompany the history – but they strike the observer as being too easily aroused, and they disappear as quickly. She tends to be egocentric in personal relationships, showing too little attention to other people's feeling to form any very deep relationships. Indeed, although she tends to be sexually provocative her own sexual relationships tend to be unsatisfactory, and she tends to be both frigid and sexually naive. She is often an attractive girl, who has learned to be flirtatious as a way of gaining her own ends rather than as a way of initiating a sexual relationship.

DIAGNOSTIC CRITERIA

The label tends to be fixed on to any female patient who succeeds in irritating the (male) medical staff, by giving an exaggerated account of her symptoms, or who behaves in a manipulative way. This is a pity, since if the term is used in this way it becomes meaningless. In this one case we will therefore give some simplified diagnostic criteria.

All three of the following should be present:

1. Attention-seeking or histrionic behaviour.
2. Demanding interpersonal behaviour.
3. Displays of emotion which are easily aroused, or more intense than the circumstances require.

AETIOLOGY

Unknown. When measured as a personality trait there appears to be no genetic component, although the disorder does tend to run in families. It can probably best be thought of as a set of behaviours that are learned by some immature girls who have been starved of parental affection. It is difficult to escape the impression that these patients use their behaviour to gain attention and admiration from older men: but there have been no systematic studies on this point.

MEDICAL RELEVANCE

The concept came about as a way of describing those thought to be at high risk for hysteria: thus the original name. Although these girls are at higher risk for conversion phenomena than those without such traits, it is now recognized that the majority of those with hysterical illnesses do not have such personalities.

You are far more likely to meet these patients in the accident room than in the neurological wards. They are certainly at very high risk for manipulative and attention-seeking interpersonal behaviours, and they will arrive in hospital having poisoned themselves with drugs, or having made superficial cuts on their forearms. You should be on your guard when someone begins to behave in this way for the first time in adult life: the diagnosis is much more likely to be an affective illness than a personality disorder!

Obsessional personality (F60.5)
(also called 'anankastic personality')

DESCRIPTION

Feelings of personal insecurity, doubt, and incompleteness lead to excessive conscientiousness, checking, stubbornness, and caution. There is perfectionism and meticulous accuracy and the need to check repeatedly in an attempt to secure this. The patient may become indecisive. There may be an unreasonable insistence that others do things their way; or an excessive devotion to work to the exclusion of leisure and friendships. There may be restricted expressions of affection and lack of generosity. Rigidity and excessive doubt may be conspicuous, and there may be insistent and unwelcome thoughts. The patient may be unable to discard worthless or worn-out items.

AETIOLOGY

Twin studies have shown that genetic factors are important in determining obsessional traits, and that there is an association between such traits and 'neuroticism' – which together may manifest as obsessional symptoms.

Ritualistic behaviour and excessive orderliness appear to be a normal developmental stage in childhood. There is no association between such traits and coercive toilet training, although there is some association between such traits in mothers and children. One study showed that parenting practices characterized as 'restrictive warmth' were associated with children who were submissive, dependent, polite, neat, and obedient: but that is about as near as the various studies of child development seem to get to 'obsessional personality'.

MEDICAL RELEVANCE

People with obsessional traits are especially likely to develop obsessional symptoms during episodes of depressive illness: in such patients special treatment for the obsessional symptoms is not required since they will respond to anti-depressants. Obsessional personalities are commonly observed in the pre-morbid personalities of those with obsessional illness (see p. 228).

Dependent personality (F60.7)
(includes asthenic personality; passive-dependent personality)

DESCRIPTION

The patient has always let others make decisions for him, and has few resources of his own. He has difficulty initiating projects or doing things on his own. He will agree with people with whom he disagrees to avoid disturbing a relationship, and will remain in a relationship in which he is mistreated for fear of being left alone. When a close relationship ends he is devastated and helpless, as he is often preoccupied with a fear of being abandoned. He constantly seeks reassurance and approval from others, and is easily hurt by disapproval.

AETIOLOGY

No systematic studies have been reported. Authoritarian parents, who enforce rules and edicts without discussion, have been shown to produce children who are miserable, are socially withdrawn, and have low self-esteem. It is possible that this might form the basis of the adult disorder, marked as it is by resourcelessness and a desire to please dominant people.

MEDICAL RELEVANCE

These people are at high risk for depressive illness when they lose the dominant person by death or separation. Left to themselves, they may drift down the social scale and become unemployed or homeless.

EXAMPLE OF AETIOLOGY

Now let's return to Mrs Woods – whom we last met in Chapter 3 – for an example of how to write an account of aetiological factors.

> Mrs Woods appears to be predisposed to the development of depressive illness due to the **family history** of depressive disorder in her mother and her own **bereavement** in childhood (death of her father when she was aged eight). She has marked **obsessional personality traits** (has always been a perfectionist, checked excessively, and was house proud to a fault) and appears to have had **difficulty in adapting to change or loss**, e.g. when her daughter left home to go to university. She had a close and **over-dependent relationship with her mother**, whom she phoned daily throughout her life but could never please, and this has made

*her particularly vulnerable to the loss of her mother. The present illness has been precipitated by the discovery of her mother's **terminal illness six months ago and death** three weeks ago. Mrs Woods felt unable to express her anger or grief whilst nursing her mother through this illness, or to express her ambivalent feelings since the bereavement: this has resulted in the process of **introjection** (giving rise to her perception of chest pains) and subsequent **idealization** of the mother.*

Notice that these factors are not independent. Although Mrs Woods has always been of impeccable character, and a dutiful daughter, her early experience of bereavement has left her vulnerable to loss, and her relationship with her mother has made her particularly vulnerable to the loss of her mother.

Notice also that although she describes both obsessional *traits* and dependent *traits*, she does not have enough features to satisfy the requirements for either type of personality *disorder*. However, she adapts poorly to change due to her obsessional traits and her dependent relationship with her mother will make her especially vulnerable to loss. Thus the gun is primed and waiting to go off. It only needs the mother's terminal illness to pull the trigger.

Her inability consciously to accept the negative aspects of her ambivalent feelings towards her mother results in *denial* of such feelings.

This example demonstrates another feature in the aetiology of mental illness: the interaction of **nature** and **nurture.** To some extent Mrs Woods' predisposition to depressive disorder may be genetically determined (suggested by the family history) although social and psychological factors have also played their part.

6 / INVESTIGATIONS

So far we have seen in the earlier chapters that the data collected from the history and mental state examination are used to formulate hypotheses about the differential diagnosis and aetiology. The next logical step is to start to test these hypotheses by planning the investigations. These provide additional data which will either support or fail to support our initial hypotheses.

The **purpose** of investigations can be summarized as follows:

1. To support the preferred **diagnosis** if possible and rule out the alternatives.
2. To confirm the identified **aetiological factors** if possible or, if this is obscure, collect new data which will lead to new hypotheses about aetiology.
3. To assess **change**, e.g. to monitor progress in response to treatment.
4. To assess likely response to treatment.

The investigations are therefore planned for each patient according to their particular needs. There are no 'routine' investigations. In this chapter we will consider how to plan investigations and then go on to describe a few special procedures which the houseman should know about. Investigations that are particularly relevant to individual diagnostic categories are noted in Part 2.

Although in many branches of medicine it is customary to think of investigations mainly as those sources of data derived from laboratory or radiological procedures, in psychiatry we also include all additional sources of information that are required after the initial history and mental state examination. For example, these will include interviews with other informants, examination of past medical records, in-patient observations of mood, sleep pattern, and weight chart, or a home assessment.

You will already be familiar with most of the physical investigations that may be needed but a number of procedures mentioned above will almost certainly be new. However, the following procedures require further explanation.

THE FAMILY TREE

When there is a possibility that a patient is suffering from a familial disorder (genetic or otherwise), it is often helpful to draw up a family tree. The data are gathered from interviews with the patient and relatives. They can be supplemented, if it is thought necessary, from hospital and general practice health records and from death certificates. The tree should include all consanguineous relatives for whom accurate data are available.

Figure 6.1 is an example for a patient, Jane Smith, aged forty-three, who has been referred on account of memory difficulties and involuntary movements. It illustrates the spread of a disorder through a family in a manner consistent with autosomal dominant inheritance.

The following conventions are used:

> The **patient**, Jane Smith, is indicated with an arrow.
> **Marriages are joined by horizontal lines**, e.g. Simon Smith and Ellen.
> A **marriage ended by death** can be indicated by a double sloping line, e.g. John Smith and Mary.
> A **marriage ended by divorce** can be indicated by a double cross, e.g. William and Elizabeth Morris.
> **Children** are shown joined to parents by vertical lines and siblings to each other (in chronological order) by horizontal lines.
> **Abortions and still births** are included, as shown for Mary Smith's first two pregnancies.
> **Twins** are indicated by a vertical line which branches at an acute angle, e.g. Keith and Lawrence Morris.
> For each person the year of birth (and death) is shown.
> **Death** is also indicated by a sloping line through the idiogram, e.g. Simon Smith, Fred Jones, and the cause of death is given.
> Important illnesses are also shown for living relatives.
> Those with illnesses (possibly) related to that of the patient are shown by a shaded idiogram, e.g. Fred Jones, Mary, Jane, and Philip.
> Any other information that might be useful can be added such as place and date of birth or occupation.

PSYCHOMETRIC TESTING

Psychologists have devised standardized tests to measure virtually every conceivable aspect of human thought and behaviour. Although many, such as personality tests, have no place in clinical psychiatry, others make a valuable contribution to the process of

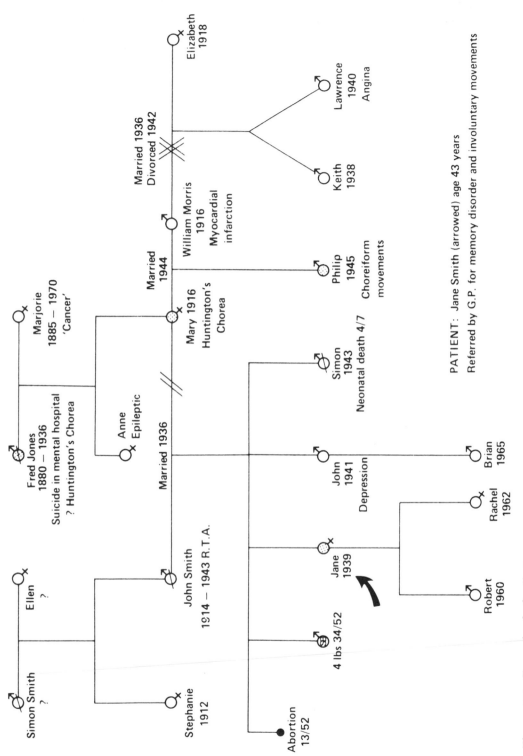

Figure 6.1 *Example of a family tree*

PATIENT: Jane Smith (arrowed) age 43 years

Referred by G.P. for memory disorder and involuntary movements assessment: particularly in differentiating patients with organic brain disease from those with affective disorders or without mental illness.

Assessment of cerebral organic disease

Many standardized tests are available to detect deterioration in brain functions that occurs in the presence of organic disorders. Some of these are designed to assess specific functions, for example, the visual–spatial functions of the parietal lobe or visual memory function of the non-dominant temporal lobe. Others are more general and include tests of a range of aptitudes such as those found in intelligence tests. Whilst you are doing your psychiatry clerkship try to arrange to watch a clinical psychologist carrying out some of these tests.

INTELLIGENCE TESTS

The most widely used intelligence tests are the **Mill Hill Vocabulary Test, Raven's Progressive Matrices**, and the **Wechsler Adult Intelligence Scale**. These provide an intelligence quotient (IQ), in which the scores obtained by the subject are expressed as a percentage of the mean scores obtained by the samples on which the tests are standardized. It is usual to subdivide the test score results and express these as two separate IQs, one for verbal tests and the other for 'performance' (that is, non-verbal) tests.

Intelligence tests can contribute to the identification of organic brain disease in the following ways:

1. Testing on one occasion may reveal an IQ which is well below the past level of attainment as suggested by the history of educational and professional achievement. For example, an overall IQ of 100 would be definitely suggestive of possible organic damage for a physicist but not for a shop assistant.

2. A gross disparity between a higher verbal IQ and a lower performance IQ (in the order of 20 or more) is suggestive of organic deterioration because verbal functions tend to be preserved longer than non-verbal functions. The reverse discrepancy is not usually of significance in this respect. Vocabulary is particularly well preserved in early organic damage, and vocabulary tests are therefore sometimes used to estimate pre-morbid ability.

3. Repetition of intelligence tests over a period of months or years may show a deterioration which usually provides a much better guide to the effects of organic cerebral disease than tests on a single occasion.

TESTS OF MEMORY

Tests of memory are used to assess the ability to register, retain, and recall new material. They include tests of verbal learning, which are affected particularly by dominant hemisphere disease, and visual memory, which is mainly a non-dominant hemisphere function.

An example of a verbal learning test is the **Synonym Learning Test**. The subject is given definitions of ten words previously unknown to him, but related to his vocabulary level, and then asked to recall their meanings. The definitions are repeated and the subject retested. Scoring is based on the number of trials required. This test has proved moderately successful in differentiating between patients with dementia and those who have affective disorders or are not mentally ill.

In the **Benton Visual Retention Test** the subject is shown a card with a design for ten seconds and then asked to draw the design. The procedure is repeated with other cards. Scores are based on the number of cards correctly reproduced and the number of errors made. The perceptual and constructional skills involved can be separated from the effects of memory deficit by getting the subject to copy the cards whilst they are in front of him. This too has proved to be a useful test in discriminating between brain-damaged and non-brain-damaged subjects although there is some overlap in the scores obtained.

This is of course only a very brief account of a few of the many tests that are used in the assessment of organic brain disease. The important point is that abnormal findings help to increase the probability of an organic disorder, and the pattern of test findings may help to localize it. These tests are only carried out if there is already some other evidence suggestive of a possible organic disorder.

The findings have to be interpreted in the light of other data, both from the history and examination and from other special investigations.

Mood assessments

Mood assessments are based on standardized self-rating questionnaires such as the **Beck Depression Inventory (BDI)** or the **State-Trait Anxiety Inventory (STAI)**, which can be easily administered and scored. However, they are not diagnostic instruments: for example, the BDI can provide a measure of the severity of depressive symptoms but cannot differentiate between the affective symptoms that may occur in the setting of a depressive illness, dementia, or schizophrenia. It does not take into account objective signs of illness but is based on the patient's subjective experience. It does not differentiate between mood 'state' and 'trait', although the STAI does attempt to do this. Despite these limitations they provide a useful measure, particularly if administered repeatedly in order to assess change, for example, to monitor the response to treatment. Mood scales are also available for both depression and mania based on observations by the nurses looking after the patient.

THE ELECTROENCEPHALOGRAM (EEG)

This is essentially a voltmeter which measures changes in potential transmitted from the brain to the scalp. Electrodes (usually eight or sixteen) are placed bilaterally on the scalp in standard positions and simultaneous tracings are made on a polygraph. The healthy adult, relaxed, awake, and with eyes closed, shows a characteristic **alpha rhythm** of about ten cycles per second and low frequency. On opening the eyes, or with increased mental activity, the tracing flattens. The records of young children normally show **delta waves** which are much slower (fewer than four cycles per second) and of greater amplitude. During adolescence these are replaced by **theta waves** (four to seven cycles per second). These slow waves are not usually present in the adult except during sleep.

The most valuable contribution of the EEG is in the diagnosis of **epilepsy**. 'Spikes' (brief high-amplitude discharges) or 'sharp waves' (more prolonged but also high amplitude) are characteristic. Alternating spikes and delta waves at three cycles per second are a classic feature of generalized absence attacks.

The EEG may be a valuable adjunct in identifying the presence of organic brain disease. In delirium there is usually an irregular slow wave pattern. In dementia the most useful findings are the loss of normal alpha activity and the emergence of delta activity in the waking state. These changes also tend to occur gradually in the normally ageing brain so they have to be interpreted with care. Negative findings do not exclude the possibility of organic disease but a grossly abnormal record is very highly suggestive. It can therefore be valuable in helping to differentiate between dementia and depressive pseudo-dementia, particularly as it is relatively cheap, non-invasive, and painless. The EEG can also be useful in helping to localize a lesion because the abnormal findings may then be limited to tracings from a few leads rather than appearing as a generalized abnormality. A major limitation is the non-specific nature of the abnormal findings, which tend to be similar regardless of the underlying pathology.

BRAIN IMAGING

Neuro-imaging techniques may be divided into structural and functional, according to whether they yield an anatomical or a physiological representation of the brain.

Computed tomography (CT) and **magnetic resonance imaging (MRI)**, sometimes called **nuclear magnetic resonance imaging (NMR)**, are the two major structural techniques. They have replaced the use of skull X-rays and pneumo-encephalography in the detection of brain abnormalities. CT scanning is cheaper and more widely available. It is better than MRI at detecting calcified lesions, but it has a poorer resolution, particularly for smaller lesions. Visualization of the posterior and temporal fossae is also inferior with CT although the latter can be improved by using reverse gantry (tilted angle) views of the temporal lobes. The use of a peripherally injected contrast medium also enhances the quality of CT scanning.

In neuropsychiatry, CT and MRI scanning is used to detect the possibility of underlying brain tumours as, for example, in the evaluation of patients with epilepsy, or in patients with a history suggestive of organic brain disorder. They may also detect the cerebral atrophy which can occur in various dementias, such as the generalized atrophy of Alzheimer's disease, or the caudate nucleus flattening of Huntington's chorea. They are useful too in the diagnosis of the cortical and/or white matter lesions which occur in multi-infarct dementia, or cerebro-vascular disorders. They may show residual lesions in cases of head injury, which is useful in the assessment of the organic component of post-traumatic disorders.

Single photon emission (computed) tomography (SPECT or **SPET)** and **positron emission tomography (PET)** are the two main types of functional neuro-imaging techniques. SPECT scanning is by far the cheaper technique and has thus made an impact on clinical management, despite its inferior resolution power. The wonders of high-resolution PET scanning images, however, are largely confined to research.

Both techniques can be used to demonstrate patterns of cerebral blood flow or, with the injection of radio-labelled markers, to identify particular neurotransmitter systems in the brain. PET scanning may also be used to demonstrate patterns of cerebral metabolism, such as glucose consumption, which are disrupted in diseased tissues. The great advantage of these techniques is that they are proving useful in the detection of cerebral abnormalities which occur before the development of, or in the complete absence of, any structural abnormalities detected by CT or MRI scanning. This occurs, for example, with some types of frontal lobe dementia: more controversial are the functional abnormalities reported in some cases of schizophrenia or affective disorder. Functional neuro-imaging is also proving that the functional impairment which accompanies a lesion, such as a tumour, stroke, or epileptic focus, is often much wider than CT or MRI scanning would suggest.

HOW TO PLAN INVESTIGATIONS

It is best to plan the investigations methodically. First consider whether it is necessary to get further information about the history and then remember the familiar categories of **biological**, **psychological**, and **social** factors. *Table 6.1* shows some examples of the commoner investigations that are needed together with some of their indications. As usual, this is only a guide: it is not intended to provide an exhaustive list of all possible investigations. Now let's find out how to apply this procedure: back to Mrs Woods.

*First consider the **history**. We already have an independent account from the husband which is consistent with that of the patient so we probably don't need to see other informants. However, it would be helpful to find out more from the general practitioner about the episode when he prescribed medication for her 'nerves', and we must certainly send for her mother's psychiatric case records.*

*Next we have to sort out the **differential diagnosis**. In this case the possibilities are limited as she seems to have a wide range of depressive symptoms and some features of a morbid grief reaction. However, she has been complaining of chest pain.*

***Biological** investigation will certainly have to include physical examination and an ECG, if only to provide an informed basis for reassuring her (and ourselves) that she does not have heart disease. As we examine Mrs Woods we note faded bruising on her left upper arm and left thorax. She reminds us that she fell down stairs three weeks ago, after taking the sedative prescribed by her GP.*

*At this stage **social investigations** do not seem to be indicated.*

Table 6.1 *Examples of investigations*

---

1. *history*

Always at least one additional **informant**, but sometimes others.

Include employers or teachers if likely to be useful *(with patient's consent)*.

Patient's past **general medical and psychiatric records**, and information from general practitioner.

Relatives' medical records, if there is positive family history of mental illness.

2. *biological*

Includes any necessary assessment of physical disease (whether or not related to the mental state) including:

Physical examination: (if not yet done).

Haematology: e.g. ESR, white cell count in infections.

Biochemistry: liver function tests – alcoholism; thyroid function tests – hyperthyroidism; electrolytes – delirium or anorexia nervosa.

Bacteriology, virology, serology: for urinary tract infection, herpes zoster, neurosyphilis.

Electroencephalogram: epilepsy, delirium, dementia.

Radiology: CAT scan – dementia or space-occupying lesion.

3. *social*

Assessment of family members: by interview (alone or with patient) to see what they are like and how they relate to each other.

Home assessment: (*if necessary*) by psychiatric social worker or others to determine adequacy of accommodation and services and home atmosphere.

Financial assessment: (*if appropriate*) balance of family income from all sources, expenses, and debts.

Occupational: by occupational therapist, to determine nature and severity of disablement, in self-care or employment.

4. *psychological*

Exploratory psychotherapy (see p. 110).

Standardized psychometric tests: organic psychosyndromes, mood disorders.

Behavioural assessment: to identify maladaptive behaviours and their environmental reinforcers, e.g. in agoraphobia or obsessive compulsive disorder.

---

*Psychological investigations might include serial observations of her mood and other aspects of the mental state, and if she is an in-patient we will want to ask the nurses to observe the daily pattern of her mood, sleep, and appetite and to keep a weight chart. This will help to confirm the presence of depressive illness as the preferred diagnosis. Later on these will also provide a base line for assessment of change in response to treatment. Further interviews with Mrs Woods in order to explore her relationship with her mother and her reaction to the mother's illness and death may help to confirm their central importance as **aetiological factors** (and may also be therapeutic).*

THE CONTRIBUTION OF OTHER PARAMEDICAL WORKERS

Psychiatric social workers

PSWs have special training in the management of the mentally ill and their families. They contribute to the social aspects of assessment and treatment with regard to material welfare such as financial status and living conditions; the impact of the mentally ill and their families on each other; and the patient's social interactions, sources of support, and satisfaction. In addition some social workers have **approved social worker** status which carries particular responsibilities with regard to the Mental Health Act (1983) (see p. 331).

PSWs may contribute to assessment, for example by interviewing family members to collect additional histories or to assess the attitudes of the relatives to the patient; or by carrying out a home assessment to determine the adequacy of material resources and to observe the nature of family relationships within the home environment.

Psychiatric nurses

Psychiatric nurses have received a special training in mental nursing and play a major part in the care of severely ill patients. It is unwise to judge patients entirely on what you observe at interview: the nurses observe the patient closely for long periods of time in a variety of settings, and regularly provide invaluable additional information about patients. They are responsible for administering medications and they participate in group therapy on the ward as well as providing intensive care for individual patients. **Community psychiatric nurses** are trained to provide nursing care in people's homes.

Occupational therapists

OTs have special skills in the management of disability in the mentally ill. They help those with acute illnesses regain their self-confidence and interact with others. They discover a patient's assets and exploit them, as well as helping patients to cope with disabilities. They may be involved in the assessment of 'activities of daily living' which include the essentials of self-care such as washing, dressing, cooking, and the use of public services; in the assessment of work, leisure, and recreational activities; and in the assessment of psychological problems through the use of 'projective techniques' such as art and drama. The contribution of OTs is particularly valuable in the rehabilitation of those with chronic disorders, and much useful work can be done by **community OTs** developing rehabilitation programmes in their patients' homes.

7 / TREATMENT

In the chapter that follows we shall give *more information than you need to pass* your Finals Examination. For Finals, you merely need to know the indications and side-effects of the more important psychotropic drugs, the indications, contra-indications, and side effects of ECT, and some idea of the principal varieties of psychotherapy. However, we make no apology for giving you more information than you are going to need before you qualify, since we are sure that you will return again and again to this chapter when you have patients under your care.

Treatment in psychiatry should always be considered under the headings **physical**, **psychological**, and **social**. This may seem different to treatments in general medicine but the example of epilepsy will serve to illustrate the model:

Physical: anticonvulsants, and folic acid if necessary.

Psychological: supportive psychotherapy and reassurance about the diagnosis and its implications; advice about avoiding stressful situations and alcohol if these precipitate fits; appropriate treatment for depression or anxiety if these occur.

Social: counselling the patient about employment, driving, marriage, and having children, helping the family coping with the epileptic fits. The person may require being registered as disabled.

Doctors vary in their inclination to regard the psychological and social aspects of treatment as important. For example, anxiety, depression, and sexual problems frequently follow mastectomy and can respond to appropriate treatment. However, some surgeons are more likely than others to detect and treat these symptoms among patients who have undergone the operation. We give separate accounts of physical treatments and psychological treatments. Some forms of social help are included in the latter section, while other forms depend upon local resources and on the needs of the individual patient: you should always seek advice from the **medical social worker.**

PHYSICAL TREATMENTS: DRUGS

Although is has been known since time immemorial that chemical agents can induce perceptual, cognitive, and affective changes, and can grossly modify human behaviour, it is only for the past forty years that the use of drugs has become generally established in the treatment of psychiatric disorders. Drugs used therapeutically fall into two major categories:

1. Drugs that have primarily a direct action on the central nervous system (CNS).

2. Drugs that have an indirect action on the CNS due to their influence on other organ systems of the body.

In this latter group we find drugs which act primarily on the cardiovascular, respiratory, alimentary, or endocrine systems, and thereby can correct a hypoxic or metabolic disturbance of the brain (for example, the beneficial effect of diuretics in a toxic confusional state caused by cardiac failure).

However, we shall restrict ourselves to the drugs that have a primary action on the central nervous system, and these are summarized in *Table 7.1*. The discipline dealing with these drugs is called **neuropharmacology**; **psychopharmacology** is the branch of neuropharmacology concerned with the effects of drugs on behaviour.

The two major classes are **non-selective** and **selective** drugs. Non-selective drugs have an action on every neurone in the brain and spinal cord: they either decrease ('CNS depressants') or increase ('CNS stimulants') neuronal excitability. Selective drugs, on the other hand, affect only certain groups of neurones or only some aspect of nervous function.

It is obvious that all neuropharmacological agents have to be able to pass through the blood–brain barrier. An important consequence of this feature of these drugs is that they can pass through other lipid membranes, such as the placenta: all centrally acting drugs have a ready access to the foetus. Therefore the general rule is that all these drugs should be avoided during the first trimester of pregnancy, and should be used with great caution during the rest of the pregnancy (see pp. 292–3).

In this chapter we shall concentrate on the discussion of centrally acting drugs which have important roles in the treatment of psychiatric disorders.

Barbiturates

Barbiturates are general, non-selective depressants of central nervous system activity. These drugs were the most important therapeutically used psychoactive agents during the first half of this century; however, their use has become very limited over the past

Table 7.1 *Classification of neuropharmacological agents*

I. non selective agents

    A. general CNS depressants
        1. anaesthetic gases and vapours (nitrous oxide, ether, halothane)
        2. aliphatic alcohols (ethanol)
        3. barbiturates
    B. general CNS stimulants
        1. convulsants (strychnine, picrotoxin)
        2. xanthines (caffeine)

II. selective drugs

        1. anticonvulsants (phenytoin; carbamazepine)
        2. centrally acting muscle relaxants (mephenesin)
        3. centrally acting antihypertensives (clonidine)
        4. narcotic analgesics (opiates)
        5. analgesic antipyretics (aspirin)
        6. anti-Parkinsonian drugs (L-Dopa; central anti-cholinergics)
        7. psychopharmacological drugs ('psychotropics')
            a. neuroleptics (chlorpromazine; haloperidol)
            b. anxiolytics (benzodiazepines)
            c. anti-depressants (imipramine; phenelzine)
            d. psychostimulants (amphetamine; cocaine)
            e. hallucinogens (LSD; psilocybin)
            f. other drugs (lithium; tryptophan)

---

twenty years or so. In small doses, they cause a degree of psycho-stimulation and euphoria; in higher doses, however, they cause sedation, and eventually coma. Tolerance readily develops to all barbiturates.

Tolerance means that, on repeated medication, the same dose becomes gradually less and less effective (or that increasing doses are needed to evoke the same effect). The tolerance is partly **pharmacokinetic** (*drug disposition tolerance*: the metabolic removal of the barbiturate becomes more effective due to the induction of microsomal enzymes in the liver) and partly **pharmacodynamic** (adaptation of the nervous tissue to the presence of the drug). It is important that while tolerance can develop to the hypnotic effect of the drug, this is not accompanied by an increase in the lethal dose. Both psychological and physical dependence can develop in patients taking these drugs: withdrawal is accompanied by a rebound hyperexcitability of the brain, leading to convulsions. Therefore the use of barbiturates should be avoided for the treatment of insomnia and anxiety; for these indications the benzodiazepines are safer drugs (see below). Barbiturates are often abused by drug addicts, especially in combination with amphetamine since a barbiturate can reduce the unpleasant excitement produced by amphetamine and also enhance the euphoria. **Phenobarbitone** is still used therapeutically as an effective anticonvulsant in generalized epilepsy, and lipid soluble barbiturates (for example, thiopentone) are used as intravenous anaesthetics. Barbiturates, especially amylobarbitone, still have some limited use in psychiatry:

1. For *abreaction* (induction of a state of clouded consciousness in which a skilled interviewer can induce the patient to reveal suppressed psychological material).

2. For *activation of the EEG* (a small dose of barbiturate increases the amplitude of high-frequency waves and can provoke the appearance of seizure activity).

Anticonvulsants

Epilepsy is a common disorder with psychiatric complications; therefore patients suffering from epilepsy are often referred to psychiatrists. The psychiatrist has to be familiar with the pharmacological management of epilepsy, the side-effects of the drugs, and also possible interactions between anti-epileptic drugs and other psychoactive medication.

Although general depressants of the central nervous system have anticonvulsant properties (for example, barbiturates), their clinical use is seriously hampered by their sedative properties. Thus only phenobarbitone has survived as a useful drug, but even with this barbiturate daytime sedation and impairment of psychomotor performance can be a problem. The ideal anticonvulsant has a selective effect on the seizure focus without affecting other parts of the CNS. None of the existing anticonvulsants satisfies completely this requirement: apart from an effect on the focus, they also influence other neurones, usually preventing the spread of epileptic discharge through the brain.

PHENYTOIN

Phenytoin (diphenyl-hydantoin) is chemically related to barbiturates. It is a broad-spectrum anticonvulsant with effectiveness in all types of epilepsy with the exception of absence seizures. There are great inter-individual variations in plasma levels on the same dosage, and the determination of plasma concentration is important in selecting a clinically effective non-toxic dosage regimen. Although the drug does not cause sedation, there are some other adverse effects which have been described in patients on chronic medication:

1. Cerebellar-vestibular effects (ataxia, nystagmus).
2. Psychiatric symptoms (a toxic delirium).
3. Gastro-intestinal symptoms (nausea, vomiting, diarrhoea, gingival hyperplasia).
4. Impaired calcium metabolism resulting in osteomalacia.
5. Megaloblastic anaemia.
6. Hirsutism.
7. Swollen gums.

Other drugs can influence the plasma concentration of phenytoin:

1. Phenobarbitone and carbamazepine reduce phenytoin plasma levels due to the induction of microsomal enzymes in the liver.
2. Ethanol increases plasma levels due to reduction of phenytoin inactivation.

CARBAMAZEPINE

Carbamazepine is chemically related to the tricyclic anti-depressants. This drug is used for the management of both generalized and partial seizures. Plasma level assessments help in selecting the appropriate oral dosage. The drug is generally well tolerated; toxic effects include *diplopia, blurred vision, drowsiness, dizziness, ataxia, nausea*. The most severe, albeit rare, side-effect is *aplastic anaemia*; patients on this drug require regular haematological monitoring. Carbamazepine is also used in the prophylaxis of recurrent manic-depressive episodes, especially in patients who do not respond to lithium (see p. 96).

VALPROIC ACID

Valproic acid (sodium valproate) is a branched chain carboxylic acid with well-documented efficacy in generalized grand mal, myoclonic-atonic and absence seizures; it is less effective in partial seizures (for example, temporal lobe epilepsy). It is believed that the drug acts by *enhancing GABA-mediated inhibition* in the CNS.

BENZODIAZEPINES

Although most **benzodiazepines** have anticonvulsant properties, clonazepam and diazepam are the two most frequently used drugs in the management of epilepsy. These are broad-spectrum anticonvulsants with effectiveness in most types of epilepsy. Both diazepam and clonazepam, in the form of intravenous injection, are the first line of treatment in major status epilepticus; clonazepam is used to treat absence and myoclonic seizures in children; diazepam can be used in alcoholic withdrawal states for sedation and prevention of fits.

ETHOSUXIMIDE

Ethosuximide is the primary drug for the treatment of absence seizures.

LAMOTRIGINE

Lamotrigine is an anticonvulsant which appears to work by diminishing the release of glutamate, an excitatory amino acid. It has appreciably fewer adverse effects than phenytoin.

VIGABATRIN

Vigabatrin is an irreversible inhibitor of the enzyme which degrades GABA, an inhibitory amino acid. This is presumed to enhance GABA ergic neurotransmission. It triggers psychotic reactions and this is a well-known side-effect. It can be minimized by careful dose adjustment.

TREATMENT OF EPILEPSY

The modern treatment of epilepsy involves clinical and electroencephalographic identification of the type of seizure involved, selection of an appropriate drug, and continuous monitoring of the clinical response, side-effects, and plasma concentration of the anticonvulsant.

It is especially important to monitor serum levels of phenytoin. The aim is *monotherapy*, that is, the control of seizures with one anti-epileptic drug. Drug combinations should be avoided because of complex pharmacokinetic interactions between anti-epileptic drugs and difficulties in identifying adverse effects attributable to a particular medication.

Anti-Parkinsonian drugs

Parkinsonism is an extra-pyramidal syndrome consisting of the triad of *hypokinesia*, *rigidity*, and *tremor*. Parkinsonism can be defined neurochemically as a **striatal dopamine-deficiency syndrome.** The syndrome can be brought about by a reduction in the dopaminergic input to the striatum in the following ways:

1. Destruction of the nigro-striatal pathway: Parkinson's disease, postencephalitic Parkinsonism, manganese poisoning.
2. Depletion of nigro-striatal neurones of dopamine by reserpine, tetrabenazine.
3. Blockade of striatal dopamine receptors by neuroleptics.

It follows from this model that **dopaminergic drugs** restoring the functional integrity of dopaminergic neurotransmission in the striatum will be beneficial in treatment. It has been found that **anti-cholinergic drugs** can also alleviate the symptoms of Parkinsonism, suggesting that there may be a functional antagonism between dopaminergic and cholinergic influences in the striatum. Thus anti-Parkinsonian drugs fall into two major categories:

1. Dopaminergic drugs.
2. Centrally acting anti-cholinergics.

The dopaminergic drugs comprise:

1. *Dopamine dispensers* (precursor: L-Dopa; releaser: amantadine).
2. *Dopamine mimetics* (e.g. apomorphine, bromocriptine).
3. *Dopamine conservers* (e.g. selegiline – a centrally acting monoamine oxidase-B inhibitor which prevents the degradation of dopamine).

Of these drugs, **L-Dopa** is the primary agent in the treatment of Parkinsonism due to the degeneration of the nigro-striatal system; the other dopaminergic drugs are useful adjuncts in management. L-Dopa is usually administered together with a peripheral aromatic-L-amino-acid decarboxylase inhibitor: the use of the enzyme inhibitor prevents the conversion of L-Dopa to dopamine in the periphery, thereby reducing peripheral side-effects and enabling a reduction in the dosage of L-Dopa. The use of L-Dopa, and to some extent of the other dopaminergic drugs, is associated with important psychiatric side-effects:

Mild side-effects (anxiety, insomnia, daytime sedation) are very common but subside with time.

Severe side-effects occur in about 15 per cent of patients treated with L-Dopa and comprise:

1. Acute brain syndrome.
2. Affective psychosis (depression leading to suicide, hypomania).
3. Paranoid psychosis.

The centrally acting anti-cholinergics readily pass through the blood–brain barrier and can produce effective central muscarinic receptor blockade with relatively little effect on peripheral muscarinic receptors. These drugs have only a limited use in the management of Parkinsonism resulting from the degeneration of the nigro-striatal system, but they are the treatment of choice in managing neuroleptic-induced Parkinsonism. In neuroleptic-induced Parkinsonism the symptoms are due to the blockade of striatal dopamine receptors by the neuroleptic drug, and thus dopaminergic drugs, whose action relies on the activation of these receptors, are ineffective. The most commonly used centrally acting anti-cholinergics are **benzhexol, benztropine, procyclidine**, and **orphenadrine**. These drugs can be useful in alleviating the symptoms of neuroleptic-induced Parkinsonism, and procyclidine in injection form can relieve the symptoms of neuroleptic-induced *acute dystonic reactions*.

The routine use of these drugs should be avoided since they can reduce the effective concentration of the neuroleptic in the body and may also promote the development of tardive dyskinesia. The *side-effects* are the same as those of atropine: dry mouth, cycloplegia, constipation, urinary retention; in susceptible individuals or on high doses an *atropine psychosis* (a toxic delirium) may develop.

Anti-cholinergic drugs can produce *euphoria* in some individuals, and thus these drugs have some abuse potential.

Neuroleptics

The term **neuroleptic** was coined by Delay and Deniker in 1952 to describe the characteristic pattern of sedation ('neuroleptic syndrome') caused by these drugs: *psychomotor slowing, emotional quieting, and affective indifference without any clouding of consciousness and/or ataxia.*

These drugs are also called 'major tranquillizers' and 'anti-psychotics'. They are called 'major tranquillizers' to distinguish them from the minor tranquillizers – benzodiazepines – which have hypnotic effects. The term 'anti-psychotic' refers to the ability of these drugs to affect some target symptoms of psychotic states, such as hallucinations, delusions, and thought disorder. The sedative and anti-psychotic effects can be separated: while tolerance develops to the sedative effect, this is not the case with the anti-psychotic effect. The classification of neuroleptic drugs is shown in *Table 7.2*.

Neuroleptics of different classes have a common mode of action: they *block transmission through dopaminergic synapses*. Most neuroleptics achieve this by their ability to block post-synaptic dopamine receptors, whereas rauwolfia alkaloids, together with some synthetic drugs such as tetrabenazine, impair dopaminergic transmission due to their ability to deplete presynaptic stores of dopamine (and also of noradrenaline and 5-hydroxytryptamine). Thus the central effects of the neuroleptics are related to the four areas of the brain where dopaminergic synapses, and thus dopamine receptors, are located:

Table 7.2 *Classification of neuroleptics*

I. *tricyclic neuroleptics*

    A. phenothiazines

        1. with aliphatic side-chain (e.g. chlorpromazine)

        2. with piperidine side-chain (e.g. thioridazine)

        3. with piperazine side-chain (e.g. trifluoperazine)

    B. thioxanthines

        e.g. flupenthixol, clopenthixol

    C. azepines

        1. dibenzoxapines (e.g. loaxapine)

        2. dibenzodiazepines (e.g. clozapine)

II. *butylperidines*

    A. 'butyrophenones'(phenylbutylperidines)

        e.g. haloperidol, droperidol, spiroperidol

    B. diphenylbutylperidines

        e.g. pimozide, fluspiriline

III. *other heterocyclic compounds*

    A. indoles

        e.g. oxypertine

    B. substituted benzamines

        e.g. sulpiride

IV. *rauwolfia alkaloids*

        e.g. reserpine

[Handwritten annotations:]
↑↑ sedative effects   ↑ antimusc SE   +↑ EPSE
↑ sedative effects   ↑↑ antimuscarinic SE
most freq cause   EPSE ↑↑
stellazine
fluphenazine (Modecate depot)
depixol   oral
depot
most freq. cause EPSE
benzisoxazole deriv.
eg. resperidone

1. **Limbic system and neocortex.** Dopamine-containing neurones in the midbrain project to the limbic system ('mesolimbic pathway') and to some areas of the prefrontal cortex ('mesocortical pathway'). It is believed that the blockade of dopamine receptors at these sites is the basis of the anti-psychotic effect of the neuroleptics.

2. **Striatum.** Dopamine-containing neurones in the pars compacta of the substantia nigra project to the striatum ('nigro-striatal pathway'). The blockade of striatal dopamine receptors is thought to be the basis of neuroleptic-induced Parkinsonism.

3. **Hypothalamus.** Dopamine-containing neurones in the arcuate nucleus project to the infundibulum of the third ventricle ('tubero-infundibular pathway'). The blockade of infundibular dopamine receptors is thought to be the basis of neuroleptic-induced hyperprolactinaemia.

4. **Brain stem.** Dopamine receptors have been identified in an area of the lower brain stem which lies outside the blood–brain barrier ('chemoreceptor trigger zone'). Neurones in this area project to the dorsal nucleus of the vagus, and their stimulation can result in vomiting. It is believed that the anti-emetic effect of neuroleptics is based on the blockade of dopamine receptors in the chemoreceptor trigger zone.

There are three major uses for neuroleptics in psychiatric treatment:

1. **Acute calming of agitated patients:** an injection of a potent short-acting neuroleptic (e.g. droperidol) can be very effective.

2. **Treatment of acute psychotic states.** Both organic psychoses (including most drug-induced states) and functional psychoses (acute schizophrenia, mania, psychotic depression) can respond to treatment with neuroleptics. Apart from a psychomotor calming effect, the drugs help to abolish specific 'psychotic' symptoms (hallucinations, delusions, thought disorder). As the psychosis subsides, the patient becomes more responsive to the environment, and amenable to other forms of treatment (for example, occupational and social therapy).

3. **Maintenance treatment** in chronic and recurrent psychotic states. This form of treatment is especially important in schizophrenia where symptoms can persist or recur over many years. Maintenance treatment helps to control the psychotic symptoms and to maintain the patient's social functioning at its optimum level, and can prevent the recurrence of acute psychotic episodes.

The choice of drug and form of administration depends on the indication and on the clinical features of the individual patient. For the treatment of acute psychoses oral medication on the ward can be used; drugs can be administered in the form of syrup. **Chlorpromazine** is the oldest and best-known phenothiazine, and it is usually a safe choice in most cases. **Thioridazine** has more anti-cholinergic and anti-adrenergic side-effects, but is less likely to produce extra-pyramidal side-effects, probably due to its 'built-in' central anti-cholinergic anti-Parkinsonian property.

Trifluoperazine, haloperidol, and **pimozide** are potent neuroleptics: these drugs are not sedative, and are relatively free from autonomic side-effects, but can produce trouble-some extra-pyramidal syndromes. These drugs can be used in small doses on an out-patient basis in the management of **chronic paranoid states.** Although drugs in tablet form are suitable for long-term maintenance treatment, depot injections are usually preferred for this purpose since they help to ensure patient compliance. The depots are usually oily injections of esters (decanoates or enanthates) of drugs; the active drug is gradually released from the injection site into the blood stream. There are depot injections for **fluphenazine, flupenthixol, clopenthixol, haloperidol,** and **fluspirilene.** Injections are administered every one to four weeks, usually at a 'depot clinic' or in the patient's home.

Clozapine appears to have a different therapeutic action to other dopamine receptor antagonists. There is good evidence that the drug is effective in some patients who have not responded to other forms of neuroleptic treatment. It has the unfortunate side-effect of causing fatal bone marrow depression. It can only be dispensed if the patient and the psychiatrist are first registered with the Central Patient Monitoring Service. Each week's medication is dispensed only when the blood test has been received by the Monitoring Service, and treatment is stopped if white cells decline in three successive samples.

There is much interest in the possibility of developing new neuroleptic drugs based on clozapine. Unfortunately, clozapine has many actions and it is not known which, or which combination, is responsible for clozapine's especial therapeutic actions. Recent molecular biological studies reveal the existence of at least five dopamine receptor subtypes. Conventional neuroleptic drugs are thought to work by blocking the dopamine D2 receptor subtypes. Modern imaging techniques reveal that recommended doses of neuroleptics achieve near-complete receptor occupancy. In keeping with this finding recent clinical trials suggest that high doses of neuroleptic drugs confer no additional therapeutic threat over conventional doses. Clozapine has anti-psychotic actions out of proportion to its D2 receptor affinity. However, the drug is unusual in having appreci-able affinity for the D4 receptor. D4 receptors are concentrated in mesolimbic areas of the brain and in contrast to the low concentration in the basal ganglia. The latter may account for the low incidence of extra-pyramidal side-effects induced by the drug and tardive dyskinesia, whereas its anti-psychotic activity may be due to D4 receptor antagonism.

The neuroleptics are relatively safe drugs: they have a high therapeutic index (toxic dose/therapeutic dose), and as they have a shallow dose–response curve, they can be administered over a wide dosage range. A rare but serious complication is the **neuro-leptic malignant syndrome.** This, together with the side-effects and drug interactions of neuroleptics, are shown as *Table 7.3.*

Anxiolytics

There are three main pharmacological treatments for anxiety: anti-depressants, benzo-diazepines, and beta-blockers. Anti-depressant drugs are considered further below. They exert anxiolytic effects even when symptoms of depression are not prominent. Like the anti-depressant effect, anxiolytic actions take a week or two to begin to emerge and treatment needs to be sustained for some weeks before the degree of response can be

Table 7.3 *Side-effects of neuroleptics*

central side-effects		
extrapyramidal syndromes	Parkinsonism	hypokinesia, rigidity, and tremor (alleviated by centrally acting anti-cholinergic drugs
	akathisia	'inability to sit still', inner restlessness, and compensatory foot-shuffling
	acute dystonic reactions; oculogyric crises	spastic contractions of the muscles of the neck and shoulders; relieved by an injection of procyclidine
	tardive dyskinesia (late onset)	orofacial dyskinesia whole body chorea
	neuroleptic malignant syndrome	rigidity, hyperpyrexia, and coma (extreme dopamine receptor blockade: potentially lethal); treat with bromocriptine (dopamine receptor stimulant) and dantrolene (muscle relaxant)
lowering of the seizure threshold	fits	
central autonomic side-effects		
	thermoregulatory failure	body cools in cold temperature → dangerous hypothermia in heat → heat stroke
	orthostatic hypotension	partly central origin (see below)
endocrine complications		
	hyperprolactinaemia	galactorrhea, gynaecomastia, impotence, and infertility
	reduction in gonadotrophins, oestrogens, and progesterone	amenorrhoea and infertility
psychiatric complications		
	apathy, lassitude, lack of initiative	(like chronic schizophrenia!)
	disturbance of the sleep/wakefulness cycle	
	depression	
	acute brain syndrome ('atropine psychosis')	esp. potent anti-cholinergic drugs (like thioridazine)
peripheral autonomic side-effects (phenothiazines > butyrophenones)		
	blockade of muscarinic receptors	cycloplegia, dry mouth, constipation, urinary retention
	blockade of α_1-adrenoceptors	miosis, orthostatic hypotension, nasal stuffiness, ejaculatory incompetence

Table 7.3 *Continued*

hypersensitivity reactions		
	cholestatic jaundice	
	blood dyscrasias	agranulocytosis
	allergic skin reactions	urticaria, dermatitis
skin reactions		
	contact dermatitis	affects nurses handling phenothiazine solutions
	photosensitivity	problem in sunny climates
	patchy hyper-pigmentation (long-term medication)	
drug-interactions		
	blockade of uptake of drug into peripheral noradrenergic neurones	inhibition of the anti-hypertensive effect of guanethidine
		potentiation of the effects of sedative drugs (including ethanol and opiates)

gauged. Older anti-depressants such as clomipramine and amitriptyline have sedative effects which may be useful in treating agitation and insomnia in anxious patients. Trazodone also has useful sedative and hypnotic actions. There is good evidence that drugs acting on the 5-hydroxytryptamine (5HT) system – for example, clomipramine and the new specific 5HT re-uptake blockers – are particularly effective in the treatment of panic disorder. Benzodiazepines have an immediate anxiolytic action but it is probable that tolerance develops with rebound exacerbation upon the withdrawal of treatment. Beta-blockers are useful in the treatment of anxiety states particularly when associated with somatic symptoms.

BENZODIAZEPINES

These drugs are also called 'minor tranquillizers'; they are effective in reducing pathological anxiety, tension, and agitation without general depression of the CNS (cf. barbiturates). They are also devoid of any anti-psychotic activity (cf. neuroleptics).

The mode of action of benzodiazepines is closely related to GABA-mediated inhibition in the CNS. Specific binding sites for benzodiazepines ('benzodiazepine receptors') have been demonstrated in most parts of the neuraxis; the highest concentrations have been found in the neocortex, limbic system, and cerebellum. The benzodiazepine receptor is closely associated with the GABA-receptor ('GABA-benzodiazepine receptor complex'), and the activation of the benzodiazepine receptor results in potentiation of GABA-mediated responses. The anti-anxiety effect is thought to be mediated via the enhancement of GABA-mediated inhibition of 5-hydroxytryptamine – and noradrenaline-containing neurones; the integrity of the monoamine-containing neurones is believed to be essential in mediating the suppression of certain behaviours and increased arousal associated with fear responses. Similarly, the enhancement of GABA-mediated neuronal inhibition in certain neuronal circuits has been related to the anticonvulsant and central muscular relaxant effects of benzodiazepines.

Each benzodiazepine possesses, to greater or lesser extent, five important pharmacological effects:

1. Anxiolytic.
2. Hypnotic.
3. Muscle relaxant.
4. Anticonvulsant.
5. Amnestic.

The **anxiolytic effect** is utilized in the management of anxiety states. While these drugs are effective and relatively harmless in the treatment of short-lived situational anxiety, their use in the management of anxiety neurosis is more controversial. The current recommended practice is to use these drugs for only a limited period (two to four weeks) during which the patient will become more amenable to other (e.g. behavioural, social) forms of treatment. The long-term use of these drugs should be avoided because of the possibility of development of tolerance and dependence. **Diazepam**, a long-acting drug, may be more suitable for the management of persistent high levels of anxiety, whereas shorter-acting drugs (e.g. **lorazepam, oxazepam**) can be used for the management of episodic or situational anxiety.

Several benzodiazepines are suitable **hypnotics**: temazepam is a short-acting drug suitable to *induce sleep and relatively free from hangover effects during daytime*, whereas longer-acting drugs, such as diazepam, nitrazepam, and flurazepam, can both *induce sleep and maintain sleep throughout the night*.

Diazepam is used as an effective **muscle relaxant** in the treatment of spasticity, and diazepam and clonazepam are established **anticonvulsants** (see p. 81).

Some benzodiazepines (e.g. diazepam, lorazepam, midazolam) can produce **anterograde amnesia**; this property of the drugs is utilized in pre-anaesthetic medication and in performing minor surgical or diagnostic interventions (dentistry, endoscopy).

Almost all the **side-effects** of the benzodiazepines are related to their actions on the CNS. Daytime sedation, drowsiness, and impairment of psychomotor performance can occur in conjunction with both anti-anxiety treatment and the use of long-acting hypnotics ('hangover effect'). Increased hostility and aggressive behaviour can occur as a rare but unpleasant complication. Physical dependence has been reported, especially in association with large-dose, long-term medication.

Withdrawal symptoms are common; these are more severe following the use of short-acting potent drugs (e.g. lorazepam) than of long-acting drugs (e.g. diazepam). Withdrawal symptoms include increased anxiety, rebound insomnia, dysphoria, anorexia; rarely, more severe symptoms (severe agitation, panic, depression, delusions, hallucinations, convulsion) can occur. Triazolam, a short-acting benzodiazepine, has been withdrawn because of consistent reports of amnesia and rebound symptoms. These withdrawal symptoms can take a few weeks to resolve, and patients must be encouraged to persevere if they are not to continue their dependence. The benzodiazepines are relatively safe drugs in overdosage; fatalities are usually due to the concomitant use of CNS depressants (ethanol, barbiturates).

Anti-depressants

These drugs are effective in treatment of the neuroses including depressive disorders, anxiety states, and obsessional compulsive disorder. There are two major groups: **re-uptake inhibitors** that work by blocking the re-uptake of monoamines into the synaptic cleft, and **MAO inhibitors** that inhibit the degradation of monoamines by inhibiting the enzyme monoamine oxidase; finally there is a small group of atypical drugs that have anti-depressant properties.

RE-UPTAKE INHIBITORS

The primary pharmacological action is to inhibit the active re-uptake of monoamines back into presynaptic terminals. Re-uptake into nerve terminals is the normal mechanism for eliminating the actions of monoamines that have been released from the terminal into the synaptic cleft. When the re-uptake site is blocked then monoamines accumulate in the synapse. However, it is clear that this cannot be their sole mechanism of action. Monoamine neurones are sensitive to the concentration of monoamines around the terminals and dendrites, which they detect with monoamine receptors on their surface called auto-receptors. Consequently, when extra-cellular concentrations begin to rise due to re-uptake blockade, terminal auto-receptors suppress further release of monoamine, and dendritic auto-receptors decrease the firing rate. This effectively neutralizes the increase in synaptic monoamine content. It is thought that auto-receptors may desensitize so that neurones come to tolerate higher concentrations of monoamine in the synapse and around the dendrites. This process of desensitization takes some time and may account for the delayed therapeutic effect of re-uptake inhibitors. In addition to monoamine re-uptake inhibition these drugs antagonize some post-synaptic monoamine receptors, including α receptors and some 5HT receptor subtypes. This may be relevant to their therapeutic actions – by correcting imbalances between α and β noradrenergic neurotransmission or between different subtypes of 5HT receptors.

There are three major groups of re-uptake inhibitors: an older group that acts on both noradrenaline and serotonin; a group that predominantly acts on noradrenaline; and one that specifically inhibits serotonin:

1. Mixed monoamine re-uptake inhibitors (MARIs) are generally older drugs and include 'tricyclics' such as **clomipramine, amitriptyline**, and **imipramine.**
2. Noradrenaline re-uptake inhibitors (NARIs) include drugs such as **prothiaden, lofepramine**, and **maprotiline.**
3. Serotonin-specific re-uptake inhibitors (SSRIs) include drugs such as **fluoxetine, fluvoxamine**, and **paroxetine.**

The **mixed monoamine re-uptake inhibitors (MARIs)** or tricyclics have been in use for almost thirty years and they are still the most important anti-depressants. There are a large number of tricyclic anti-depressants available on the market. **Imipramine** is the prototype drug which established effectiveness. **Desipramine** is less sedative than imipramine and has more marked sympathomimetic activity. **Amitriptyline** is a widely used and effective drug with marked sedative and peripheral anti-muscarinic and adrenolytic properties. **Clomipramine** has been claimed to have beneficial effects in obsessional states. Some of the side-effects of MARIs are attributable to their antagonism not only to post-synaptic receptors of monoamines but also to acetylcholine receptors and histamine receptors. The blockade of central α_1-adrenoceptors, muscarinic, and histamine receptors is believed to be responsible for the sedative effects of tricyclic anti-depressants; the blockade of these receptors in the periphery results in characteristic autonomic side-effects. The side-effects are summarized in *Table 7.4*.

Table 7.4 *Side-effects of anti-depressants*

central neurological side-effects	
	fine static tremor
lowering of the seizure threshold	convulsions
peripheral autonomic side-effects	
anti-muscarinic	cycloplegia, mydriasis, tachycardia, constipation, urinary retention
sympathomimetic (due to noradrenaline uptake blockade)	mydriasis, tachycardia
adrenolytic (α_1-adrenoceptor blockade)	miosis, orthostatic hypotension, nasal stuffiness, ejaculatory difficulties
cardiovascular side-effects	
	tachycardia orthostatic hypotension arrhythmias
reduction in cardiac contractility	reduced cardiac output
psychiatric side-effects	
	hypomania paranoid–hallucinatory states
potent anti-cholinergics like amitriptyline	acute brain syndrome ('atropine psychosis')
hypersensitivity reactions (relatively rare)	
	cholestatic jaundice blood dyscrasias allergic dermatitis

Noradrenaline re-uptake inhibitors (NARIs) developed from attempts to isolate re-uptake inhibition from the many other pharmacological properties of the MARIs. Noradrenaline-selective drugs are less sedative than MARIs and the newer ones lack anti-cholinergic side-effects.

More potent and selective serotonin-specific re-uptake inhibitors (SSRIs) have been developed, and are almost devoid of other pharmacological actions and lack the side-effects listed in *Table 7.4*. There are three major side-effects. Nausea is quite marked early on in treatment but tends to improve after the first week. A second important side-effect is failure of orgasm in both males and females. In the first week of treatment there may be a transient exacerbation of anxiety symptoms. These drugs have the important advantage that they alone amongst anti-depressant drugs do not cause weight gain. They are non-cardiotoxic and safe in overdosage.

MONOAMINE OXIDASE INHIBITORS

The anti-depressant action of these drugs has been directly related to their main pharmacological action – the inhibition of the enzyme monoamine oxidase: enzyme inhibition results in an increased concentration of cerebral monoamines which would correct the neurochemical deficiency underlying depressive illness (see 'monoamine theory of affective disorders', p. 196). Older MAO inhibitors bind irreversibly to the enzyme. The return of normal activity requires the synthesis of the new enzyme. There are three older monoamine oxidase inhibitors in clinical use, **phenelzine, tranylcypromine,** and **isocarboxazide.**

The clinical uses of these drugs are:

1. As a *second line of treatment* in the case of patients whose depression does not respond to treatment with tricyclic anti-depressants.

2. They have been recommended for some *atypical forms of depression* characterized by features such as 'reversed diurnal variation', weight gain, or histrionic or hypochondriacal features.

3. *Phobic anxiety states,* in which they are as effective as tricyclics. Relapse is common on withdrawal of the drug.

4. *Narcolepsy.*

These are potentially toxic drugs, and **side-effects** are common and troublesome. These are excessive central stimulation (agitation, hypomania, convulsions); orthostatic hypotension (probably due to sympathetic ganglion blockade); and hepatocellular jaundice (as a rare but severe hypersensitivity reaction).

Drug-interactions are important and basically of two kinds:

1. Potentiation of the effects of **monoamine precursors** (e.g. L-Dopa) and indirectly acting sympathomimetic amines (e.g. tyramine, amphetamine). The potentiation of the effects of sympathomimetic amines can lead to a hypertensive crisis (as in the

cheese reaction following the ingestion of tyramine-containing foodstuffs, such as cream cheese, broad beans, pickled herrings, avocado pears, Marmite, and Chianti).

2. **Inhibition of the detoxification** of a number of drugs (barbiturates, ethanol, centrally acting anti-cholinergics, tricyclic anti-depressants).

REVERSIBLE INHIBITORS OF MONOAMINE OXIDASE A (RIMAs)

Meclobamide is the first of this class and there are likely to be more. In contrast to the older MAOIs, RIMAs are competitive antagonists of the enzyme monoamine oxidase-A. This means that treatment with trycyclics and other anti-depressants can begin within a day or two of stopping meclobamide. The relative clinical efficacy of the RIMAs has yet to be clearly established. Meclobamide has minimal sedative and anti-cholinergic side-effects. It lacks the cheese reaction because it is a selective MAO-A inhibitor, leaving MAO-B to metabolize tyramines in food.

ATYPICAL ANTI-DEPRESSANTS

Trazodone and **mianserin** are sedative anti-depressants which significantly inhibit the re-uptake of monoamines. They are antagonists at 5HT2 receptors but it is not clear whether these actions are relevant to their anti-depressant effects. At first sight 5HT antagonism at 5HT receptors would seem to be opposite to the primary actions of SSRIs and therefore countertherapeutic. However, it may be that both actions serve to correct an imbalance in functioning between 5HT2 and 5HT1 receptor subtypes. Trazodone and mianserin also block α-noradrenergic auto-receptors. This promotes noradrenaline release and this is another possible mechanism of action. Neither drug is widely used and mianserin causes blood dyscrasias.

Buspirone mimics the action of 5HT at 5HT1A receptors. It is effective in the treatment of generalized anxiety but not in panic disorder. It appears to have weak anti-depressant activity, which is probably of theoretical interest only. It is thought that targeting the 5HT1A receptor may be productive of new anti-depressants.

TRYPTOPHAN

Tryptophan is the amino-acid precursor of 5-hydroxytryptamine. It is believed that the administration of tryptophan results in increased 5-hydroxytryptamine synthesis in the brain, which in turn would lead to the replenishment of presynaptic stores. Tryptophan has only weak anti-depressant properties, and is usually administered as an adjunct to enhance the effectiveness of tricyclic anti-depressants or monoamine oxidase inhibitors in the case of treatment-resistant depression. An outbreak of a dangerous eosinophilia-myalgia syndrome was attributed to tryptophan. Although the cause was probably a contaminant from a single manufacturer, the drug is only available on a named-patient basis.

MANAGING ANTI-DEPRESSANT TREATMENT

The therapeutic effect appears gradually, usually after one to three weeks on the drug; therefore in severe retarded or psychotic depression a faster-acting treatment, such as ECT, may be more appropriate. It is important to administer a therapeutically effective dose, and plasma level assays may be helpful in dosage selection. It has been recommended that the anti-depressant medication should be continued after remission of the depressive symptomatology since there is an increased risk of relapse for the first six to twelve months following a depressive episode.

TREATMENT-RESISTANT DEPRESSION

Treatment with re-uptake-inhibiting anti-depressants should be continued for at least six weeks to see the full therapeutic effect. If there has been only a partial response, the addition of lithium (see below) can potentiate the effect of the anti-depressant. This has proved to be a very useful combination. Caution is required when using lithium in combination with SSRIs because there is a very small risk of CNS depression, myoclonic jerking, and hypothermia.

More aggressive combination therapy is best reserved for in-patients. The combination of a monoamine oxidase inhibitor, lithium, and the 5HT precursor, tryptophan, has been advocated by some authorities.

Psychostimulants

These drugs increase the level of alertness, stimulate mental activity, and suppress fatigue in the normal person. The two major classes of psychostimulants are the **amphetamines** and **cocaine**; the **xanthines** (e.g. caffeine) are classified as non-selective CNS stimulants (see *Table 7.1*). Both the amphetamines and cocaine exert their alerting effects by increasing the central actions of monoamines: amphetamine releases both noradrenaline and dopamine (and at higher doses 5-hydroxytryptamine) from presynaptic stores; cocaine blocks the (re-)uptake of noradrenaline. These drugs also possess powerful sympathomimetic effects. Of these drugs only the amphetamines have therapeutic uses.

AMPHETAMINES

The most important amphetamines are:

1. Amphetamine.
2. Methamphetamine.
3. Methylphenidate.
4. Fenfluramine.

Apart from a psychostimulant/anti-fatigue effect, these drugs also have anorectic (appetite-suppressant) properties. However, they have no place in the treatment of obesity, since they are not effective and produce dependence.

Before the advent of the tricyclic anti-depressants, amphetamine was the most popular drug for the treatment of depression. The current clinical use of these drugs is limited, and it includes the treatment of the following:

1. **Narcolepsy** (alerting effect).
2. **Hyperkinetic children** (a paradoxical 'calming' effect of amphetamine and methylphenidate).
3. **Nocturnal enuresis** (partly a central alerting effect, partly a direct effect on the bladder sphincter).

SIDE-EFFECTS

1. Excessive **central stimulation** (anxiety, over-activity, insomnia).
2. **Paranoid psychosis** (especially on larger doses). Since most of the amphetamines cause euphoria, they have an abuse potential; **psychological dependence** rapidly develops on these drugs (see p. 220).

Lithium

Lithium cannot be classified with other psychoactive drugs: it is a unique drug which has no psychotropic effect in normal individuals. However, it has remarkable effectiveness in manic-depressive psychosis (acute 'anti-manic' effect and 'mood-stabilizing' effect on maintenance treatment). Lithium is a monovalent cation which is available for clinical use in the form of carbonate or citrate salts. The most important cellular effects are:

1. Competition with sodium ions for the *sodium pump:* interference with the maintenance of membrane potential and action potential generation in neurones.
2 Increase in the *uptake of catecholamines* into nerve terminals.
3. Reduced effectiveness of the *activation of central α_1-adrenoceptors and muscarinic receptors.*
4. Inhibition of the activation of *adenylate cyclase*
   - by antidiuretic hormone (ADH) in renal tubules;
   - by thyroid-stimulating hormone (TSH) in the thyroid gland.

The first three effects have been related to the anti-manic and mood-stabilizing properties of lithium, whereas the effect on adenylate cyclase activation seems to be the basis for some side-effects (nephrogenic diabetes insipidus; hypothyroidism).

The elimination of lithium from the body is almost entirely through the kidneys. In steady state, the serum lithium concentration is determined by the ratio of the *daily lithium intake* and the *renal lithium clearance*. Renal lithium clearance is the produce of the fractional tubular excretion of lithium and the glomerular filtration rate. The elimination of lithium through the kidneys can be impaired if either of these components is reduced: fractional tubular excretion of lithium will be reduced if the serum sodium concentration declines (e.g. as a result of thiazide diuretics, Addison's disease); glomerular filtration rate can be reduced as a result of dehydration, cardiac failure, kidney disease.

Lithium can be used clinically both in acute affective episodes and in prophylactic maintenance treatment. The oldest use of lithium is in the treatment of mania. The therapeutic (anti-manic) effect of lithium does not appear for about a week, therefore the additional use of neuroleptics is often required. The plasma concentration aimed at is higher than in maintenance treatment (0.6–1.2 mEq/1); thus there is an increased risk of lithium toxicity. In general, a neuroleptic is more effective and safer for the management of acute mania.

There is increasing evidence that lithium has an **anti-depressant effect,** and its use has been recommended to treat depressive states unresponsive to tricyclic anti-depressants. The most important use of lithium is the **prophylactic maintenance treatment of recurrent manic-depressive psychosis**. Patients with both bipolar (manic and depressive) and unipolar (only depressive) episodes can respond to maintenance treatment: relapses may be completely prevented or their frequency and/or intensity reduced. Patients with frequently alternating mood states (*'rapid cycling manic-depressive psychosis'*) usually respond only poorly to lithium; such patients may benefit from maintenance treatment with **carbamazepine** (see 'Anticonvulsants', p. 81). Patients on lithium maintenance treatment are usually followed up at 'lithium clinics' where plasma concentration of lithium, therapeutic response, and side-effects can be monitored. This is done monthly until a steady state has been achieved; three-monthly thereafter. The recommended plasma level is 0.4–0.8 mEq/1 for maintenance treatment.

Lithium maintenance treatment is contraindicated in the following conditions:

1. Renal and cardiac insufficiency.
2. Addison's disease.
3. Hypothyroidism.
4. Pregnancy.

It is usual to measure/assess **blood urea** before starting lithium; other tests only if clinically indicated. Lithium has a low therapeutic index, and **toxicity** quickly appears as the plasma concentration rises above 1.2 mEq/1.

SIDE-EFFECTS

Side-effects can occur even at 'therapeutic' plasma levels:

1. **Gastro-intestinal side-effects** are common, especially early in treatment, and include nausea, vomiting, indigestion, metallic taste, diarrhoea.
2. Of the **neurological side-effects** a fine static tremor is the most common; the appearance of coarse tremor, ataxia, fasciculations are the signs of intoxication.
3. Of the **metabolic effects** a nephrogenic diabetes insipidus (polyuria, polydipsia),

increased water retention leading to ankle oedema, and an increase in weight are the most important.

4. An important **endocrine side-effect** is the development of hypothyroidism.

Drug-interactions involve:

1. **Thiazide diuretics** (these can lead to sodium loss and thus to lithium toxicity).
2. **Neuroleptics** (these can increase the neurotoxicity of lithium).

PHYSICAL TREATMENTS: ELECTROCONVULSIVE TREATMENT (ECT)

The use of electroconvulsive therapy has been the cause of much controversy both in psychiatry and among the general public. This is partly because the treatment has been used outside those situations where its use is appropriate and partly because there has been difficulty in performing accurate research. Several large studies have established that ECT is superior to anti-depressant drugs, and far superior to placebo, in the treatment of depression. The necessity of the seizure has now been proven by studies comparing the effects of ECT with 'simulated' ECT (administration of the anaesthetic and muscle relaxant but without the electric shocks).

The relative effects of treatments for severe depressive illness were demonstrated in a study some years ago:

> After four weeks over 70 per cent of those receiving ECT had few or no symptoms (they had received four to eight treatments during this time). Just over one half of those receiving imipramine had made a similar response, to be compared with 39 per cent of the placebo group and only 30 per cent of the phenelzine group.

Mode of action

It is highly probable that grand mal seizure activity is necessary for the anti-depressant effect, and there is some evidence that seizures elicited by higher currents have greater anti-depressant activity than those elicited by lower currents. Thus, attempting to minimize confusion and memory loss by minimizing the current may reduce the therapeutic efficacy. However, unilateral ECT to the non-dominant hemisphere evokes a bilateral seizure with much less confusion but with reduced efficacy: it requires on average between two and four additional treatments.

ECT potentiates behaviour mediated by serotonin (5HT) and there is neurochemical evidence from work with experimental animals that this is due to an increase in post-synaptic 5HT receptor numbers. Behaviours mediated by dopamine are also enhanced by ECT, and there are influences too on noradrenergic functions similar to those described for anti-depressant drugs (see p. 91). In particular, it has been shown that ECT has an effect in down-regulating β receptors. The neurochemical and behavioural effects of ECT parallel its anti-depressant actions since the changes emerge after several treatments and sub-seizure currents are ineffective.

Clinical uses

The principal use of ECT is in severe depressive illness. Features of that illness that predict a good response to ECT are:

1. Severe weight loss.
2. Pronounced early morning wakening.
3. Psychomotor retardation.
4. Psychotic features – especially depressive delusions.

In clinical practice ECT is used:

1. When a **depressive illness with the appropriate features fails to respond** to anti-depressant treatment.
2. In psychotic depression where suffering is severe, especially when **depressive delusions** are present.
3. In **depressive stupor.**
4. In **catatonic stupor.**
5. In **puerperal psychoses**, especially those with clouding, perplexity, and marked affective features.

More controversial indications include:

6. *Acute schizophrenia* with clouded consciousness and perplexity.
7. *Schizophrenia* where there are pronounced depressive features.
8. *Mania* when neuroleptic and lithium have failed to control persistent over-activity.

Administration of ECT

ECT requires a general anaesthetic and the usual precautions are observed. The treatment is usually given early in the morning so the patient is starved from midnight. Atropine is administered as pre-medication to dry up bronchial and salivary secretions and also to prevent an extreme bradycardia. A short-acting anaesthetic is administered together with a muscle relaxant to modify the fit. Following ventilation with oxygen (this has been shown to reduce amnesia afterwards), the electrodes – moistened to ensure good contact with the skin – are placed one on the temporal region and one near the vertex of the side of the non-dominant hemisphere for unilateral ECT. (For bilateral ECT the electrodes are placed on each temporal region.) Treatment is given twice a week with two clear days between treatments until a satisfactory response has been obtained: this is usually after six to eight treatments.

Unwanted effects

ECT is a safe treatment. The mortality rate is similar to that of a brief anaesthetic when used for dental or investigative procedures. The largest series demonstrate a mortality of 1 death per 20,000 treatments.

The treatment causes *alteration of pulse rate, a rise in blood pressure*, and *a great increase in cerebral blood flow*.

The **contraindications** are therefore illnesses affecting the cardiovascular and central nervous systems:

> Cerebral and aortic aneurysms.
>
> Recent cerebral haemorrhage.
>
> Myocardial infarction.
>
> Cardiac arrhythmias.
>
> Raised intracranial pressure and brain tumour.
>
> Acute respiratory infections form a contraindication to the anaesthetic and require treatment before ECT is given.

Physical side-effects following ECT are rare. However, *physical problems following the anaesthetic* may include:

> Myocardial infarction.
>
> Cardiac arrhythmias.
>
> Pulmonary embolism.
>
> Pneumonia.

If the *muscle relaxant has not been properly given* the following may occur:

> Dislocations.
>
> Fractures (and consequent fat embolism).

Increased blood pressure during the fit itself may occur, causing:

> Cerebral haemorrhage.
>
> Bleeding from peptic ulcer.

PSYCHOLOGICAL SEQUELAE

Mania is precipitated by ECT in approximately 5 per cent of cases. This figure is similar to that found with tricyclic anti-depressants and occurs in those patients known to have, or be vulnerable to, bipolar manic-depressive illness.

A post-ECT **confusional state** usually lasts for about half an hour. A headache may also occur but is usually short-lived.

Memory loss is a more important side-effect. There is a short and rapidly dwindling amnesia for the time preceding each treatment (retrograde amnesia) and a longer post-ECT (anterograde) amnesia. Patients may also complain of *subjective difficulty in remembering* previously well-learned material, like telephone numbers or addresses. These problems are usually hard to demonstrate with objective tests of memory. However, the following factors will reduce the memory problems:

1. Unilateral shock to the non-dominant hemisphere.
2. Not giving too many treatments.
3. Not giving treatment too frequently.
4. Oxygenating the patient well before the shock.
5. Not using an unnecessarily big shock.

COGNITIVE AND BEHAVIOURAL TREATMENTS

These treatments involve the manipulation of the patient's thought processes (cognitions), overt behaviour, physiological responses (autonomic functions), and environment in order to bring about positive change and alleviation of the identified problem. These manipulations or therapeutic tactics can vary depending on the problem and the results of the behavioural analysis, but will make up a treatment programme or therapeutic strategy which will have predefined goals. Cognitive-behaviour therapy is not necessarily antagonistic to physical approaches to treatment: rather the two approaches can be complementary. Many patients derive benefit from a combination of the two types of treatment.

Theoretical foundations

The fundamental principles of change in psychological treatments based upon cognitive-behaviour therapy are:

1. **Classical (Pavlovian) conditioning**. This is the process by which a neutral stimulus (the 'conditioned' stimulus, or CS) acquires the ability to elicit an involuntary response (a CR) as a result of association with a stimulus (the 'unconditioned' stimulus, or UCS) which normally evokes that response. Pavlov's famous experiments on gastric acid and salivary excretion in dogs exemplify this form of learning. Thus the sight of food (UCS) usually evokes salivation, and by initially pairing this with a bell (CS) Pavlov was subsequently able to make the dog salivate (CR) when the bell rang in the absence of food.

    A clinically relevant example of classical conditioning would be the hypothetical explanation of the origin of phobic anxiety, whereby the phobic object (for example, spiders) acts as a CS eliciting a fear response because of earlier pairing with such responses.

2. **Operant (instrumental) conditioning**. This is the process whereby voluntary behaviours are strengthened ('reinforcement') or weakened ('punishment') because of their consequences. Skinner's experiments in which rats pressed levers for food

reinforcement typify this type of learning in animals, while a clinically relevant example in humans would be the engendering of temper tantrums in a young child when he discovers that such behaviour is particularly effective in obtaining his parents' undivided attention.

3. **Vicarious learning**. This refers to the process by which learning occurs through symbolic representations by exposure to instructional, observational, or imaginal material. Learning is thought to occur through the informative and instructional function of reward. For example, many childhood fears are thought to be acquired through the child's observing other people's reaction to the feared situation and hence building up expectations about it. This process is known as modelling and can be used as a powerful therapeutic tool as well as a process through which disorders are acquired. The action of the therapist modelling appropriate coping responses during a stressful situation, or appropriate management strategies with a difficult child, are good examples of this.

4. **Cognitive processes**. These refer to the way that information is detected (perception and attention) and then organized, stored, and retrieved from memory. This flow of information is manifest in conscious thought, processes of attention and interpretation, and underlying beliefs and attitudes. There is a subtle interplay between such cognitive processes, physiological processes, and overt behaviour in all human actions, but they are especially important in abnormal behaviour and emotional disorders. For example, certain types of information may be more accessible and hence come to the fore under certain conditions, such as low mood or high levels of physiological arousal. A clinical example would be the patient who suffers panic attacks because he over-attends to minor physical sensations which when detected are catastrophically interpreted as being the sign of a major illness. Small changes in heart rate or difficulty in breathing due to tension are interpreted as an indication of an imminent heart attack, resulting in the sudden upsurge of anxiety characteristic of panic attacks.

Both classical and operant conditioning tend to be situationally specific (that is to say, the learned responses occur most readily in situations similar to those prevailing when the conditioning took place). Both types of conditioning are deemed to be reversible. Thus a classically conditioned fear of crowded places would be expected to **extinguish** as a result of repeated visits to busy shops, while tantrums cease when they no longer elicit the same parental attention.

Many pathological behaviours involve a complex interplay between classical and operant conditioning. For example, although phobic **anxiety** may arise from a classical learning experience, phobic **behaviour** is more likely to be maintained by operant conditioning – that is, the reinforcement of avoidance behaviour by anxiety reduction.

Contemporary thinking incorporates all of these principles into explanations of abnormal behaviour and psychological disorders, although the emphasis given to the balance of the different contributions of each can vary across different disorders.

General principles of cognitive-behaviour therapy

All cognitive and behaviour therapies start with a cognitive-behavioural analysis. The objective symptomatology or problem area is clearly defined, and details of the frequency, duration, and intensity of the symptoms are recorded together with events that occur at the time when symptoms are experienced. This is usually accomplished by asking the patient to keep a diary for a week or so before any formulation is attempted. It is frequently helpful to describe the patient's problem in terms of their thoughts (cognitions), actions (overt behaviour), and physical sensations (physiological reactions). Although practical considerations usually mean that it is the patient's subjective account of their cognitions, behaviour, and physiological reactions that are used in the cognitive-behavioural analysis, if possible the patient's behaviour should be observed and their physiological responses measured directly through non-invasive methods. Such a formulation must take account of:

A. The Antecedents – the environmental context in which the symptom occurs.

B. The Behaviour – the problem itself.

C. The Consequences – events which may contribute to the maintenance of the behaviour.

The formulation constitutes a **hypothesis** about the nature and origin of the symptom. The hypothesis will usually suggest appropriate treatment strategies: for example, the hypothesis that a patient's withdrawal from social contact is maintained by anxiety reduction might suggest a different type of intervention from the hypothesis that it stems from an inadequate repertoire of social skills. The treatment thus constitutes a test of the hypothesis, which itself may require modification in the light of the success or failure of the treatment.

Cognitive-behavioural treatment invariably involves a clear objective goal based on the formulation derived from the cognitive-behavioural analysis and agreed upon by the patient. Most therapists also use **intermediate goals** or 'targets', the attainment of which provides an important source of reinforcement for the patient.

Specific techniques

RELAXATION

Since the conditioned response in so many of the above states is one of anxiety, the patient must first be trained to produce the opposite response, relaxation. This is done initially well away from any anxiety-provoking stimulus. The patients are first taught to recognize the signs of tension in their body and how these can be altered by voluntary control. They are then taught a series of exercises by which they can learn to reduce physiological arousal, and they may also be given an audiotape of these exercises which they can use for regular home practice. The technique of relaxation must become sufficiently rehearsed so that it can be applied even in situations which have previously caused anxiety. There are a number of different methods of relaxation, such as **progressive muscle relaxation (PMR)**, in which the patient is taught a series of exercises during which muscle blocks are alternatively tensed then relaxed to achieve a relaxed state, or

autogenic relaxation, in which muscle tension is released without the muscle block first being tensed. Other variations include the speed at which training in relaxation progresses and the application of relaxation skills to stressful situations. It is generally accepted that learning to relax is a skill and includes cognitive aspects such as a sense of control over difficult situations. It is also worth noting that some patients find it very difficult to relax, or even find it anxiety-provoking because the feeling of 'letting go' of tension fuels their fear of 'being out of control'.

Breathing exercises are also important, especially for patients who hyperventilate, such as some who have panic attacks.

EXPOSURE

Many of the treatments used in cognitive-behaviour therapy require an **exposure** to the feared or conditioned stimuli. This is to allow the **habituation** of the emotional response conditioned to that set of stimuli. It is thought that exposure may also serve the function of **disproving** the expectations or beliefs held by the patient about specific situations and their consequences. There are a number of variations to exposure-based treatments which depend on the mode and speed of exposure (that is, whether exposure is carried out gradually or not and whether it is carried out in imagination or *in vivo*). In some circumstances, such as exposure to traumatic memories, as in the treatment of post-traumatic stress disorder (see p. 191), by the nature of the disorder exposure has to be imaginal. Similarly, in cognitive-based treatments irrational thoughts are challenged by the patient exposing themselves to situations which indicate that these thoughts are untrue or unrealistic. Some examples of exposure-based treatments are given below.

DESENSITIZATION

With the therapist's help, the patient constructs a hierarchy of anxiety-provoking stimuli. These stimuli are then presented to the patient, starting with the most innocuous. As each stimulus is mastered, the patient progresses to the next one. The stimuli may be presented in one of two ways:

Desensitization in imagination consists of the patient imagining anxiety-provoking scenes while in a relaxed state.

Graded exposure (or *in vivo* desensitization). This treatment consists of the patient having to encounter anxiety-provoking stimuli in real life, starting with those which provoke least anxiety. This procedure is favoured by most therapists since confrontation with stressors in real life is always the eventual goal of treatment, and it is more effective.

Here is an example of graded exposure:

> *Mrs X presented with a moderately severe fear of wasps. On occasion this resulted in her running away leaving her baby and pram unattended in the street. A twelve-step hierarchy of increasingly anxiety-provoking wasp-related stimuli was constructed and this determined*

a programme of graded exposure, starting with reading about and looking at pictures of wasps in books, and ending with killing a wasp trapped against a window. Initial exposure to each item took place in the clinic, the patient then being encouraged to complete similar assignments at home without the therapist. The duration of each exposure to an item was dependent on the rate of habituation of the anxiety response: exposure was discontinued when the patient described a significant reduction in anxiety. In practice this was rarely more than fifteen minutes per item. Usually more than one item was completed at the same appointment. After only five treatment sessions, the patient completed the hierarchy, and remained anxiety-free in the presence of wasps at a six-month follow-up point.

FLOODING

Whereas desensitization is a 'little-by-little' approach, flooding plunges in at the deep end. The patient is confronted with a situation at the top of her hierarchy (for example, shopping in a crowded department store, or travelling on a bus in the rush hour), and is required to remain in that situation until her anxiety has spontaneously dissipated ('habituation'). Although it is often difficult to persuade patients to undergo flooding, it is a rapid and a generally more effective treatment than desensitization.

Mrs Y had not ventured more than one quarter of a mile from her home and had completely avoided all shopping areas for more than a year, because of agoraphobic anxiety difficulties. The patient and therapist travelled by car into the city centre on a Saturday afternoon and spent two and a half hours in a crowded shopping mall. Initially the patient complained of extreme panic, the therapist both reassuring and prompting her to remain in spite of an intense desire to exit from the situation. These feelings began to subside after about thirty minutes, and by the end of the session the patient was euphoric. Two further sessions of the same took place, and these were characterized by even more rapid habituation of anxiety. Subsequently, Mrs Y was encouraged to travel alone to the same shopping centre, and this was accompanied by a generalization of the treatment effect to other public situations. After only three weeks from the commencement of treatment she was able to travel to and shop in local supermarkets and city centre departmental stores.

BIOFEEDBACK

Many visceral and neuromuscular activities of which we are normally unaware can be brought into consciousness by providing an auditory or visual 'feedback' signal (for example, a tone whose pitch varies with frontalis muscle tension). This technique is often used as an adjunct to relaxation training, but can also be used in the treatment of specific symptoms such as tension headache, or in the treatment of hypertension.

SOCIAL SKILLS TRAINING

Sophisticated social behaviour is largely acquired by learning. Many people cope poorly with social situations because they have never acquired a full repertoire of appropriate social responses. Social skills training is usually undertaken with groups of patients, and aims to provide explicit training of such social responses. Mock social situations are set up, and the patients practise by **role-playing**, after the therapist has provided a **model** of the appropriate behaviour ('modelling'). The patient's performance may be videotaped, so that particular problems can be discussed and corrected in debriefing sessions.

BELL AND PAD TRAINING

This is a behavioural treatment for nocturnal enuresis. A pad containing electrical contacts is placed under a sheet on the patient's bed. If the patient urinates in the bed a circuit is completed, setting off an alarm bell which wakes the patient. This is one of the most effective treatments for enuresis, although the underlying psychological processes remain obscure. Simple classical conditioning cannot provide a full explanation for the treatment's efficacy, because the alarm bell (CS) occurs after the unconditioned reflex of micturition. It seems likely that as a result of extensive practice the patient learns to become more aware of stimuli associated with bladder distension.

RESPONSE PREVENTION

This is used in the treatment of compulsive rituals. The patient feels compelled to perform some act such as washing hands but is firmly persuaded from doing so. This must be maintained for prolonged periods to be effective. It is best performed while the person is repeatedly faced with a situation in which the compulsion occurs, such as touching dirt. In this way it is similar to flooding – the patient is faced with intense anxiety which gradually wanes as it is not relieved by the habitual means of giving in to the compulsion.

> *Mr Z presented with an obsessional preoccupation with dog excrement. After returning home from walking in the street, he would be compelled to engage in a decontamination ritual beginning with scrubbing his shoes with disinfectant (these were not normally soiled to the objective observer). He would then take all his clothes off, and place them in the washing machine, then scrub his hands, and bath himself. The ritual took more than two hours to perform. Treatment involved the patient being encouraged to deliberately soil his shoes with dog excrement and return home, leaving his contaminated shoes on the door step. The therapist then spent an hour or more with the patient, preventing any cleaning ritual from occurring and distracting him with other activities. After two months of twice-weekly visits by the therapist the patient was able to venture out alone and return without performing the ritual, apart from washing his hands in a normal fashion.*

Cognitive-behavioural approaches to severe mental disorders

DEPRESSION

In depressive illnesses cognitive approaches can be used in conjunction with pharmacological treatment, and are especially useful in milder or long-standing depressive conditions where anti-depressant drugs are either ineffective or undesirable. They are based upon the observation that depressed patients often have erroneous and highly pessimistic beliefs about themselves, their circumstances, and their future (the 'negative triad').

Cognitive therapy aims to correct these gloomy thoughts, and at the same time to demonstrate to the patient that he is capable of surmounting problems which because of his pessimistic beliefs he would not normally deal with. Although the primary focus of this type of therapy is the patient's beliefs, it can be included with behaviour therapies because of the emphasis on practical goals, and because thoughts appear to be subject to the same laws of reinforcement as acts.

> *Mr A, who six months previously had failed to obtain an important job promotion, was diagnosed as suffering from a moderately severe depressive illness. He was preoccupied with thoughts of incompetence at work and in the home, worries that nobody liked him, and ideas of low self-esteem. He was asked to keep a diary in which he recorded recurrent negative thoughts and their underlying assumptions. Treatment sessions focused on reality-testing these assumptions. For example, one recurrent thought suggested that he had been passed over for promotion because he was incompetent in his current position.*

Underlying assumptions included:

1. *His manager paid particular attention to every error that he had made over the years, no matter how insignificant.*
2. *Because of (1), the manager believed Mr A to be the most incompetent person in the firm.*
3. *It was because of (2) that Mr A had not been promoted.*
4. *Mr A would not be promoted at any future date.*

As a result of treatment sessions and reality-testing assignments, the patient began to realize that most of these assumptions were incorrect. This led to adjustments in his attitude towards his work and his career, and after three months of treatment the depression was ameliorated.

SCHIZOPHRENIA

Besides the use of social skills training, which has long been a part of rehabilitation programmes for the severely mentally ill, recent cognitive-behavioural approaches to schizophrenia have shown great promise. These have taken two forms. First, based on a recognition that stress is frequently a precipitant of psychotic relapse, interventions have focused on helping the families, relatives, or carers of schizophrenic patients to cope better with stress, especially by modifying the manner in which they interact and deal with problems and difficulties within the home situation. These methods have been termed **family management** or **family intervention**. The other approach, which is becoming more prevalent, is the cognitive-behavioural treatment of positive symptoms of schizophrenia, such as delusions and hallucinations. In cases in which medication is failing to improve residual symptoms further, or when the patient does not comply with medication, or there are reasons why medication is contraindicated, these methods have proved useful.

Indications for cognitive-behaviour therapy

It can be seen that behavioural treatments are helpful in a very wide range of psychological disorders: in **affective disorders** like anxiety, phobias, post-traumatic stress disorders, or depression; in **maladaptive behaviours** such as obsessional states and sexual problems; in **abnormal illness behaviours**; in **deficient social skills** and **nocturnal enuresis**; and as an adjunct treatment in the **severe mental illnesses**.

PSYCHOTHERAPY

The doctor–patient relationship is one in which the patient places great trust in the doctor. The patient discusses personal problems which he would otherwise keep private, and he may be prepared to comply with whatever treatment and advice the doctor prescribes. Some knowledge of how this relationship operates is essential to being a good doctor. However, it is important to realize that this relationship can be used in a therapeutic way. This is formalized in psychotherapy, in which the doctor aims to help the patient by recognizing his needs and helping him with them through the medium of the therapeutic relationship.

Types of psychotherapy

Psychotherapy may be divided according to the type of recipient: thus **individual, marital, family, and group psychotherapy**; or it may be divided according to the kind of technique used. We will now consider first, the kinds of psychotherapeutic techniques that should be possessed by every doctor; and second, techniques which are used by those with greater experience.

Ingredients of psychotherapy relevant to general medical practice

There are many different forms of psychotherapy, but even in a crowded general practitioner's surgery or a busy out-patient clinic there are a number of techniques that a doctor will find helpful. Taken together they are sometimes described as '**supportive psychotherapy**'.

ACTIVE LISTENING

Students are often surprised to find that taking a full history in the psychiatric out-patient clinic leads to the patient saying that he feels much better! The patient will probably have never before had such an opportunity to review all aspects of his life and to express emotions associated with events in his life. In addition the student's intense interest in what the patient is saying demonstrates a concern which the patient appreciates.

Active listening is an important part of the therapeutic process. There is no need for such listening to be a time-consuming business – in fact it can save time. The patient with a sexual problem, for example, can spend many fruitless consultations with the doctor who is not skilled in gaining her confidence and listening for clues as to the nature of the underlying worry.

VENTILATION OF FEELINGS

Allowing expression of feeling is an important aspect of the therapeutic relationship. It is especially useful to be able to express anger, frustration, or grief that has previously been suppressed. This is particularly important following bereavement or where the doctor has just had to give 'bad news'. For example, after the birth of a child who unexpectedly has a severe deformity the parents will often feel numb, and they will not be able to take in important factual information until after they have had a chance to express their feelings of shock, bewilderment, anger, and loss.

REASSURANCE

The patient who correctly suspects that he has cancer may ask the doctor about the diagnosis. He may well be asking for reassurance rather than for information. Even if there is nothing in the prognosis about which the doctor can reassure, listening carefully to the patient may help to understand his particular fears, such as unrelieved pain, incontinence, or the effect on his relatives. On these matters the doctor can reassure and in doing so relieve some of the patient's suffering.

It is important to realize that a properly conducted **physical examination** may be a vital ingredient in the ability to provide reassurance, and that the doctor's own behaviour during a physical examination can serve either to increase or to decrease the patient's anxiety.

A doctor frequently has to reassure a patient (especially an anxious one) that he does not have a serious disease. In spite of these efforts, attempts at reassurance may fail and the patient may seek further tests elsewhere. This is because the doctor has either not fully understood the patient's underlying worries or not explained adequately the cause of the symptoms.

EXPLANATION

The patient who fears that his headaches indicate an underlying brain tumour is less reassured by the doctor's statement '*All the tests show that nothing is wrong*' than by:

> *Your headaches are due to the muscles of your scalp tightening; this is why they also affect the back of your neck and occur when you get tense.*

Thus an explanation by the doctor can be very therapeutic, although it uses neither technological investigations nor drugs.

You may observe a patient in the out-patient clinic look greatly relieved by the consultant's authoritative statement that the patient's illness is recognized and appropriate treatment can be prescribed. The 'explanation' may just be a name for a disease whose aetiology is not understood; the 'treatment' something that is known to work, although no one is quite sure why. Yet until this time the patient has been perplexed as to what has been happening to him, and the *doctor's explanation is reassuring*.

ADVICE/GUIDANCE

Patients often turn to the doctor for advice. This may be on matters about which the doctor can be precise (such as giving up smoking, or stopping benzodiazepines), or related to problems such as leaving a job, or getting a divorce. The doctor must avoid telling people what they should do, although it is legitimate to tell them what effect a particular change might be expected to have upon their health.

Thus the doctor might advise that if the patient took time off from caring for a sick parent it would help in the treatment of the patient's own depressive illness: but whether the patient does so or not must be their own choice.

SPECIAL INTERVIEW TECHNIQUES

1. Instead of asking questions, use statements to encourage the patient to talk.
2. Be prepared to try to understand what the patient is feeling (using empathy) and then to make intelligent guesses to prompt further discussion.
3. Allow the patient to show their emotions to you, whether they be crying, anger, or distress. You can respond with a supportive comment, such as 'I can see you've been through a difficult time'; but remember that silence can also be supportive.
4. The doctor is not always right. Give the patient the chance to correct you.
5. Don't reassure too soon.

It is easier to get an idea of such techniques by looking at what might actually be said during a consultation. They are often used in an attempt to explore predisposing psychological causes which may be linked to current problems of the patient's problems, and are then described as **insight-orientated psychotherapy**. We will return to Mrs Woods, and first see how a doctor who has no knowledge of psychotherapeutic techniques might interview her, using a traditional 'question-and-answer' format:

Doctor	Mrs Woods
What is the matter?	*Nothing.*
Then why are you looking so depressed?	*Wouldn't you if your mother had just died?* (awkward silence)
Have you been taking the anti-depressant tablets?	*Yes.*
Is your sleeping improving?	*A bit.*

Doctor	Mrs Woods
Why aren't you talking much?	*Nobody understands how I feel.* (eyes fill with tears)
I do, it's normal to feel like this after a death; don't distress yourself.	

A more experienced doctor might say:

Doctor	Mrs Woods
You look very down, Mrs Woods.	*Yes.*
You look near to tears.	*I can't cry, they won't let me.*
They?	*My relatives. They say how well I've taken it, I don't want to let them see me cry.*
Perhaps your husband doesn't like you crying. (silence)	*It's not my husband, it's my sister.* *She was always mother's favourite and it upsets her too much to see me cry, it's always been my job to comfort her.*
You sound cross about that.	*Well, wouldn't you be? All those years I did far more for my mother than my sister – but my mum thanked her, never me.* (bursts into tears)
Yet you always felt that you had to do more for her.	

Distress is bound to follow a bereavement, but the doctor's comments in the second extract have led to a much fuller understanding of the patient's distress. It is this understanding, combined with familiarity with the normal grief reaction, that puts the doctor in a position to help Mrs Woods. It has become clear that she cannot cry in front of her sister, and her guilt is perhaps becoming easier to understand.

Formal exploratory psychotherapy

This type of psychotherapy is more intensive and is usually given by those who have received some special training. It aims to help the person modify long-standing aspects of their feelings and behaviour, often by modifying defence mechanisms. It is more formal in the sense that the doctor spends a specified time with the patient each week, the therapy may last for some time, and in the longer forms of treatment there is much greater emphasis on analysis of the doctor–patient relationship.

TECHNIQUES USED

Getting the patient to express their most intimate feelings and to react spontaneously within the therapy requires:

1. Careful selection of suitable patients.
2. A fixed time each week for the therapeutic session which is held in a quiet and private office where interruptions are prevented.
3. A trusting relationship in which the doctor facilitates the patient's spontaneous expression of emotion and yet makes the patient feel that it is safe for this to occur.
4. Treatment taking place in the framework of a **therapeutic contract** which makes clear to the patient how much treatment is being offered, and what should be achieved during these sessions. The doctor must be very careful not to break their side of the contract, so that if the patient breaks their side the doctor can interpret this behaviour.

INDICATIONS

This type of psychotherapy may be used as an adjunct to other treatments in anxiety disorders, depressive illness, and anorexia nervosa. It is occasionally used alone in any of these conditions and in the management of maladaptive behaviours such as self-poisoning and bulimia. Patients are selected who are well motivated to engage in this form of treatment and who can understand it. They must be able and willing to make some important changes in their lives.

Almost invariably patients who will benefit from exploratory psychotherapy will describe difficulty in relationships and problems of self-esteem even when other psychiatric disorders are present.

CONTRAINDICATIONS

This treatment is generally not recommended for patients who:

1. Are psychotic.
2. Show marked paranoid traits.
3. Are seriously dependent on drugs or alcohol.
4. Are unable to tolerate personal discomfort.
5. Are involved with an impossible life situation which cannot be expected to change.
6. Have an anti-social personality.

HAZARDS

The principal hazard is **excessive dependency**, so that the patient relies so completely on the doctor that he needs to consult him on every aspect of his life, and termination of treatment is impossible. This should be avoided by careful selection of patients for this form of treatment, by not allowing treatment to be prolonged unnecessarily, and by recognizing the early signs of dependency and dealing with them appropriately.

CONTENT OF TREATMENT SESSIONS

Psychotherapy often starts with the patient asking *'What do I talk about?'* There is usually a presenting problem to initiate the discussion but the doctor is deliberately non-directive. This is partly to ensure that the patient does the work of exploring his own feelings and partly so that the patient, not the doctor, leads the discussion.

It is assumed at the outset that the doctor and patient can together make sense of the patient's symptoms and life situation. This requires a theoretical model around which the material brought up during psychotherapy may be arranged. Any such model must enable the doctor to identify key problems, provide explanations for the present problems, and prescribe a means of change.

A case treated by formal exploratory psychotherapy will now be used to illustrate several general principles:

THE PROBLEM

A forty-year-old man presented to the neurologist with a marked tremor at times of stress. This had been present for twenty years, but was becoming more of a problem as the patient was promoted at work. Previous treatment with propranolol and tranquillizers had been ineffective and he increasingly used alcohol to suppress the tremor.

INDICATIONS FOR PSYCHOTHERAPY

He was treated with psychotherapy in view of the failure to respond to other treatments, and the evidence that the tremor was related to interpersonal conflicts. The patient also showed considerable determination to find a psychological cause for his tremor.

THE CONTRACT

It was agreed that the patient would attend six sessions of forty minutes each and progress would then be reviewed. During these sessions the patient's emotions would be explored to try and understand why the patient reacted to particular situations.

THE TREATMENT

When tackled directly no progress was made: the patient simply went over his habitual thoughts on the matter – saying that his marriage was happy, his friendships normal, and others become nervous in front of a crowd; it was inexplicable that his anxiety was so marked.

Once the patient began to trust the doctor, however, it became appropriate to point out that the patient repeated this description as though he was trying to hide his true feelings ('denial'). It eventually transpired that he felt a failure in his own eyes and that he felt he had let his parents down. This emotional arousal was accompanied by tears. Rather than trying to ignore these, he was encouraged to dwell on the feeling of failure. This sense of failure was profound and extended to another problem which had only been hinted at previously, namely premature ejaculation.

The doctor suggested that the patient normally kept such feelings well hidden, which meant that the patient lived in terror of being exposed. But the true fear of exposure did not become apparent until later, when, with great anxiety, he admitted to **dreams** of a homosexual nature. He felt enormous relief that his bisexual feelings could be accepted by the doctor as a normal part of his personality.

The whole set of problems then began to make sense. The tremor had begun soon after he had left a boys' boarding school (where homosexual activity had been common) and at a time when he was beginning to experience a sense of rejection in his heterosexual relationships. His aspirations to be a great success both socially and in his career were proving unrealistic, and those situations where he felt he was under scrutiny were the ones in which he developed anxiety.

He then felt able, for the first time, to tackle the sexual problem which had previously seemed insuperable. The anxiety symptoms did not at this stage disappear but he also felt able to tackle these, and a course of behavioural therapy utilizing relaxation and desensitization was successful.

PARTICULAR TECHNIQUES USED DURING PSYCHOTHERAPY ARE ILLUSTRATED IN THE ABOVE CASE HISTORY

Analysis of the **patient's reaction to the doctor**: the patient habitually promoted a self-confident image. When the doctor persistently suggested that this facade hid anxiety and doubt the patient became annoyed. It was analysis of this annoyance that led to exposure of the feelings of failure.

The **emotional arousal** that occurs during treatment may lead to the patient expressing strong feelings (love or hate) towards the doctor. The origin of such feelings may be in the patient's past experience and this can be pointed out. It emerged that sitting with the doctor aroused feelings of being with his father; this elicited feelings of dislike and frustration that were initially directed to the doctor.

Such **linking of the present with the past** is often helpful in psychotherapy but is most efficacious if the present is actually within the psychotherapy treatment session.

The **doctor's reaction to the patient**: in the above case the doctor felt irritated that the patient repeatedly asserted that he was really no different from anyone else. He noted that the patient was using denial too forcefully and this prevented the treatment progressing. The patient initially refuted the doctor's suggestion that he was using denial, but later said that if he had allowed himself fully to accept the need for treatment he would have crumbled into a nervous wreck.

Interpretation of dreams: this technique is simply a way of gaining access to unconscious material which is usually blocked by defence mechanisms. In the above example there had been little or no hint of the patient's homosexual feelings – he was so ashamed they had been well hidden – and it cost the patient an enormous effort to describe them to the doctor. Yet having described the dreams the patient felt enormous relief. The fact that the doctor could accept these as part of the patient's make-up without expressing the revulsion that the patient himself felt was the starting point of improvement.

Note also that in this case it was possible to move from an **initial exploratory phase** on to a more **task-orientated stage** whilst maintaining the patient's cooperation in treatment.

Group therapy

Some patients benefit from discussing their problems in a group. Groups are especially appropriate for those who have difficulty relating to other people, or for people sharing a common problem. Large numbers of specialized groups exist for helping patients with particular problems: for example, groups exist for patients who have had operations such as mastectomy or colostomy, for recovered alcoholics, and for those who have recently been bereaved. Support comes from the knowledge that others are experiencing similar problems, and learning ways of coping from other group members.

Family therapy

Working directly with a family or a couple can be particularly helpful when relationships within the family are maintaining or perhaps even causing a psychiatric disorder. For example, the family can play a significant role in anorexia nervosa especially when the patient is still adolescent, and the parents have used eating as a way of exerting control within the family. The eating problem then draws attention to the conflicts about control and the particular ways in which a particular family might express them.

PLANNING TREATMENT

Treatment should follow logically from the specific aetiology of the illness as well as from the diagnosis. A plan of treatment should be drawn up and recorded for each patient, and an outline of factors to be considered is shown in *Table 7.5* (see p. 116).

In addition to the usual categories of physical, psychological, and social aspects of treatment, it is important to consider the order in which they are appropriate. This can be divided for convenience into the earlier stages, which are concerned with arrangements for treatment, symptomatic relief, and the treatment of the underlying causes; and the later stages which include rehabilitation, prophylaxis, and arrangements for after-care.

Table 7.5 *The treatment plan*

acute illness

1. *Where will treatment take place and who will provide it?*
   Consider the extent to which supervision and physical care are required:
   Psychiatric unit as in-patient, day-patient, out-patient; or domiciliary care; general practitioner; social services; clinical psychologist.

2. *What should be done if the patient refuses treatment?*
   Is compulsory admission clinically necessary and legally justifiable? What is the risk to the patient or to others?

3. *Is urgent intervention required to relieve distressing or life-threatening symptoms?*
   For example, change of environment by hospital admission; sedation.

4. *Treatment aimed at relieving mental illness or its symptoms*

   Physical: neuroleptics, minor tranquillizers, anti-depressants, hypnotics, electroplexy.

   Psychological: psychotherapy – insight, supportive, individual or group; behaviour therapy – desensitization, flooding, response prevention, operant conditioning.

   Social: environmental manipulation, marital or family therapy or support; use of social agencies or legal advice.

   Occupational: diversionary, creative, expressive; maintenance of or training in skills or social behaviour.

5. *Treatment of associated physical disorders*
   Specific treatments for organic brain syndromes, e.g. thyroxin, vitamins, antibiotics. Correction of fluid and electrolyte balance, vitamin depletion due to malnutrition, treatment of intercurrent infection.

6. *The correction of handicaps*
   Vision, hearing, speech.

chronic illness

1. *Rehabilitation and resettlement*
   To what extent does the patient need help with accommodation, work, social interactions which may affect the long-term outcome?
   For example: psychiatric after-care or other hostel; referral to Disablement Resettlement Officer, occupational retraining, or sheltered work shop; domiciliary social services such as home help, family-aid, meals-on-wheels; community services such as luncheon club.

2. *Other prophylactic measures for those vulnerable to relapse*
   Physical: long-term depot phenothiazines, tricyclic anti-depressants, lithium.
   Psychological: supervision, support, social casework.

3. *Liaison between psychiatrist, general practitioner, community psychiatric nurse, psychiatric social worker*
   What information do they need? Who will prescribe?

FURTHER READING

Ashton, H. (1992) *Brain Function and Psychotropic Drugs*. Oxford: Oxford University Press.

Bloch, S. (1986) *An Introduction to the Psychotherapies*. 2nd edition. Oxford: Oxford University Press.

Cooper, J.R., Bloom, F.E. and Roth, R.H. (1991) *The Biochemical Basis of Neuropharmacology*. 6th edition. Oxford: Oxford University Press.

Corney, R. (ed.) (1991) *Developing Communication and Counselling Skills in Medicine*. London: Routledge.

Stern, R. and Drummond, L. (1991) *The Practice of Behavioural and Cognitive Psychotherapy*. Cambridge: Cambridge University Press.

Strange, P.G. (1992) *Brain Biochemistry and Brain Disorders*. Oxford: Oxford University Press.

8 / PROGNOSIS

The outlook for a psychiatric illness depends partly on the particular condition under consideration, but partly on factors that cut across diagnoses and will be considered in this short chapter. If you are trying to predict the future course of a particular patient's illness, read the section on prognosis in the appropriate section and then take the following factors into account as well.

GENETIC FACTORS

A patient with a strong family history of an illness known to be partly determined by genetic factors – such as schizophrenia or manic-depressive illness – can be expected to have a worse outlook than one with a slight or no family history. However, do not put much reliance on this factor, because there are exceptions in each direction: those with a strong family history can have a good prognosis, and vice versa.

EARLY CHILDHOOD FACTORS

Severe deprivation in early childhood often leaves scars for the rest of a lifetime. If your patient will need to settle down in some stable relationship in order to improve, ask yourself what experience life has so far offered your patient of such relationships. A person who has been bereaved in early childhood will always carry a greater vulnerability to losses in later life.

PRE-MORBID PERSONALITY

Don't forget that personality characteristics are by definition relatively constant, so you must not expect your patient to improve much in these respects. For example, a person who has always had depressive traits in their personality is unlikely suddenly to cheer up in middle age: in real life, Scrooge would have been found to have had a manic illness or a temporal lobe lesion!

Similarly, the damage done to dissocial personalities has been inflicted in childhood, and cannot be undone. If your patient is aged over thirty, the best level of their pre-morbid adjustment indicates the probable limits of what can be expected of them in the future.

MATURITY AND IMMATURITY

If your patient is under thirty, ask yourself to what extent they can still be expected to mature. Emotionally healthy people in our society, who have not experienced deprivation and upheaval in childhood, can be expected to have completed the greater part of maturation before the age of twenty: in developing countries, it is much earlier than that.

However, those who have had disrupted childhoods and who have had no good parental role-models may take much longer to grow up. Thus a young woman from a miserable home, who has endured divorce of her parents and has been poorly parented, may present in her twenties with episodes of wrist-cutting and self-poisoning. With sympathetic and patient handling such patients may settle down in life later on, so that the demands they have made on medical services during the time of their repeated episodes of self-injury appear, in retrospect, to have been a phase in growing up.

Try to assess your young patient's maturity by asking yourself these questions about them:

1. How physically mature do they look?
2. Are they emotionally independent of their parents yet?
3. Are they financially independent of their parents and, if they are, are they earning their own living?
4. Have they succeeded in having a lasting sexual relationship with another adult?

To the extent that your patient is still immature, there is scope for further improvement. With help, maybe they can learn to adapt more successfully.

LEVEL OF PRE-MORBID ACHIEVEMENT

Ask yourself what your patient has been able to achieve in their life before they became ill. Those who have achieved much – emotionally and occupationally – have a much sounder basis to build on after an episode of psychotic illness or head injury. Try to identify any ways in which your patient was disadvantaged **before** he became ill: these are his **pre-morbid handicaps**, and it may be very important to help him with them during rehabilitation. But to the extent that they may be severe and irremediable, the prognosis is poor.

PREVIOUS PSYCHIATRIC HISTORY

This is critically important. As any actuary can tell you, if you want to know about the future, look at the past. One saying has it that in psychiatry 'the diagnosis is from the mental state, but the prognosis is from the history'.

If your patient has never been ill before, there is a much better chance that he will recover completely. If a patient tells you that they have been depressed off and on for the past twenty years, the chances are that they will continue to have episodes of depression in the future.

PRECIPITATING FACTORS

To what extent can your patient's illness be understood as a reaction to a stressful environment? To the extent that it can, and provided that the patient has a good record of pre-morbid adjustment, the future is likely to be good.

CURRENT LIFE ADJUSTMENT

What sort of social environment has your patient got to go back to in the community? Has the patient someone in whom they can confide, and how much support does this confidant provide at times of crisis? What are the living conditions like? And is there financial hardship?

These factors seem especially important in determining the course of non-psychotic affective illness.

MODE OF ONSET

How did the illness begin? Generally speaking, psychological illnesses that begin suddenly have a much better outlook than those with a gradual onset. The best combination is to have a severe stress followed by an illness with an acute illness, while the worst is to have an unprovoked illness of insidious onset.

LENGTH OF PRESENT ILLNESS

Once more, on actuarial considerations: the longer, the worse.

COMPLIANCE WITH TREATMENT

Is the patient likely to comply with treatment? Some people with eccentric personalities, and many of those with dissocial personalities, are less likely to accept any treatment which requires prolonged cooperation.

If they have had previous episodes of illness, to what extent have they complied with treatment in the past?

THE NATURE OF THE DISORDER ITSELF

Generally speaking, the majority of patients with psychiatric illnesses will recover, and a substantial proportion may never have another episode of illness. Even major psychoses like schizophrenia and psychotic depression can have wide variability in their course, with some patients getting completely well, some having only a partial recovery, some having a fluctuating course, and others having a progressive course.

Remember that disorders like manic-depressive psychosis are known to be remittent so that although you can assure your patient that they will get well, they are actually very likely to have further episodes of illness.

Other disorders – like Alzheimer's disease and Huntington's chorea – are progressive and incurable: details will be found in the appropriate sections.

When considering an individual patient's prognosis, avoid such uninformative terms as 'guarded'. Weigh up the different factors which suggest a good or bad outcome for that particular patient. Remember that the expected outcome may vary according to which aspects of the case we are considering: for example, we might predict:

Complete recovery from florid symptoms, but will probably fail to return to work and there is a high probability of further episodes.

9 / FORMULATION

THE PURPOSE OF THE FORMULATION

The formulation is the method used to integrate all the clinical data that are required in order to treat the patient and evaluate the outcome: *it is not a case summary*. It follows a logical sequence which we have dealt with in turn in the preceding chapters. The purpose of this chapter is to show how these are integrated, and why.

No doubt you will by now be in the habit of making and using diagnoses and may wonder why that isn't good enough for psychiatry, but we have already noted in Chapter 4 that diagnoses have important limitations. A diagnosis involves a *nomothetic* (literally 'law-giving') process. This means that all cases included within the identified category have one or more properties in common. For example, all those with a diagnosis of pulmonary tuberculosis will have an infectious disease of the lungs caused by the tubercle bacillus. Whilst this is useful information it is quite inadequate as a basis for management. It tells us little about the clinical state, which might range from a chance radiological finding in an apparently healthy person to a fulminating pneumonia, and it certainly won't help us to decide which are the appropriate drugs to use.

By contrast the formulation is an *idiographic* process (literally 'picture of the individual'). This means that it includes the unique characteristics of each patient's case which are needed for the process of management. So, while nomothetic processes are the only way we can advance knowledge about *diseases*, we use idiographic methods to understand and study the *individual*.

To pursue the example of pulmonary tuberculosis, the additional information that is taken into account might include the subject's previous state of immunity, nutrition, and the state of health of those with whom he lives. It would also take into account the varieties of clinical presentation, sensitivities of the tubercle bacillus, the extent to which he is likely to be compliant with medication, and the risk of relapse through cross-infection.

THE FORMAT OF THE FORMULATION

Demographic data

Begin with the name, age, occupation, and marital status.

Descriptive formulation

Describe the nature of onset, for example acute or insidious; the total duration of the present illness; and the course, for example cyclic or deteriorating. Then list the main phenomena (that is, symptoms and signs) that characterize the disorder. As you become more experienced you should try to be selective by featuring the phenomena that are most important, either because of their greater diagnostic specificity or because of their predominance in severity or duration. *Avoid long lists* of minor or transient symptoms and negative findings. These basic data are chiefly derived from the history of the present illness, the mental state, and physical examinations, and are used to determine the syndrome diagnosis in the next section. Note that this is not usually the place to bring in other aspects of the history: that comes later. If we know the diagnosis of a previous episode of mental illness, this should also be taken into account, but remember, the present disorder may not be connected and the diagnosis may be different.

Now let's return to Mrs Woods for an example. We have already seen most of the history and examination findings in earlier chapters, but this is how it would be used in the formulation.

FORMULATION 1

> *Mrs Woods is a forty-five-year-old married housewife. Three weeks ago, following the death of her mother, she experienced an acute onset of an illness characterized by depressed mood, anhedonia, poor sleep and early morning waking, poor appetite and weight loss, poor libido and constipation. She has had intermittent left chest pain. On examination she shows mild retardation of movement and speech, weeps frequently, and appears depressed. Her thought content is focused on the death of her mother and she has the delusion that she is responsible for her mother's death. Physical examination reveals recent and older bruising.*

Differential diagnosis

List in order of probability all diagnoses that should be considered and include any disorders that you will wish to investigate. These will usually be syndrome diagnoses based on the descriptive formulation above. Give the evidence for and against each diagnosis that you consider. Include any current physical illness which may account for some or all of the phenomena. A common error is to include, for example, thyroid function studies in the investigations without including thyroid disease in the differential diagnosis. If you think a condition is worth investigating then you are obviously including it in your differential diagnosis; if it's not worth mentioning don't bother to investigate it.

Remember that in addition to the primary diagnosis you may need to consider a supplementary diagnosis, for example alcoholism in a patient presenting with delirium, or a personality disorder in a patient with an anxiety state. Regarding Mrs Woods:

1. *Depressive illness: morbid grief reaction* (preferred diagnosis). *The symptoms and signs are essentially those of a depressive illness, with depressed mood, depressive thought content, and neuro-vegetative features. This has developed in the setting of bereavement and the content of abnormal beliefs and perceptions is limited to the bereavement.*

2. *Manic-depressive disorder: in view of the psychotic symptoms it is necessary to consider the possibility that this is a depressive episode in a bipolar affective disorder. However, there is no evidence of manic episodes in the past.*

3. *Angina pectoris: the distribution of chest pain is more characteristic of anxiety than of myocardial insufficiency, but this possibility will have to be investigated before it can be excluded.*

Aetiology

The various factors that have contributed should be evident mainly from the family and personal histories, the history of previous illness, and the pre-morbid personality. Remember you should aim to answer these questions: why has this particular patient developed this particular illness at this particular time? If necessary look back to *Table 5.1* for the systematic method used to identify the relevant factors. We have already considered the aetiology of Mrs Woods' case in some detail (p. 67) but this is how it might be presented in the formulation:

Predisposing factors include a family history of depressive illness in her mother, the death of her father during her childhood, and marked pre-morbid obsessional and dependent traits. The illness has been precipitated by the illness and subsequent death of her mother and her inability to face the ambivalent nature of that relationship.

Investigations

List all investigations that are required to support your preferred diagnosis and to rule out the alternatives and also any that you think are required to improve your understanding of the aetiology. Give reasons for investigations if they are not self-evident. Include all sources of additional information. Have another look at *Table 6.1* to remind yourself about how to plan investigations systematically.

Investigations should include contacting her general practitioner to find out more about her past history of mental illness and review of her mother's hospital records. She also requires physical examination, chest X-ray, and an ECG. It will be important to observe her mood state through the day, sleep, and appetite, and to keep a weight chart. Insight-orientated psychotherapy may help to determine the aspects of her bereavement that have determined morbid grief.

Treatment

Outline the treatment plan that you wish to follow. This should stem logically from your discussion of the aetiology as well as from the diagnosis. Consider each stage of management in turn as described in Chapter 7, starting with the preliminary arrangements and finishing with the possible need for prophylaxis.

> *Treatment: It is preferable initially to provide treatment on an in-patient basis in view of the severity of Mrs Woods' depression and self-neglect and this should be on a voluntary basis. If the physical investigations confirm that there is no evidence of cardiac disease she should be told of this and the ways in which psychological factors can give rise to chest symptoms should be explained. If the depressive symptoms persist in hospital following a few days' observation she should then be started on a tricyclic* **anti-depressant drug** *with sedating properties, e.g. Amitriptyline, increasing to a full dose of 150 mg at night after a few days. If no improvement occurs within two to three weeks it may then be necessary to consider* **ECT**. *She should be encouraged to attend occupational therapy in order to maintain social and occupational skills.* **Psychotherapy** *should initially be supportive and, although some insights may be obtained, it should not be interpretive – at least until her depressive symptoms are much improved. It is too early to predict how much help she will need to adjust to her mother's death in the longer term.*

Prognosis

Describe the expected outcome of management of this illness episode, with regard to both the symptoms and also subsequent function, e.g. self-care and return to the community. Consider the risk of subsequent relapse. Give your reasons for these predictions based on the principles described in Chapter 8.

> *Prognosis: Mrs Woods is likely to make a complete recovery from her present illness because it is an affective disorder (and these generally result in recovery); it had an acute onset and a specific precipitant; and she has a supportive husband and no material hardship. The prominence of neuro-vegetative symptoms suggests a good response to tricyclic anti-depressant drugs. However, she is likely to have some continuing difficulty in adjusting to her mother's death. She is constitutionally predisposed to suffer from depressive illness and is likely to suffer further episodes in the future, particularly when she experiences bereavement or other loss.*

HOW TO USE THE FORMULATION

Aim to write up formulations for each patient you clerk during the psychiatric attachment and discuss them with the medical staff. The formulation should be written up as soon as you have clerked the patient and written up the record of the history and mental state examination. Of course you will probably want to modify your formulation later on when you have additional information.

The formulation is not an alternative to the history and mental state examination. In many departments you will be expected to present the history and mental state followed by the formulation, but this will depend on local practices.

We have referred in earlier chapters to the hypotheses that are an intrinsic part of the clinical approach, and this requires explanation. In the formulation the clinical data are used to set up hypotheses concerning the diagnosis and aetiology of the case. The investigations, and even more important the response of the illness to the treatment, provide the method for testing them. By observing the outcome of investigations and management we are able to discover whether our initial hypotheses were correct, but we can only do so if we recorded them in the formulation.

If our hypotheses are not supported, for example the patient has failed to improve with the planned treatment, then we have to review the accuracy of the original data. This will require reappraisal of the history and mental state and possibly further investigations.

Now we are going to look at two further formulations which illustrate this process, based on two very different clinical problems. They should help you to start to integrate what you have learnt from the previous chapters in this section of the book and give you an idea of what to aim at when you are writing up your own formulations. They also illustrate points about the assessment and management of several different disorders which are described in the following chapters.

FORMULATION 2: PSYCHOSIS

Demographic data

Mr Alan Reeves is a twenty-four-year-old unmarried graduate who is unemployed.

Descriptive formulation

He was admitted as an emergency one week ago after being taken to the casualty department by his flat-mates. He had shown increasingly disturbed behaviour in the last three months, with persecutory delusions of being followed by the CIA, and believed that they were using laser beams to control his actions. He had heard voices discussing plans to kill him, and on the day of admission had destroyed most of his possessions whilst apparently searching for a video-camera which he thought had been 'planted' in his room. He had started to become withdrawn socially four years previously, in his final year at university, and despite graduating had not worked since. He had cared for himself adequately but showed little motivation or interest except for playing the guitar and taking a variety of non-opiate drugs, including cannabis and amphetamines, regularly since then.

On mental state examination he appeared fully conscious, his clothes were dishevelled, he was suspicious in manner, and he paced the room. There was no spontaneous speech and he appeared secretive when answering questions, but talk was coherent and relevant. His mood was subjectively 'all right' but he appeared tense and frightened and sweated profusely. He was secretive about the recent destruction of his possessions. During the interview he appeared to be distracted, listening and talking to voices on several occasions, but denied this when asked. He was correctly orientated in time and place. He would not cooperate with formal tests of cognitive function but correctly identified and had learnt the names of the ward staff and gave an accurate account of a recent visit from his parents. He thought he was not ill but needed help – 'probably police protection' – and was willing to remain in hospital because he said he felt safer.

On physical examination he was thin, with evidence of self-neglect, but no other abnormality.

Differential diagnosis

1. **Paranoid schizophrenia.** This is characterized by the persistent delusions of persecution, control, and auditory hallucinations discussing the patient. The history prior to this suggests the insidious development of 'negative' symptoms, with apathy, lack of volition, marked social deterioration, and gradual development of hallucinations. There is no evidence at present of clouding of consciousness, cognitive impairment, or persistent mood disorder. Drug abuse may be secondary to schizophrenia.

2. **Psychotic disorder due to drug abuse (symptomatic schizophrenia).** The symptoms that have occurred in the last three months are consistent with the acute psychoses which are associated with both amphetamines and cannabis, particularly following heavy or prolonged abuse. The chronic social deterioration during the preceding four years may be due to the 'amotivational syndrome' which is associated with chronic ingestion of cannabis. These states commonly occur in clear consciousness. The possibility of other drug and alcohol effects must also be considered despite the patient's denial of abuse.

3. **Psychosis secondary to other organic conditions.** Many other intracranial or systemic disorders (e.g. cerebral tumours, endocrine disorders) can present with a paranoid psychosis but the absence of physical abnormalities on examination together with the long duration make this less likely. Some evidence of clouding of consciousness or intellectual impairment would be likely and these have not yet been excluded, due to the patient's limited cooperation.

4. **Drug abuse with psychological dependence.** This is an additional rather than differential diagnosis, which does not in itself account for the psychotic features. It is based on evidence of the prolonged use of, and strong desire to continue taking, cannabis and amphetamines; the neglect of other activities; and continuation of the habit despite evidence of harm.

Aetiology

Predisposing. There is a non-specific family history of a maternal uncle who is said to have lived for many years in a mental hospital, and one of his brothers has shown social deterioration similar to the patient's, so there may be a genetic predisposition to schizo-phrenia. There is no evidence of perinatal or developmental problems, or of personality problems before the last four years.

Precipitating. The social withdrawal and deterioration started in his final year at university when he had the stress of impending Final Examinations and the disappoint-ment of a broken engagement (although the latter may have been secondary to his disorder). The more recent deterioration followed within weeks of the arrival of a new flat-mate who wanted the patient to move out.

Maintaining. Contributory factors are likely to be drug abuse, increasing social isolation, and failure to receive treatment.

Investigations

1. **Medical records** of the uncle and brother.

2. **Further history** from his parents, particularly concerning his family history, child-hood development, and pre-morbid personality, and from his flat-mates about his recent state.

3. **Psychological**. Observations on the ward of his beliefs, perceptions, and behaviour – including possible drug or alcohol ingestion. Examination of cognitive aspects of the mental state and, if performance is impaired, psychometric testing for an organic disorder. Later, it will be necessary to assess his insight into psychosis and drug abuse and his likely compliance with their management.

4. **Physical investigations** should include haematology, electrolytes, and liver function tests in view of self-neglect and possible effects of drugs and alcohol; urine drug and alcohol screen. If there is evidence in his mental state of a possible organic disorder then electroencephalogram and computerized axial brain scan.

5. **Social**. Observation of the extent of his social withdrawal on the ward and of relationships with his family and flat-mates when visiting – consider whether there is evidence of 'high expressed emotion'. When his mental state improves, assess his abilities and strengths in occupational therapy and other settings in order to plan aspects of rehabilitation, including self-care, occupation, and recreation.

Treatment

Initially he should receive in-patient care, in view of his self-neglect and destructive behaviour. This should be as a voluntary patient as he was willing to be admitted and accept treatment.

Physical. It is best to observe him for one to two weeks without medication to see if the psychosis starts to resolve spontaneously when he is drug free, although a neuroleptic such as chlorpromazine or haloperidol may be given if he is otherwise difficult to supervise on the ward, for symptomatic control. If there is no obvious improvement then he should be started on regular doses of an oral neuroleptic, the dose of which will have to be adjusted depending on response and possible unwanted effects. In view of chronicity, it is very likely that subsequently he will require long-term neuroleptics, preferably with depot injections to improve compliance. He will need counselling regarding the effects of drug abuse and encouragement to remain abstinent.

Psychological and social. Initially he should be allowed to avoid the pressures of involvement in group activities, but as psychotic symptoms settle down there should be increasing emphasis on rehabilitation. This should include individual and group activities, which build on past interests and achievements and encourage self-care, and social activities, initially in hospital and then increasingly in the community. He will then need help to find suitable accommodation, possibly in a supervised hostel or sheltered housing for the mentally ill. Alternatively it may be possible for him to return to live with his family, who will need information about his disorder and how they can contribute. He will also need arrangements for day-care, in either a day hospital or a social services day-centre. Subsequently it may be possible for him to do voluntary work, or retraining for work might be arranged through the Disablement Resettlement Officer.

Long-term care may involve follow-up at the psychiatric out-patient clinic and/or the clinic for depot medication, or this may be provided by the general practitioner and community psychiatric nurse.

Prognosis

Factors suggesting a poor outcome include insidious onset, prolonged duration, and 'negative symptoms'. However, there are also some favourable factors – the lack of problems in his pre-morbid personality, his good educational record, and continuing contact with and support from a caring but not over-involved family. If drug abuse has been an important cause and he becomes abstinent this will greatly improve the outcome.

FORMULATION 3: SOMATIZATION

Demographic data

Mrs Mary Green is a forty-eight-year-old married woman with two children who is in receipt of disability allowance.

Descriptive formulation

Mrs Green was referred from the Orthopaedic Surgery Department with a three-year **history** of back pain for which no relevant organic disorder has been found on repeated investigation. Pain developed following a minor accident at work. It is mainly in the lumbar region but also spreads up to both shoulders and down both legs. Despite seeing five consultants, pain has been unrelieved by analgesics, acupuncture, or osteopathy, and she says it was made worse by facet nerve and joint injections, laminectomy, and a transcutaneous nerve stimulator. She describes depressed mood for up to a day at a time, but no diurnal mood variation or suicidal thoughts; her sleep is disturbed by pain although she sleeps seven hours on most nights; she has poor appetite but weight gain. She has not worked since the accident, has given up previous interests, feels tired, and spends most of the day 'resting'. She is cared for by her husband, who has taken early retirement, and by her fourteen-year-old daughter, who often stays off school.

On **mental state** examination, she arrived in a wheelchair pushed by her husband, but was able to walk unaided and showed a good range of movement. She sat in a normal posture but rubbed her back and grimaced frequently. Although she appeared co-operative, she made repeated, disparaging comments about previous doctors whom she said had neglected her care. Talk showed preoccupation with her physical complaints, and she appeared to idealize past and present relationships. Her mood was mildly anxious and not depressed. She had an over-valued idea that a physical disorder had been missed but would be found on further investigation, and her perceptions were dominated by pain. There was no evidence of other abnormalities of belief or perception, and cognitive functions were intact. Her insight was that she was suffering from an undiagnosed physical disorder which caused depression.

On **physical examination**, she stood stiffly, walked hesitantly, but showed a full range of movements in her spine and upper and lower limbs. She complained of wide-spread pain on palpation of her back and there was mild, bilateral wasting in the lower limbs. Otherwise, in the central nervous system, cranial nerves, sensory and motor functions, and deep reflexes were intact. There were no other abnormalities.

Differential diagnosis

1. **Somatoform pain disorder**, suggested by the chronic pain and severe disability for which there has been no evidence of relevant physical pathology on examination or extensive investigation. Depressive features are mild and likely to be consistent with present life circumstances.

2. **Somatization disorder**. The present episode of pain appears to be part of a long-term history of somatization, with multiple, recurrent physical complaints and invalidism, starting at the age of ten, with little objective evidence of physical disease. This includes past consultations and investigations for abdominal pain (diagnosed as irritable bowel syndrome), headaches and menorrhagia (resulting in a hysterectomy at the age of forty-three). These have usually coincided with stressful life events, particularly in family relationships.

3. **Depressive disorder** must also be considered in view of the subjective complaints of depressed mood, fatigue, poor interest, and sleep and appetite disturbance. However, there is little objective evidence for these and characteristic neuro-vegetative changes and depressive cognitions are absent.

4. **Personality disorder** is an *additional diagnosis*, characterized by anxious, depend-ent, and histrionic traits. Although she had a good work record, she has always tended to worry excessively, particularly about the family's health and safety, has been unusually dependent on her mother, husband, and daughter, and never had close relationships outside the family or interests outside the home.

Aetiology

Predisposing. Her mother, with whom she closely identified, was abused by her alcoholic father, was frequently unwell, and served as a model for the benefits of chronic invalidism. Mrs Green was herself often away from school, maintaining a close and mutually dependent relationship with her mother by caring for her. These early experiences have resulted in the personality problems and tendency to somatize which have already been described. She has perpetuated this pattern by becoming a professional carer, and also by marrying a weak man who abused alcohol and was physically violent.

Precipitating. During the year prior to the onset of her symptoms she had been distressed when her son married and moved away from home. A few weeks prior to the accident she learnt of her husband's extramarital affair, but consequently he has remained at home to care for her and has stopped drinking. In addition she had found it difficult to adapt to the expectations of a new work supervisor and new work practices.

Maintaining. Somatization has resulted in the denial of psychosocial problems and now she regards all distress as due to a physical disorder. The gains which result from and perpetuate her symptoms include the avoidance of marital and work problems; the closer and attentive relationship with her daughter (in whom this cycle is starting to be repeated); and the financial gains of permanent disability payments and the outstanding claim for compensation from her past employers. There is also an important iatrogenic contribution – her doctors have spent three years treating non-existent physical disorders, told her she 'will never work again', and failed to identify a treatable mental disorder until it has become chronic.

Investigations

1. Examination of patient's and mother's past **medical records** from general practitioners and hospitals.

2. **Interviews with husband**, to obtain further details of history, to determine his knowledge of the patient's disorder, his attitudes and beliefs about her health problems and their marital difficulties, and whether he is willing to cooperate with psychological treatment.

3. **Psychological**. Interviews with the patient to explore past and recent experiences (described above) and her feelings about these, and the extent to which she is able to engage in psychological treatment. Assessments of the patient's skills, interests, and other assets will also be needed in planning treatment.

4. **Physical**. If records confirm that all appropriate investigations have been completed, the patient should be informed of the results and all further investigation should be avoided.

5. **Social**. Home visits will indicate the extent to which the home has been adapted to the needs of an invalid. Joint interviews with the patient, husband, and children are likely to be necessary to assess family relationships and the family's possible involvement in treatment.

Treatment

First, the agreement of all health professionals to end inappropriate physical interventions will be essential. The patient should be provided with an explanation of how stress can lead to physical symptoms, and helped to recognize the relevance of past experiences. Her agreement will be needed if **psychological treatment** is to be pursued, and this may take the form of a 'contract' regarding the ending of other consultations, limiting unhelpful medication, and regular attendance at the psychiatric department. She will have to be introduced to an active model of rehabilitation rather than the curative model of treatment in which she has previously been a passive recipient of care.

Medication is unlikely to help, but it may be worth trying a tricyclic anti-depressant, building up to a full dose for one month, in view of the possibility of depressive symptoms and also because of the analgesic effects of this group of drugs.

Out-patient treatment may include **exploratory psychotherapy,** but this may be difficult because she is a somatizer. Other approaches which may be more acceptable include stress management using **relaxation techniques,** or **cognitive therapy** which may be provided by a clinical psychologist. Another possibility will be a **behavioural programme**, with structured and increasing activities, which may initially involve in-patient treatment in a specialized unit, subsequently progressing to day-patient and out-patient management. Her family and doctors will need to be involved in this in order to stop reinforcing invalidism and to start reinforcing appropriate activities and achievements, and the husband and daughter are also likely to require attention for their own needs. (For further details about the management of somatization, see Chapter 15.)

Prognosis

The outcome is likely to be poor because of the past history of somatization and personality problems; the prolonged duration of the present episode and the continuing gains from invalidism; and the uncertain cooperation of other doctors and family members. However, the patient has attended the department of psychiatry for the first time and appears willing to consider alternative approaches.

FURTHER READING

Greenberg, M., Szmukler, G. and Tantam, D. (1986) *Making Sense of Psychiatric Cases.* Oxford: Oxford Medical.

PART 2
THE SYNDROMES
OF PSYCHIATRIC
DISORDER

10 / PSYCHIATRIC ASPECTS OF PHYSICAL DISEASE

This chapter will first consider the kinds of relationships which can exist between psychological and physical ill-health, and will then consider the psychological manifestations of various physical illnesses, and we will include psychiatric aspects of epilepsy. A final section will deal with acute and chronic pain.

Numerous studies have shown that there is a strong relationship between physical and psychological illness, which cannot be accounted for by chance association. All too often, doctors in hospital practice consider the possibility that there is something psychologically wrong only when they have failed to find a physical cause for their patient's symptoms. This is a very bad policy since most psychologically disturbed patients on the medical wards *have a physical disorder as well*. Nor is it true that patients in whom we have failed to make a physical diagnosis necessarily have psychological disorders! *Psychiatric diagnoses should be made on positive evidence of disorder, and not by exclusion.*

At one time it was usual to divide physical diseases into those in which psychological factors were thought to be relatively unimportant, and others called 'psychosomatic diseases' which were thought to be partly caused by psychological factors. Eczema, asthma, coronary heart disease, diabetes, and ulcerative colitis were thought to be examples of such diseases. However, the term is no longer used since no one now supposes that diseases can be divided up in this way. It is impossible to think of a disease which is not affected in some way by psychological factors, and to the extent that the word 'psychosomatic' is still used it refers to the systematic study of psychological factors in physical disease processes.

RELATIONSHIPS BETWEEN PHYSICAL DISEASE AND PSYCHIATRIC ILLNESS

There are in fact five kinds of relationship between psychiatric disorders and physical symptoms which account for the high rates of psychiatric illness seen on surveys in general medical settings:

1. **Psychiatric disorder may provoke or release physical disease**. Depression is the illness most likely to do this. In surveys of psychiatric illness in medical in-patients, a proportion of cases will be found where the sequence is:

   stressful life event → episode of depression → physical ill-health

   It is possible that these apparently causal sequences are just part of the tendency for illnesses to come in clusters in people's lives, rather than at random time points. There is no doubt that illnesses like asthma and migraine are more likely to occur when patients are psychologically unwell, and there is some evidence that the same is true for conditions such as eczema and carcinoma of the cervix.

2. The **psychiatric symptoms may be the presenting symptoms of a physical disease**. This is not all that common, but it happens. Thyrotoxicosis may present as an anxiety state, myxoedema and pernicious anaemia may present as depression, myasthenia gravis may be mistaken for neurosis. A full account of such disorders is given later in this chapter (see pp. 138–41).

3. **Psychiatric illness may be the direct consequence of a physical disease**. If the physical disease had not occurred, the psychiatric illness would not have done so – at least, not at that particular time in the patient's life. This is a common relationship, and is perhaps the easiest one to understand. A patient who has noticed a potentially serious symptom like a breast lump or an episode of rectal bleeding may become anxious about the possible cause; a patient who knows he has cancer may become depressed. It is important to recognize these illnesses, since they cause much suffering and respond well to treatment.

4. **Psychiatric disorder may exacerbate the pain of a physical disease**. Patients who are depressed experience pains and discomforts more severely than when they are well, and the experience of anxiety has been shown to lower the pain threshold. This general relationship holds for any chronic pain, from sciatica to malignant disease. When a patient who is known to have some chronic disease complains of an exacerbation of their pains it is tempting to conclude that the underlying disease has deteriorated: but it is often not true.

5. **Psychiatric illness may present to doctors with physical symptoms which have no organic basis**. This phenomenon is called the 'somatization' of psychological distress, and its existence explains why some clinicians consider psychological causes only when they have failed to make a physical diagnosis.

However, as we shall see, somatization can be expanded to cover cases where there is undoubted physical disease, but this disease does not really account for the patient's physical symptoms. We give an extended account of somatization in Chapter 15 (see pp. 233ff.).

TREATMENT OF PSYCHIATRIC ILLNESS ASSOCIATED WITH PHYSICAL DISEASE

Psychiatric symptoms as presenting symptoms of a physical disease

Treatment will of course be directed at the underlying disease. However, do not forget to explain to your patient that their disease has been responsible for the psychiatric symptoms described to you, and ask the patient to let you know if these symptoms do not remit.

Psychiatric disorder secondary to physical disease

Allow the patient to ventilate his anxieties, and be sure to correct any fears that are unrealistic or just wrong. If it is not possible to reassure the patient, give information about the investigations that are to be carried out, and promise to keep the patient informed. If the patient has a depressive illness an anti-depressant should be prescribed. Tetracyclic anti-depressants such as mianserin, trazodone, or maprotiline are better tolerated by patients with physical illnesses, since they have fewer side-effects than tricyclic anti-depressants. Sedating anti-depressants are also effective in anxiety, and will not lead to dependence.

Psychiatric illness exacerbating symptoms of an undoubted physical disease

Treatment of such affective illnesses is an extremely important part of your general management plans for the patient's illness. However, the principles are the same as those described already: see p. 193 for anxiety states, and p. 201 for depressive illnesses with anxiety.

PSYCHIATRIC PRESENTATIONS OF PHYSICAL DISEASE

Many physical diseases have psychological symptoms as part of their presentation. This is true of most endocrine disorders, many metabolic disorders, and some neurological diseases.

ENDOCRINE DISORDERS

Hypothyroidism

Mental symptoms are as prominent as physical symptoms in myxoedema, and take the form of memory loss, somnolence, and depressed mood. The cognitive changes may be so severe that the patient is thought to have a **chronic brain syndrome**: since the condition is reversible in its early stages, **thyroid function tests** should be done in all cases of **pre-senile dementia** (see pp. 161–5). The patients complain of lethargy: they feel slowed up, are disinclined to undertake even familiar tasks, and are unable to concentrate. Patients are often diagnosed as depressed, and the hypothyroidism is missed. Major psychotic illness may also occur.

Hyperthyroidism

Patients are over-aroused, distractible, and anxious. The presentations may be irritable, show easy startle responses, and be intolerant of frustration. They can therefore closely resemble **anxiety states,** but the additional feature of hyperthyroidism should allow the correct aetiology of the anxiety to be diagnosed. There may be histrionic disturbed behaviour, and sometimes excitement is such that the patient satisfies the criteria for a **manic illness.** As with myxoedema, other psychotic illnesses, including agitated depression and schizophreniform illnesses, have also been reported. The thyroid disease is presumably releasing psychosis in vulnerable people.

Cushing's syndrome

Depression is easily the commonest psycho-syndrome seen, ranging in severity from mild to severe with paranoid features. Well over 50 per cent of patients with Cushing's syndrome may be expected to have depressive symptoms. These symptoms are directly due to the increased level of corticosteroids, since treatment of the hormonal disorder causes the depressive symptoms to disappear, yet they reappear if the Cushing's syndrome relapses. In theory one might expect manic syndromes since exogenously administered steroids produce euphoria: but such syndromes are rare.

Hypopituitarism and hypoadrenalism

The psycho-syndrome consists of weakness, lack of energy, tiredness with defective memory, and poor concentration. The patient may be somnolent and self-neglectful, so the condition can be misdiagnosed either as depression or as dementia.

Sheehan's syndrome

This is a post-partum necrosis of the pituitary. There is chronic ill-health with lack of energy, depression, and sensitivity to cold: think of it if lactation did not occur and menstruation did not resume after the post-partum haemorrhage; confirm by the absent pubic and axillary hair, followed by appropriate biochemical investigations.

Acromegaly

Earliest symptoms often include apathy and loss of initiative. Some become depressed and irritable, while others show lability of mood.

Parathyroid disease

The commonest psychological disorder is **depression,** which tends to be both marked and early. It occurs in both hypo- and hyper-parathyroidism and appears related to calcium rather than to parathormone levels.

Diabetes mellitus

Listlessness, irritability, and confusion may usher in diabetic coma. Late complications include some degree of chronic brain syndrome if there have been cerebrovascular accidents, or if there has been damage secondary to prolonged hypoglycaemia.

Hypoglycaemia

This may occur with diabetes mellitus or with an insulinoma ('spontaneous hypo-glycaemia'), or it may be provoked by alcohol. Early psychological symptoms are anxiety or panic, weakness, and sometimes depersonalization. This may be followed by ataxia or clouding of consciousness, or by peculiar and uncharacteristic behaviour. The patient may be aggressive and noisy, and there is usually some degree of motor incoordination. If treatment is delayed, irreversible brain damage will result. When hypoglycaemia is provoked by alcohol a malnourished person takes a large quantity of alcohol and lapses first into stupor, then coma. Surrounding drinkers assume he is 'dead drunk'. Unless the true diagnosis is made, death is indeed a possibility.

METABOLIC DISORDERS

Electrolyte imbalance

These are shown in *Table 10.1*.

Renal failure

Mental clouding, poor concentration, and listlessness lead to drowsiness and disorientation. 'Uraemia' may thus present as **delirium,** or it may aggravate a mild dementing illness in an elderly patient. Depression can be marked and require treatment. Symptoms are not due to urea itself, but to electrolyte imbalance and toxic levels of drugs.

Table 10.1 *Metabolic disorders*

Electrolyte imbalance

Alkalosis	Dulling of perception, confusion, and tetany
Acidosis (includes hypercapnia)	Dulling of mental functions, drowsiness, impaired consciousness, eventual papilloedema
Hyponatraemia	lassitude, weakness, irritability, confusion
Hypokalaemia	apathy, lethargy, confusion
Hypomagnesaemia	depression, disorientation, delirium

RENAL DIALYSIS

This is associated with three psychological problems: patients often complain of *anxiety and depression;* rapid reduction of urea may lead to *headache, muscular twitches, fits,* and *confusion* – perhaps because of cerebral oedema; and a *progressive dementia* has been described associated with high brain aluminium concentration ('dialysis encephalopathy').

Hepatic failure

The features of hepatic pre-coma are psychological and motor, and are due to nitrogenous substances derived from food. The patient may be noted to have a fixed, staring appearance with a reduction of spontaneous movements.

There are periods of clouded consciousness with perplexity, forgetfulness, dysarthria, and ataxia. Hypersomnia occurs, and the characteristic flapping tremor can be elicited. There is sometimes a fatuous personality change similar to a frontal lobe disorder (see p. 171).

Acute intermittent porphyria

This is a rare disorder, but psychotic symptoms may be prominent, in association with unexplained abdominal pain. Histrionic behaviour and emotional lability are common. It is beginning to look as though George III did not suffer from it.

TOXIC STATES AND DEFICIENCIES

Carbon monoxide poisoning

This is a cause of a severe amnestic syndrome. Extra-pyramidal damage may also occur: personality changes include impulsiveness, moodiness, and aggression.

Thiamine

Depression, irritability, lassitude, and anorexia occur in those deprived of dietary thiamine. Vague somatic complaints and forgetfulness occur as deficiency becomes more severe; finally Korsakow's syndrome (see pp. 168–9). Acute depletion will cause Wernicke's encephalopathy (pp. 168–9).

Nicotinic acid

Pellagra has prominent psychiatric abnormalities, of which the most dramatic is a *paranoid hallucinatory psychosis*. However, other psychological manifestations include disorientation and confusion; excitement with outbursts of violent behaviour; and depression.

Vitamin B₁₂ and folic acid

Amnestic syndrome, subacute delirium, and chronic brain syndrome may either antedate or accompany the megaloblastic anaemia, and are reversible with treatment. *Vitamin B₁₂* deficiency has been said to lead to depressive symptoms, but the evidence is unclear. *Folic acid deficiency* is associated with depressive symptoms accompanied by low drive and anergia, and also with chronic brain syndrome in the elderly (see pp. 159, 300).

ACQUIRED IMMUNE DEFICIENCY SYNDROME (AIDS)

AIDS is caused by infection with *human immunodeficiency virus (HIV)* and at present is a fatal illness. The virus is thought to be neurotropic and symptoms can arise from any site in the central nervous system. In addition to the direct effect of the virus, there may be effects on the central nervous system caused by intercurrent infections and neoplasia. The organic effects, the psychosocial consequences, and the anticipated fatal outcome all contribute to the high psychiatric morbidity.

Epidemiology

The world-wide distribution of HIV infection and AIDS is thought to vary considerably. In the United Kingdom high-risk groups include intravenous drug abusers, homosexual men, and haemophiliacs, and infection may be increasing in heterosexual men and in women. A high risk for mental disorders arises due to AIDS and also to the increased psychiatric morbidity associated with substance abuse and homosexuality.

Psychiatric syndromes

CHRONIC BRAIN SYNDROME

Chronic brain syndrome occurs eventually in at least two-thirds of patients with AIDS, in whom it has been called *AIDS Dementia Complex (ADC)*. The early stages may not be obvious on routine clinical examination but defects on complex mental and motor tasks are evident on psychological testing. The disorder usually develops gradually over months, with increasing cognitive impairment, focal neurological signs, and sometimes psychotic symptoms. More rapid deterioration may be due to infection or malignancy. Computerized tomography or magnetic resonance imaging usually show cortical atrophy.

ACUTE BRAIN SYNDROME

Acute brain syndrome results commonly from the various physical disorders that occur in the course of AIDS, and from their treatments. It presents in the same way as in other medical disorders.

AFFECTIVE DISORDERS

Depressed and anxious mood are common in all the groups that are at high risk for HIV infection, even if they are HIV negative, but tend to be increased in those who are HIV positive. There are many factors that contribute. Depressed mood is often found in patients with ADC and is also thought to occur as a *symptomatic mood disorder* due to HIV infection, in the absence of cognitive impairment. Suffering from a socially stigmatizing, terminal illness often leads to *major depressive disorders* or *generalized anxiety states*, and in others there are *adjustment disorders* with depressive and anxiety symptoms, anger, and hostility. Most patients are likely to go through a process of *grief*. Investigation of haemophiliac men has demonstrated the effect of *predisposing factors* in addition to the effects of infection, diagnosis, and their consequences. Those who are HIV positive are particularly susceptible to disorders of mood if there is a past or family history of mental disorder, poor social support, or recent life events involving loss.

Treatment

Antiviral treatment, for example with zidovudine, can result in improved cognitive function in those with ADC. *Neuroleptic drugs* may be needed to control psychotic symptoms but should be used with particular caution because HIV appears to result in supersensitivity to the dopamine blocking effects and there is particular risk of extra-pyramidal symptoms as well as neuroleptic malignant syndrome. The use of *anti-depressants* should be based on the same criteria as in other disorders, although there are reports of increased sensitivity to anti-cholinergic side-effects so that it is preferable to start with relatively small doses which should then be increased. 5-hydroxytriptamine re-uptake inhibitors may be better tolerated than tricyclics.

Psychosocial approaches to treatment should be made available to all patients and contributions to compassionate care can be provided effectively by voluntary and self-help organizations as well as by professional multi-disciplinary services. Individual and group support can help patients and carers and some may benefit from psychological approaches to anxiety management.

Prevention of spread of infection is a major priority. Measures include education and counselling for sexually active heterosexuals and homosexuals about 'safe sex' and also the availability of uncontaminated syringes and needles for intravenous drug users.

NEUROLOGICAL DISEASE

We deal with cerebral tumours and dementia in Chapter 11. Two neurological illnesses are strongly linked with *affective illness*:

Parkinson's disease

There is an important association with **depression**, which often follows the onset of Parkinsonian symptoms. Treatment of the depression may dramatically alleviate the motor symptoms.

Multiple sclerosis

At one time students were taught that patients tended to develop euphoria. This can happen when there is general cerebral impairment, but it is not common. Most patients will describe symptoms of **anxiety and depression**, and such symptoms can greatly add to the burden which their disease imposes.

EPILEPSY

Most of those prone to epilepsy are psychiatrically normal, and are not at particular risk for chronic brain syndromes, for major mental illness, or for personality disorder. However, there is an increased risk for such disorders in those whose epilepsy is symptomatic of some organic cerebral disorder, and pathology in the temporal lobe seems especially important in this respect.

Nevertheless, most epileptic patients experience prejudice from others, and this may cause both social handicaps and depressive symptoms which are more disabling than the fits.

Definition

A *seizure* is an attack of *sudden* onset and usually brief duration which becomes clinically manifest through sensory, motor, psychic (affective, cognitive), or autonomic symptoms. It is associated with spontaneous abnormal electrical activity in the brain as measured by the EEG.

Every brain has a *threshold* for the development of seizures. Given the right type of stimulus, anyone could develop a seizure. These triggers include metabolic derangements, febrile illnesses, cerebral inflammatory or infectious illnesses, acute stroke or head injury, intoxication with certain drugs, and acute drug or alcohol withdrawal syndromes. The occurrence of such *symptomatic seizures* does not indicate a diagnosis of epilepsy.

Epilepsy may be defined as the occurrence of *recurrent* seizures. Although patients are not usually started on anti-epileptic drugs after an isolated spontaneous seizure, the other factors that are taken into account in estimating the risk of further seizures are: age of onset (children and old adults being more at risk), partial seizures, structural or congenital brain lesions, neurological disorder, and an abnormal EEG. However, an abnormal EEG is not by itself sufficient for a diagnosis of epilepsy, since 'epileptiform' EEG abnormalities may also occur in seizure-free individuals.

Epidemiology

The prevalence of epilepsy in the general population has been estimated to be between four and six per thousand at risk, with an equal sex incidence. The lifetime risk of developing seizures is about 5 per cent and about 30 per cent of those with epilepsy will develop a mental disorder.

The incidence of epilepsy is highest in childhood and adolescence and is approximately equal in both sexes. There is a small tendency, thought to be genetically determined, for epilepsy to run in families. Among children, psychiatric disorders occur among 7 per cent of those without epilepsy, in 30 per cent of those with uncomplicated epilepsy, and among 60 per cent of those with epilepsy complicated with brain damage.

Clinical features and classification

The most important basis for the classification of seizures is whether or not they start focally in the brain. This has implications for choice of anti-epileptic drugs. *Partial seizures*, as their name implies, start focally, most commonly in the temporal lobes. *Generalized seizures* have no focal onset when recorded on the EEG.

PARTIAL SEIZURES

Partial seizures are divided into *simple* and *complex*: the former do not involve impairment of consciousness whereas the latter do. Partial seizures may spread and become generalized, a process known as *secondary generalization*. It is important to note that a partial seizure may only manifest itself clinically at the time of generalized spread, so that its focal nature may only be realized when recorded on the EEG.

In **simple partial seizures** the ictal manifestations include sensory or motor phenomena, depending upon the part of the cortex involved. Spontaneous movements may spread along a limb and then recede, while the subject retains full awareness – a sequence called a 'Jacksonian march'. The focal symptoms of which the patient is aware are called *auras*, and they may or may not be followed by a generalized seizure with impairment of consciousness. Auras last only a few seconds. This, together with their sudden onset and intense, stereotyped characteristics, helps to differentiate them from other types of mental phenomena such as anxiety attacks or other neurotic symptoms.

In **complex partial seizures** the aura is followed by impairment of consciousness, as the attack originates in areas of higher cerebral organization. In complex partial seizures of *temporal lobe* origin (previously called temporal lobe epilepsy or psychomotor epilepsy) the aura may include hallucinations of hearing, vision, taste, or smell. There may be an 'epigastric aura' experienced as a central abdominal churning feeling that spreads upwards through the chest, and there may also be feelings of flushing, tachycardia, fear, and dizziness. Particularly memorable are sudden feelings that unfamiliar surroundings are familiar (*déjà-vu*) or the reverse (*jamais-vu*) but similar experiences occur commonly in the absence of epilepsy. Automatic behaviours, such as grimacing, lip-smacking, automatisms (*p. 336) and fugues (*p. 336), may occur in a state of clouded consciousness.

GENERALIZED SEIZURES

The two commonest types of generalized seizures are *tonic-clonic* and *absence attacks*, also known as 'grand mal' and 'petit mal'.

Tonic-clonic attacks are subcortical in origin, and therefore start without warning. However, there may be ill-defined prodromata such as malaise, nausea, or headache which build up in the days before an attack. There is sudden loss of consciousness and generalized increase in muscle tone. This tonic phase is shortly followed by a clonic phase of generalized, rhythmic, muscle spasms involving all parts of the body symmetrically from the same moment. During the fit the tongue may be bitten and there may be incontinence of urine. This stage usually lasts for minutes but can last for hours ('status epilepticus'). Clinical examination during this stage reveals fixed pupillary dilatation, absent corneal reflexes, and extensor plantar reflexes. The post-ictal phase lasts for about an hour, during which time the patient may be disorientated, incoherent, or drowsy, and may complain of nausea or headache.

In **absence attacks** the patient suddenly loses touch with his environment and appears dazed. Posture and balance are maintained, but the pupils will dilate and the patient appears pale and immobile to an observer. Sometimes the head may slump forward slightly and there may be twitches round the eyes. Consciousness is deeply impaired during the attack, which typically lasts only five seconds or so, but can last longer. Attacks typically occur at least daily, and there is usually no evidence of a brain lesion.

Other types of generalized attacks include *myoclonic and atonic attacks* ('akinetic attack'). The former is characterized by generalized myoclonic jerks and the latter by an abrupt loss of muscle tone. All generalized attacks are associated with sudden loss of consciousness at the onset of the attack.

Epilepsy in childhood

Epilepsy presents in distinctive ways:

1. **Neonatal seizures** are often the presenting symptoms of serious congenital abnormalities or meningitis. Unless they are due to hypocalcaemia, the prognosis is grave.

2. **Febrile fits** are the commonest form of epilepsy, affecting 3 per cent of children at some time. They accompany fevers and are generally bilateral; brief and benign. If they take their onset in the first year of life, last for more than half an hour, or are lateralized the prognosis is more serious.

3. **Infantile spasms** take the form of recurrent forward flexion of the trunk ('Salaam epilepsy') coming perhaps three times a day. The onset is between four and eighteen months, there is an association with early infantile autism (see pp. 267), and there may be failure of normal intellectual development.

4. **The Lennox–Gastaut syndrome,** or 'atypical petit mal', is associated with four kinds of attack: generalized seizures, drop attacks, tonic attacks, and atypical absences. The EEG shows atypical, 'notched' spike and wave discharges.

5. **Petit mal** occurs in childhood: the child maintains posture, but is unconscious during attacks (which may be referred to as 'absences'). The EEG shows three per second spike and wave during an absence, and the child may have generalized seizures at other times.

6. **Petit mal status** ('status of minor epilepsy') is commoner in childhood and old age than in adult life: it can persist for prolonged periods (several months!) and although the child is conscious there is clouding accompanied by inability to concentrate and motor incoordination: school work usually suffers, and the EEG shows continuous three per second spike and wave.

7. **Generalized epilepsy** ('grand mal') is sporadic throughout childhood.

Differential diagnosis

Epileptic seizures must be distinguished from other organic causes of sudden loss of consciousness, such as simple faints (syncope), transient ischaemic attacks, and spontaneous hypoglycaemia.

Psychiatric and behavioural disorders include: temper tantrums and breath-holding attacks and night terrors in children; hyperventilation, panic attacks, aggressive outbursts in explosive personalities, and pseudo-seizures in adults.

PSEUDO-SEIZURES

Finally, epileptic seizures must be distinguished from psychologically determined simulations of fits, or pseudo-seizures. Although pseudo-seizures tend to occur in young females they can present in anybody, including those who also have epileptic seizures! The simulation may be unconscious (usually classified with dissociative symptoms – see p. 239) or conscious (that is, malingering – pp. 232, 239–41).

Pseudo-seizures are usually characterized by non-stereotyped motor activity, which does not follow closely any of the recognized patterns of epileptic fits. They tend to occur when others are present, and may involve emotionally laden cries or sexualized movements. The patient may tend to fight the examiner off, but fixed pupillary dilatation, absent corneal reflexes, and extensor plantar reflexes are not found if the examiner persists. It is rare for the patient to void urine and bite their tongue during the attack. However, they appear to be unconscious during the attack, and to thrash their limbs about in ways that can be quite convincing if they have seen others with genuine seizures. They tend to be in a bad temper when 'coming round', but they share this characteristic with patients recovering from tonic-clonic attacks.

The importance of a past history of sexual abuse is increasingly being recognized in some of these patients. These episodes are not accompanied by the typical EEG changes of epilepsy, nor is a raised serum prolactin level found subsequently.

Aetiology

In about 66 per cent of cases no cause can be found for epilepsy even after full investigation ('idiopathic'); in such cases genetic factors appear to have some importance. In the remainder the epilepsy can be shown to be secondary to some known cerebral disease: birth injury, congenital malformations, exanthemata, and metabolic disorders in children; cerebrovascular disease, head injury, and degenerative disorders in the elderly.

Drugs may cause seizures in two ways: sudden withdrawal of agents known to have anticonvulsant properties such as benzodiazepines or barbiturates; or administration of agents known to lower the convulsive threshold, such as phenothiazines and, to a lesser extent, tricyclic anti-depressants.

Withdrawal from large doses of alcohol also causes generalized seizures (see p. 145). Alcohol or drug abuse should therefore always be considered in a patient with no previous history of epilepsy who has a fit following admission to hospital.

Psychiatric aspects of epilepsy

PERSONALITY CHANGES

Attitudes of dependency and insecurity may be engendered by over-protection during childhood or by the social and occupational problems which must be faced. These may increase vulnerability to depressive illness.

Patients with temporal lobe epilepsy can exhibit explosive irritability and aggressiveness, and also may report sexual problems: either hyposexuality or deviant practices such as fetishism or transvestism.

ANXIETY AND DEPRESSION

The most common psychiatric disorders which occur in those with epilepsy are anxiety states and depressive disorders. There is an increased risk of suicide. An over-protected existence and the social handicaps that often accompany epilepsy may contribute to feelings of worry and low self-esteem, although these do not necessarily amount to psychiatric disorder.

Depression, anxiety, and low self-esteem are common, perhaps because of the social handicaps experienced by most epileptics.

PSYCHOTIC ILLNESSES AND EPILEPSY

Post-ictal psychosis is uncommon. Typically it develops following a period of lucidity, about twenty-four hours after a major attack. A florid psychosis, with schizophreniform or affective symptoms, or a mixture of these, then develops and lasts around three weeks, sometimes longer. It may take the form of a *paranoid hallucinatory state* accompanied by some clouding of consciousness ('epileptic twilight state').

Inter-ictal psychoses are uncommon but tend to develop many years after the onset, particularly of complex partial epilepsy arising from the temporal lobe. They usually present as *symptomatic schizophrenia* of chronic paranoid type. There is no clouding of consciousness. It takes its onset a decade or more after the onset of the complex partial seizures. It is thought that this is more likely to develop in patients with a dominant (usually left-sided) epileptic focus in the temporal lobe. The expectation of schizophrenia in first-degree relatives is not increased, nor is there increased expectancy of schizoid personality, suggesting that the psychosis is indeed secondary to the epilepsy. *Forced normalization* refers to the normalization of the EEG or the improvement in seizure frequency which occurs in some patients when they develop recurrent psychotic episodes.

EPILEPSY AND CHRONIC BRAIN SYNDROME

There are three possible relationships: a dementing illness may present with epilepsy; or hypoxia associated with long-standing epilepsy may cause a chronic brain syndrome; or in old age *petit mal status* may present as an apparent dementing illness of sudden onset. Diagnosis is on the EEG.

MANAGEMENT OF EPILEPSY

A full history, including an interview with anyone who has witnessed the seizures, is essential. A physical examination followed by laboratory and brain imaging investigations are necessary to exclude the possibility of symptomatic seizures. Inter-ictal EEG studies are used for the classification of epileptic seizures. Video-telemetry consists of videorecording of seizures in parallel with EEG recordings. A post-ictal EEG is invaluable in the diagnosis of post-ictal psychosis, which demonstrates generalized post-ictal slow wave changes.

Serum prolactin rises immediately after a tonic-clonic seizure and reaches a peak about twenty minutes after seizure onset. It does not, however, rise after status epilepticus and it may be equivocal following complex partial seizures.

The vast majority of patients with epilepsy can be managed with *single anti-epileptic agents*. In a minority with recalcitrant seizures, combinations of drugs may be useful, although this increases the likelihood of drug-interactions and side-effects. The drugs are described on pp. 81–3.

Counselling on social aspects, such as driving law, and on practical steps to avoid injury must not be forgotten. Relatives must be advised to ensure the safety of patients during a seizure but to avoid restraining movement as much as possible. In particular, they should be asked not to insert spoons or any other sharp objects into the mouth in misguided efforts to open the airways. Inappropriate disability is common and advice for the patient and carers is needed to avoid its development, or to reduce disability after it is established.

Neuroleptic drugs or anti-depressants may be needed for the treatment of mental disorders associated with epilepsy, but many psychotropic agents *lower the convulsive threshold*.

The treatment of **pseudo-seizures** follows the same principles as other forms of abnormal illness behaviour (Chapter 15, see pp. 230–45).

PAIN

Pain is a perception and as such is a part of the mental state. It is commonly associated with tissue damage, and peripheral nerves then play an important part in its transmission. However, central neural mechanisms play a predominant part in pain perception: pain can be caused by CNS lesions, and is also modified by CNS activity, serving both to exacerbate it (as in depressive illnesses) and to relieve it (as exemplified by the use of hypnosis for dental analgesia).

Frequency and diagnosis

Pain is the commonest symptom of which patients complain, accounting for between 50 per cent and 95 per cent of presentations in medical out-patient clinics. Frequently it remains undiagnosed: approximately half of all patients presenting with pain to neurologists, cardiologists, and gastroenterologists show no evidence of relevant organic pathology after intensive investigation and long-term follow-up. Of patients with diagnosed mental illness in general practice and psychiatric out-patient settings, about 60 per cent complain of pain. It seems likely that pain is associated as much with mental as with physical illnesses and occurs particularly in the setting of affective disorders. However, it has little diagnostic specificity and can occur as a symptom of any mental illness. As usual, diagnosis is based on the nature of associated symptoms.

Psychological mechanisms of pain

1. The physiological effects of anxiety are widespread. Increased muscle tension is believed to result in 'tension headache'; increased intestinal motility may be experienced as abdominal pain; palpitations may lead to chest pain.
2. Pain is often experienced at a site where there is, or has been, some minor organic pathology, which has not previously caused the patient distress, but serves as a focus once the patient becomes anxious or depressed.
3. Depression and anxiety result in reduced tolerance of pain, whatever its origins.
4. Somatization frequently presents as pain and may result from the use of other defence mechanisms, such as introjection. It is a common feature of anxiety states, depressive disorders, and morbid grief reactions.

5. The awareness of pain becomes more intense and the associated illness behaviours (see *Table 15.1*) more frequent as a consequence of reinforcement by others who respond to the patient more positively when he shows such behaviours.

Acute pain

The intensity of pain associated with organic disease and trauma, including post-surgical pain, is related particularly to anxiety. Patients in hospital may experience anxiety for many reasons but much is often due to lack of familiarity with investigation and treatment procedures and the extent to which pain should be anticipated. Pre-surgical preparation which includes careful explanation of the procedures that the patient will experience and the availability of post-surgical analgesia has been shown to reduce both the post-surgical pain experienced and the need for analgesia.

Female patients and those with higher scores on measures of neuroticism tend to complain more about post-surgical pain and receive more analgesics from ward staff; others suffer pain of similar intensity but complain less and consequently suffer more because staff are unaware of their pain and fail to give analgesics. It is important to ask patients routinely about pain in order to determine the appropriate management.

Chronic pain patients

Patients with chronic pain (usually defined as of more than six months' duration) may suffer from a wide range of physical and mental disorders. It is a common error to suppose that such patients can be divided into those with 'real' or 'organic' pain and those with 'imaginary' or 'psychogenic' pain': first because both organic and psychological factors often play a part in the same patient, and second because pain is primarily a subjective experience and, if perceived, is always 'real', whatever its origins. Any combination of the mechanisms described above may play a part and many aspects of illness behaviour associated with the pain may appear inappropriate. Drug abuse is often an important secondary problem which may be iatrogenic.

Surveys of patients attending pain-relief clinics show that at least half are suffering from mental illness, diagnosed using standardized methods, but few of these disorders are recognized by the anaesthetists who run the clinics and few are referred to psychiatrists. About two-thirds of those with mental illness have depressive disorders, most of the remainder having primary hypochondriasis.

FURTHER READING

Eastwood, M. (1975) *The Relationship between Physical and Mental Illness*. Toronto: University of Toronto Press.

Kleinman, A. (1980) *Patients and Healers in the Context of Culture*. London: UCLA Press.

Williams, P. and Clare, A. (1979) *Psychosocial Disorders in General Practice*. London: Academic Press.

11 / ORGANIC BRAIN SYNDROMES

Organic brain syndromes may either involve the entire cortical canopy, in which case they are said to be **generalized**; or they may involve only a specific part of the cortex, in which case they are said to be **focal**. Generalized brain syndromes are further subdivided by their course, into **acute brain syndrome** and **chronic brain syndrome**. Even this distinction cannot always be made in a hard-and-fast way, and intermediate disorders can be referred to as **subacute brain syndromes**.

These are all syndromal diagnoses, and they will always require further investigations to establish the cause in a particular case.

DELIRIUM
(also known as ACUTE BRAIN SYNDROME)

Terminology

You may be confused by a variety of terms for an acute brain syndrome, all meaning almost the same thing. Old people are often said to present with an *'acute confusional state'*, and this term is further discussed on p. 298. A *toxic confusional state* refers to an acute brain syndrome secondary to toxic causes such as those listed in *Table 11.1*. Many clinicians use the word *delirium* to mean an acute brain syndrome with pronounced psychomotor agitation often accompanied by hallucinations and illusions, but others do not make this distinction.

Epidemiology

This is a common condition occurring in 5–10 per cent of general medical and surgical in-patients. It is common in the elderly and up to 30 per cent of the population have been estimated to suffer from this syndrome at some time of their lives. It is the most common cause of a psychotic state that occurs in the general wards. The syndrome occurs when normal brain functioning is disturbed by any one of the many causes listed in *Table 11.1*.

Table 11.1 *Causes of delirium*

	systemic	intracranial
trauma		head injury
degenerative		dementia with acute illness
epileptic		post-ictal states
		petit mal status
vascular	myocardial infarction	cerebral thrombosis or embolism
	anaemia	subarachnoid haemorrhage
	heart failure	transient ischaemic episode
	internal haemorrhage	hypertensive encephalopathy
infections	exanthemata	encephalitis
	septicaemia	meningitis
	pneumonia	rheumatic chorea
	influenza	cerebral abscess
	typhoid	
	typhus	
	cerebral malaria	
	trypanosomiasis	
metabolic	uraemia	
	liver failure,	
	alkalosis, acid-base disorders	
	acidosis, hypercapnia	
	electrolyte disturbances	
	remote effects of carcinoma	
	anoxia	
	CVS, chest disease, and anaemia	
endocrine disorders	hyperthyroid crises	
	myxoedema	
	Addisonian crisis	
	diabetic pre-coma, hypoglycaemia	
	parathyroid disease	
toxic	drugs: see text, pp. 154–5	
	alcohol: delirium tremens	
	Wernicke's encephalopathy	
	heavy metals: lead, arsenic, mercury	

Clinical features

Despite the plethora of aetiologies shown in *Table 11.1* the clinical picture is relatively constant. It is characterized by:

1. **Clouding of consciousness** (see p. 36) which has an acute onset and a fluctuating course – being worse at night, better during the day, and improving as the underlying pathological process resolves. Minor degrees of clouding of consciousness may be difficult to detect unless the patient is examined at night or when he is fatigued. Poor attention and impaired thinking may only be evident with persistent cognitive testing. In severe cases it may be impossible to gain the patient's attention at all as he is responding only to hallucinatory experiences and his speech is an incoherent rambling totally incomprehensible to the observer.

2. **Disorientation in time** (see p. 35) occurs first, followed by that of **space and person**. The disorientation fluctuates with level of consciousness and the person may be orientated by day and disorientated by night.

3. **Impaired thinking** ('confusion') occurs in conjunction with clouding of consciousness. Thinking may be slowed initially but progressively reasoning becomes less clear and incoherent.

4. **Disturbance of registration, retention, and recall** occur.

5. **Perceptual abnormalities** often make the staff first aware of the patient's abnormal mental state. *Illusions and misinterpretations* may dominate the picture. Unfamiliar objects and people are at greatest risk of being misinterpreted. Members of staff may be regarded by the patient as enemies or involved in a plot. Drugs may be misinterpreted as poison and these will be refused. *Visual hallucinations* are common though *auditory and tactile hallucinations* also occur.The hallucinations may form complex scenes in which the patient feels he is involved and by which he may be terrified.

6. **Emotional changes**. Anxiety, irritability, depression, and apathy occur first but frank fear may occur with or without the hallucinatory or persecutory phenomena described above. The patient may attempt to leave the ward in order to escape the frightening scenes he is experiencing.

7. **Psychomotor changes**. Either change may occur: *psychomotor retardation* may be evident with apathy and withdrawal from the patient's surroundings; but in the more severe forms *restless over-activity* is more common, with the patient plucking at the bedclothes or attempting to get out of bed. The latter pattern is seen in *delirium tremens* (see p. 157).

The failure to learn new material is usually evident on recovery when a dense amnesia for the duration of the delirium is evident. Occasionally there have been lucid intervals when the patient's conscious level returns to normal and there may be fragmented but vivid memories of emotionally charged scenes.

Diagnostic criteria

The following criteria may be used for research purposes:

A. **Clouding of consciousness** of acute onset, accompanied by *reduced capacity for attention,*

B. and TWO or more of the following:

    1. **Disorientation** or **memory impairment**.

    2. **Perceptual disturbance** (misinterpretations, illusions, or hallucinations).

    3. **Incoherent speech**.

    4. Disturbed **sleep–wakefulness cycle** with insomnia and daytime sleeping.

    5. Increased or decreased **psychomotor activity**.

Aetiology

The syndrome is produced by any cause that disrupts total brain functioning, and is the same irrespective of whether the exciting cause is intracranial (such as encephalitis or subdural haematoma) or systemic (such as pneumonia or uraemia). More than one factor may be present, and factors may contribute to the aetiology that have not been listed as 'main causes'. For example, following an operation residual anaesthetic, pain, mild respiratory problems, toxins from blood transfusion, opiate analgesic drugs, dehydration, anxiety, and unfamiliar surroundings may each be insufficient in itself, but together account for delirium.

Examination of the time of onset of the condition may provide a clue to the principal factor; this may coincide with the onset of a pyrexia, the changing of a drug, or development of dehydration.

TOXIC EFFECTS OF DRUGS

A wide range of drugs is capable of causing an acute brain syndrome, particularly:

1. **Dopamine agonists** (especially in combination):
   Benzhexol.
   L-Dopa.
   Amantadine.

2. **Anti-depressants**, notably Amitriptyline (especially when used in patients with severe physical illness or in large doses).

3. **Tranquillizers and hypnotics**:
   Barbiturates.
   Benzodiazepines.
   Phenothiazines.

4. **Anti-cholinergic drugs**:
   Atropine.
   Hyoscine.

5. **Anti-tuberculous drugs**:
     Isoniazid.
     Cycloserine.

6. **Cytotoxic drugs**.

7. **Anticonvulsants** (especially in high dose).

Alcohol and **barbiturates** can cause toxic symptoms either by acute intoxication or by withdrawal. Thus, an acute brain syndrome developing twenty-four to seventy-two hours after admission may result from the sudden cessation of regular alcohol intake or a drug upon which the patient is dependent.

Differential diagnosis

CHRONIC BRAIN SYNDROME

A previously undetected chronic brain syndrome can present for the first time as an acute brain syndrome if the patient develops some intercurrent infection which produces a state of acute cerebral decompensation. As the infection resolves, the chronic brain syndrome becomes apparent. The same can happen if there is some sudden change in the patient's environment, such as death of a spouse or moving to a new house. In either case, such a transient acute brain syndrome is sometimes referred to as a *decompensated dementia*.

FUNCTIONAL ILLNESS

Depression in the elderly (see p. 303) may present with clouding of consciousness and impaired ability to concentrate. The acute onset of *mania* or *schizophrenia* may be accompanied by perplexity, clouding, and impaired ability to think in addition to more typical schizo-phrenic phenomena.

   In these functional conditions clouding, disorientation, and impaired concentration will generally be less pronounced than other features of the mental state. Thus in severe depressive illness depressed mood and psychomotor retardation will predominate over the cognitive changes, and in schizophrenia the psychotic features will become clear with time.

Investigations

These will be ordered according to the abnormal physical findings present. Unless a likely cause is evident from your physical examination:

A useful first round of investigations would be:

   Full blood count
   ESR

   Urea and electrolytes

Liver function tests
Thyroid function tests
Blood sugar
Serology for neurosyphilis

Urine for microscopy and culture
Urine for drugs or porphyrins

Chest X-ray

To distinguish between delirium and functional illness:

EEG – shows slow waves in delirium

The following may be necessary:

Serum B$_{12}$ and folate
Lumbar puncture
CAT scan

Treatment

The patient must be investigated in hospital.

TREATMENT OF THE UNDERLYING CAUSE

Correction of the underlying physical abnormality is the primary goal of treatment. It may be necessary to correct a number of factors. Any abnormalities of fluid or electrolyte balance, or haematological and nutritional factors, should be corrected. *Any drugs that are not essential should be stopped.*

SYMPTOMATIC AND SUPPORTIVE MEASURES

Tranquillizers may be necessary if the patient is otherwise unmanageable. Since such medication can itself cause delirium it should be kept to a minimum and only used if the nursing procedures described below are unsuccessful.

Haloperidol is preferable to chlorpromazine as it tranquillizes without sedating, is less hypotensive, and has fewer adverse effects on the liver. It does not accumulate in the body like diazepam, nor is it likely to release clouding and disturbed behaviour in the same way as benzodiazepines.

Chlormethiazole is useful in delirium from any cause in which epileptic fits might occur, such as delirium tremens.

These drugs are particularly useful at night, as sleep deprivation can exacerbate the delirium.

In order to minimize misinterpretations the patient should be nursed in a room that is *well lit during the night* and by a small number of staff whom the patient can easily recognize. The patient will require *frequent reassurance* because of his fear, and *repeated explanation* by calm members of staff can reduce the need for sedation.

Early detection of acute brain syndrome may avoid the necessity for sedation, so any reports by the night staff of mild degrees of clouding or disturbed thinking in seriously ill patients should be investigated fully.

It is essential that a patient with an acute brain syndrome be kept in hospital for treatment. Occasionally this requires use of Section 5(2) of the Mental Health Act (see p. 333).

Course and prognosis

Following resolution of the underlying disorder, the delirious state may linger for days. In one study of delirium the majority of patients had either cancer or serious heart disease and the mortality rate during the index admission was 20 per cent and by one year nearly 50 per cent. However, the prognosis in cases due to drug intoxication or withdrawal is much better than for those in whom an underlying potentially fatal illness causes the delirium.

SUBACUTE DELIRIOUS STATE
(also known as SUBACUTE BRAIN SYNDROME)

This is a state intermediate between an acute and a chronic brain syndrome: the onset will have been less sudden than is usual in delirium; there will be a combination of features of the two; and the course is also intermediate. Wernicke's encephalopathy (see p. 168) often presents in this way.

DELIRIUM TREMENS

About 5 per cent of patients admitted to hospital with physical complications of alcoholism will display delirium tremens. Typically it occurs in middle-aged men who have been drinking heavily for some years, but it can also occur after only a few months of heavy drinking.

The first twelve hours:

Mild withdrawal phenomena such as tremor and agitation occur;

Twelve to forty-eight hours after withdrawal:

Generalized epileptic seizure may occur;

Three to four days after withdrawal:

The clinical picture in delirium tremens occurs, and is similar to that in acute brain syndromes of other aetiologies, but the following features are marked:

1. Dramatic, sudden onset with restlessness, insomnia, and fear.
2. Clouded consciousness and disorientation.
3. Startle reactions, nightmares, and panic.
4. Face terror-stricken.
5. Ataxia and tremor present.
6. Perspiration, tachycardia, low pyrexia; flushing or pallor.

Later:

1. Profuse visual and tactile illusions and hallucinations (pink elephants rare; rats, snakes, and nameless small animals common, vivid, and terrifying).
2. Auditory hallucinations may be threatening or persecutory.
3. Disorientation and confusion.

Treatment

This is an urgent matter; the patient is **admitted to hospital** and:

1. **Sedation** is essential with chlormethiazole or diazepam, which have **anti-convulsant properties** in addition to being tranquillizers. These can be given four-hourly and intravenously if necessary. They should be given on a reducing regime and stopped after, at most, fourteen days.
2. Parenteral administration of **B vitamins** can prevent Wernicke's encephalopathy if instituted early.
3. **Fluid replacement** may be necessary as dehydration can be severe. Electrolyte balance must be obtained: hypokalaemia and hypomagnesaemia are common.
4. **Hypoglycaemia** is common and can cause serious cerebral damage. The infusion fluid should therefore include **dextrose.**
5. Concurrent **infection or head injury** often accompany the delirium and treatment is instituted as necessary.
6. Once the acute phase is over the patient will require continuing **sedation at night** when vivid nightmares result from REM rebound. To avoid dependence on the sedative drug a *reducing regime lasting for approximately ten days* is used.
7. Upon recovery, the patient must be examined for all the *effects of alcohol* including evidence of chronic alcoholic brain damage (see p. 163). Assess motivation for treatment of alcoholism.

Course

Delirium tremens usually resolves in three days but continuing high levels of anxiety may continue for weeks or months afterwards. These require treatment as they contribute to the risk of the patient rapidly returning to alcohol.

Mortality of DTs has been 10–15 per cent with death due to epileptic fits, heart failure, infection, or self-injury during the most disturbed phase.

DEMENTIA
(also known as CHRONIC BRAIN SYNDROME)

Although some clinicians use these terms interchangeably, others reserve the term 'dementia' for those chronic brain syndromes which are irreversible.

Epidemiology

It is estimated that 10 per cent of the population over sixty-five years are affected by dementia. This figure rises to 22 per cent in the over eighty-year-olds (see p. 300). The majority remain in the community and less than one-fifth of the severe cases are admitted to hospital or live in an old people's home.

Terminology

Chronic brain syndromes require investigation to establish their cause, as some are reversible. Those chronic brain syndromes presenting before the age of sixty-five years are known as the **pre-senile dementias,** while **senile dementia** applies to syndromes occurring over the age of sixty-five years. **Senile dementia of Alzheimer's type (SDAT)** and **multi-infarct dementia** are the commonest forms. **Pick's disease** is less common and **Huntington's chorea** and **Creutzfeld–Jacob disease** are least common.

Clinical features

PRESENTATION

Failure of memory may be so insidious that it does not attract medical attention until it is very pronounced. There may be progressive failure to cope with social situations, or matters may come to a head when normal routines are disturbed, and the patient is unable to cope.

FEATURES

1. **Memory impairment (amnesia)** without clouding of consciousness is the hallmark of the syndrome. This is often first noticed by relatives and workmates rather than the patient himself, who may even deny the impairment. It may be so gradual that it is difficult to date the onset. Minor forgetfulness, failure to remember names and appointments, lead on to more definite evidence of amnesia. The patient may lose his way in familiar territory, a decline in performance at work may become evident, and the patient may become hopelessly mixed up with complex tasks at home such

as cooking from a recipe. Leaving the gas on, wandering at night, and forgetting the day are common ways in which the memory loss is brought to the attention of others. The impairment of memory is global, but loss of short-term memory is a conspicuous early sign with relative preservation of long-term memory initially. Recall is affected and the person may need prompts even for previously well-established memory traces. Some patients conceal their memory loss by using lists and sticking to a strict daily routine. A spouse or other close relative may have tolerated and helped to compensate for the patient's memory loss, in which case the death or move of the relative will bring the difficulties to light.

2. **Personality deterioration** reflects both intellectual deterioration and changes in social awareness. The earliest change may be an exacerbation of personality traits producing obsessional or hypochondriacal symptoms. Loss of manners may occur; the person ignores the feelings of others and becomes increasingly stubborn, irritable, and withdrawn. In later stages personal care and hygiene deteriorate with food stains on clothing and chaotic living conditions resulting. Eventually urinary and faecal incontinence occur but the patient may have become so apathetic that he appears unconcerned by this.

3. **Thinking** becomes slowed and restricted with a tendency to brood on a few themes from the past. Perseveration occurs. The dementing person cannot cope with new ideas and abstract thinking is lost. Concentration is impaired and the person becomes easily fatigued. Judgement is impaired, and ideas of reference or even delusions develop because the power to reason is lost. Thus an item which is lost through forgetfulness and later found is regarded by the person as evidence that an intruder has been in the house. In later stages thinking is confined to very few themes and may become incoherent. These abnormalities of thinking are reflected in the speech of the dementing person, which is slow, impoverished, and may eventually become a series of incomprehensible words and phrases.

4. **Psychiatric symptoms**, traditionally associated with the functional psychoses, can occasionally occur as the presenting sign of an organic brain syndrome. Between one-third and one-half of patients with Alzheimer's disease will have such a symptom at some stage in their illness. They include: delusions, paranoid ideas, hallucinations (mainly visual or auditory), misidentifications (of other people, of themselves in a mirror, of events on television; or a belief others are in the house), affective disturbance (usually depression but occasionally mania), and behavioural disturbances (such as aggression, wandering, sexual disinhibition, and eating disorders). Some changes may be understandable in the light of amnesia (accusing a relative of stealing a handbag when in reality it has been lost). Irritability occurs and occasionally emotional lability (unprovoked outbursts of anger, distress, or laughter) but these are said to be commoner in vascular dementia. Occurring during cognitive testing, an outburst of frustration and tears is deemed a **catastrophic reaction**.

5. **Aphasia, apraxia, agnosia**. These are signs of cortical dysfunction. Aphasia is usually a mixture of receptive and expressive and may be manifest as an inability

to name objects on confrontation (anomia). Apraxia indicates an inability to carry out a motor task, despite intact motor and sensory symptoms, and is manifest by an inability to dress properly or to use a knife and fork. Agnosia reflects an inability to recognize people or objects. Occasionally, the presenting symptom of dementia may be an inability to recognize a close friend or relative.

Diagnostic criteria

Dementia may be defined as an acquired global impairment of intellect, memory, and personality without impairment of consciousness.

For research purposes it can be diagnosed when there is **loss of intellectual abilities** sufficiently severe to interfere with social or occupational functioning, memory impairment, and at least ONE of the following, in the absence of clouding of consciousness:

1. Impairment of **abstract thinking**.
2. Impaired **judgement**.
3. **Aphasia, apraxia, agnosia,** or **constructional difficulty**.
4. **Personality change**.

Aetiology

Senile dementia will be discussed in Chapter 19 (see p. 300); we will here consider *chronic brain syndromes occurring before the age of sixty-five*.

The degenerative causes of such chronic brain syndromes (sometimes called **pre-senile dementias**) are sufficiently important to be discussed separately.

ALZHEIMER'S DISEASE

This is one of the common forms of pre-senile dementia.

Familial cases have been described with autosomal dominant inheritance but generally a multifactorial inheritance is suggested. The morbid risk of first-degree relatives of patients with Alzheimer's disease is increased four times.

Onset is uncommon before age forty, and females predominate over men. In the first phase of the illness there is failing memory, muddled inefficiency over the tasks of life, and spatial disorientation. The patient may be apathetic, or perplexed and agitated. In the next stage the patient develops more rapid signs of intellectual deterioration and parietal lobe symptoms (see p. 171) and extra-pyramidal symptoms may appear. Delusions and hallucinations may occur. In the final stage there is a profound apathetic dementia with the patient bedridden and doubly incontinent. The EEG is always abnormal.

Neuropathology and neurochemistry: cortical atrophy is generalized but most marked over the frontal and temporal lobes. Loss of neurones in the neocortex, together with proliferation of astrocytes, senile plaques, and neurofibrillary tangles, are striking, and in greater number than in the normal aged brain. Clinical manifestations of dementia appear when the plaque count and neurofibrillary changes reach a certain threshold. In normal ageing the brain seems to have sufficient reserve capacity to withstand a limited amount of such changes and yet maintain normal function.

There is a **loss of cholinergic neurones** innervating the neocortex: the loss of these neurones is indicated by marked reductions in the concentration of the enzymes *choline-acetyltransferase* and *cholinesterase*. Much of the cholinergic innervation of the neocortex originates from the nucleus basalis of Meynert located at the base of the forebrain; neurones in this nucleus degenerate in Alzheimer's disease. The importance of cholinergic mechanisms has been demonstrated: cholinergic drugs, such as the cholinesterase inhibitor *physostigmine*, cause a transient improvement in memory functions in patients suffering from Alzheimer-type dementia, whereas anti-cholinergic drugs, such as the muscarinic receptor antagonist scopolamine, have the opposite effect. Since cortical postsynaptic muscarinic receptors remain relatively unaffected in Alzheimer's disease, attempts have been made to stimulate these receptors by *cholinomimetic agents* (choline, lecithin) administered to the patients: these efforts, however, have remained unsuccessful.

Apart from cholinergic neurones, noradrenergic and 5-hydroxytryptaminergic neurones innervating the neocortex can also degenerate, resulting in reductions in cortical noradrenaline and 5-hydroxytryptamine levels. Consistent decreases have been shown in the cortical levels of *somatostatin*, indicating the degeneration of nerve cells containing this neuropeptide transmitter.

MULTIPLE-INFARCT DEMENTIA (ARTERIOSCLEROTIC DEMENTIA)

This results from repeated cerebrovascular accidents, often from cerebral emboli. Other evidence of arteriosclerosis is found throughout the cardiovascular system and focal signs such as pseudobulbar palsy, increased reflexes, extensor plantar responses, and extra-pyramidal features occur more often than in Alzheimer's disease. Marked cerebral softening occurs in this type of dementia and this differentiates it from Alzheimer's disease, where senile plaques predominate.

Onset is uncommon before the age of fifty, and the sex ratio is approximately equal. The most striking difference between this type of dementia and Alzheimer's disease is the step-wise progression, and the presence of the evidence of arteriosclerosis on physical examination. Patients may complain of somatic symptoms such as headache, dizziness, tinnitus, and syncope in addition to problems with memory. There may be transient attacks of hemiparesis, dysphasia, or visual dysfunctions which are at first followed by restitution, but which eventually lead to the dementia becoming more profound.

PICK'S DISEASE

This is less common than Alzheimer's disease, but a familial pattern is also well recognized. The frontal and temporal lobes are particularly atrophied. Personality changes and dysphasia therefore occur early in the disease. Neuronal loss occurs with gliosis but plaques and tangles do not and the EEG may be normal.

HUNTINGTON'S CHOREA

This disorder is characterized by a combination of pre-senile dementia, extra-pyramidal features, and choreic movements. The transmission of this disease by a single autosomal *dominant gene* is well recognized, with half the offspring of an affected person being affected. It is now becoming possible to identify some of the carriers of the gene. Reduced levels of GABA in the basal ganglia and substantia nigra are thought to be responsible for the choreiform movements. The dementia often appears slowly and later in the disease than the neurological or psychotic features. The latter start with personality changes, such as becoming quarrelsome, slow, and apathetic, but schizophrenic symptoms and marked mood changes occur.

The frontal lobe shows greatest atrophy along with the caudate nuclei and marked dilatation of the ventricles.

CREUTZFELD–JACOB DISEASE

Cerebral atrophy is less marked in this form of dementia but a characteristic spongy appearance of the grey matter is seen microscopically along with neuronal loss and proliferation of astrocytes. This may occur in different parts of the brain, accounting for the different clinical presentations. The *EEG is always abnormal* with increased slow-wave activity and bilateral spike-wave discharges which accompany the characteristic myoclonic jerks. It has been demonstrated that this disease can be transmitted from people to primates experimentally, and some instances have occurred when there has been 'natural' transmission. It is therefore believed that a slow virus or virus-like particle is responsible, and the illness has been related to Kuru. It is probable that the virus-like particle fails to invoke the usual inflammatory response in the brain and a similar aetiological factor is being sought in other forms of pre-senile dementia.

ALCOHOLIC DEMENTIA

There is increasing evidence that cerebral atrophy occurs in a proportion of those who have drunk heavily for many years. In the early years the chronic brain syndrome associated with alcoholism appears to be reversible.

Non-degenerative causes of dementia are shown as *Table 11.2*. Four *neurological diseases* are worth highlighting.

NORMAL PRESSURE HYDROCEPHALUS

This is a form of hydrocephalus in which there is an obstruction in the subarachnoid space to the free egress of CSF from the ventricles. Memory impairment, a stiff-legged shuffling gait, urinary incontinence, and slowness develop over weeks or months. The EEG is frequently abnormal; but the diagnosis is confirmed by CAT scan, which shows symmetrical ventricular enlargement but no enlargement of the subarachnoid space

Table 11.2 *Causes of dementia*

	systemic	intracranial
degenerative		see text, pp. 161–3 boxing encephalopathy
space-occupying lesions	secondaries	cerebral tumours* subdural haematomas* normal pressure hydrocephalus*
infections		neurosyphilis* (GPI or meningovascular) chronic encephalitis
anoxic	anaemia* congestive cardiac failure* chronic respiratory failure	carbon monoxide poisoning post-cardiac arrest
metabolic	uraemia* liver failure* remote effects of carcinoma	
endocrine	myxoedema* Addison's disease* hypoglycaemia* parathyroid disease*	
toxic	barbiturates,* bromides* mananese, carbon disulphide	alcohol atrophy
vitamin deficiency	B12 and folic acid deficiency* thiamine deficiency* nicotinic acid deficiency*	

Note: * = potentially reversible cause for chronic brain syndrome.

above the basal cisterns. Treatment is by insertion of a **shunt** with a low-pressure, one-way valve between the lateral ventricle and the superior vena cava. Results are variable, but sometimes impressive.

NEUROSYPHILIS

General paralysis of the insane (*GPI*) has become something of a rarity, but was at one time an important cause of a chronic brain syndrome accompanied by highly characteristic neurological signs (Argyll–Robertson pupils, trombone tremor of tongue, dysarthria, ataxia, and upper motor neurone signs). *Meningo-vascular syphilis* presents with headache and lethargy which proceeds to a dementia: there may be a basal meningitis with cranial nerve palsies and a wide variety of other neurological signs depending on the area involved.

PARKINSON'S SYNDROME

Arteriosclerosis may underlie both the dementia and movement disorders in Parkinson's syndrome. But dementia has also been reported in cases of idiopathic Parkinsonism, the aetiology of which is uncertain.

MULTIPLE SCLEROSIS

Minor cognitive impairment can be detected in the majority of patients with multiple sclerosis. Profound global dementia is uncommon but is rarely the presenting feature of the illness.

When investigating a case of chronic brain syndrome it is especially important to detect conditions which may be either arrested or partially reversed, and these have been asterisked in *Table 11.2*.

Differential diagnosis

DEMENTIA MUST BE DIFFERENTIATED FROM FUNCTIONAL ILLNESSES

1. **Depressive pseudo-dementia.** Old patients who are depressed may appear to be demented, in that they complain of defective memory, appear disorientated, have a poor knowledge of current events, and perform poorly on cognitive tests. A detailed history from an informant should differentiate the initial depressed mood leading to later disturbance of memory from the picture of dementia which starts with memory and behavioural impairments but leads on to depression at a later stage. A past history of a depressive episode, depressive symptoms antedating other symptoms, and a more acute onset should put one on the right track.

2. **Hysterical pseudodementia.** A patient may be brought to a casualty department having been found wandering and unable to give his name and address (see **hysterical amnesia,** *p. 337). Alternatively a patient may be admitted with suspected dementia but close observation reveals inconsistencies between his poor performance on formal cognitive testing and his ability to find his way around the ward.

   The **Ganser syndrome** consists of 'talking past the point' and giving 'approximate answers':

How many legs does a horse have?
Five.
What colours are the lights on a traffic light?
Red, yellow, and blue.

The patient's answers are markedly inaccurate, yet they indicate that the question has been understood. The absurd responses are given deliberately and with apparently serious intent. The playful, childish quality of some of the patient's answers is also seen in the **'buffoonery syndromes'** associated with hebephrenic schizophrenia or chronic hypomania. The patient may also report hallucinatory experiences, have a fluctuating level of consciousness, and demonstrate other hysterical phenomena (see p. 239). Such states are most likely among those with low IQ and a history of previous head injury. Either hysterical mechanisms or conscious simulation (malingering; see p. 238) may be involved.

3. **Psychotic illness.** *Hypomania* may appear as a picture of dementia especially as formal cognitive testing is difficult or impossible. Chronic schizophrenics with prominent defect symptoms may also appear demented. The other characteristics of the illness should be clear from the history.

DEMENTIA MUST ALSO BE DISTINGUISHED FROM OTHER ORGANIC ILLNESS

1. **Korsakow's syndrome** (see p. 168). Here the disorder is confined to short-term memory and disorientation in time, whereas chronic brain syndrome is a global syndrome involving ability to think, lability of emotion, and changes of personality.

2. **Acute brain syndrome** (see p. 151). Here the onset is more acute, and there is clouding of consciousness. In chronic brain syndrome the patient is more in touch with his surroundings, and attempts to cooperate despite cognitive difficulties. In acute brain syndrome the patient fluctuates, and can sometimes be shown to be cognitively intact in lucid intervals. Severe perceptual disturbances are more likely in acute brain syndrome.

3. **Focal brain syndromes.** Focal neurological signs are of great importance in localizing disease within the brain. In the degenerative pre-senile dementias neurological signs are usually symmetrical. If dysphasia is produced by focal disease patients have as much difficulty recalling objects from sight as from memory, whereas patients with diffuse chronic brain disease do much better if they can handle and see the object.

4. **Mental retardation.** A careful history will reveal that the patient's problems are not of recent origin, and psychometric tests will show a vocabulary in keeping with verbal and performance IQ, whereas in dementia there will be relative preservation of vocabulary.

Investigations of chronic brain syndrome

CONFIRMATION OF THE DIAGNOSIS

Psychometric testing (see p. 70) when the patient is not physically ill, in pain, unduly depressed, or anxious.

INVESTIGATION OF POSSIBLE CAUSES

Interview an informant to obtain the following information:

1. Possible family history of dementia or Huntington's chorea.
2. Previous head injuries: even slight ones may be important.
3. Recent history of faints, fits, or episodes of collapse.
4. What drugs have been taken? Is there possible dietary neglect?
5. What is the patient's usage of alcohol?
6. Obtain description of the personality before illness. Ask about previous episodes of depression.
7. What is the duration of the patient's symptoms? (Short duration suggests tumour, covert infarction, or extracranial causes.)

PHYSICAL INVESTIGATIONS TO DISCOVER REMEDIABLE CAUSES

All patients should have the following:

1. Haemoglobin, full blood count, viscosity.
2. Wasserman reaction or equivalent.
3. Blood urea, electrolytes, calcium, and phosphate.
4. Liver function tests, cholesterol, and plasma proteins.
5. B_{12} and folate.
6. Thyroid function tests.
7. Urine should be examined microscopically, and cultured if necessary.
8. Chest and skull X-ray.
9. EEG.
10. CAT scan (if available).

THE FOLLOWING MAY BE CARRIED OUT IF INDICATED

1. Lumbar puncture (if no cause has been found from other tests).
2. Anti-nuclear antibodies.
3. ECG.

Treatment

This depends upon the aetiology. **Reversible causes** (see *Table 11.2*) must be **detected as early as possible** and vigorously treated.

Non-progressive disorders such as trauma may show improvement over the year following injury; and share with reversible causes a need for active rehabilitation. A decision on long-term care should only be taken when the patient has reached his optimal level of function.

Progressive causes of dementia (for example, Alzheimer's disease) will inevitably cause deterioration, requiring progressive care facilities in the community and eventual residential care.

GENERAL MEASURES

Any physical illness that is present (this is common in the elderly) must be treated, and **hearing or visual deficits** corrected as far as possible. **Anti-depressant treatment** is indicated if depression is severe. **Sedation** may be required for behavioural disturbance, but should only be prescribed if the patient is disruptive or is a danger to others. It may make matters worse.

Continuation of normal life at home should be aimed at if it is possible, since this provides sufficient stimulus and the familiar surroundings which help to preserve functions. Increased social support will become necessary and attendance at a day-centre or day-hospital can provide further systematic assessment and stimulating daily routine. The needs of relatives at home must be considered if they are to be able and willing to continue the care of an increasingly dependent person.

Course and prognosis

The course of dementia is variable. Creutzfeld–Jacob disease leads to the most rapid deterioration, with half the patients being dead within nine months. Alzheimer's disease usually leads to death within two to five years. With multi-infarct dementia the course is variable, with many patients dying within five years of the diagnosis. The latter dementia often has a step-wise deterioration determined by further cerebrovascular accidents.

FOCAL BRAIN SYNDROMES

Wernicke's encephalopathy and Korsakow's syndrome

Wernicke's encephalopathy is a subacute brain syndrome caused by a deficiency of thiamine. **Korsakow's syndrome** is a chronic brain syndrome with the same cause. The acute symptoms of the former syndrome may incompletely resolve leaving the clinical picture of the latter.

EPIDEMIOLOGY

The condition is found throughout adult life, most often in the forties and fifties, and is twice as common in men as in women.

CLINICAL FEATURES

Wernicke's encephalopathy is a subacute brain syndrome accompanied by ocular palsies (especially abducent palsies, conjugate deviation gaze palsies, and nystagmus) and ataxia of gait. There may be prodromal nausea and there will usually be a marked memory disorder.

It is not confined to alcoholics, and can occur with thiamine deficiency from any cause (that is, dietary, carcinoma of the stomach, toxaemia of pregnancy, pernicious anaemia).

Korsakow's syndrome refers to the selective memory disturbance that is revealed once the generalized cognitive impairment of the acute state clears. Immediate recall (registration) is intact, but the *ability to form new memories* is grossly deficient (see p. 37). The patient is, usually *disorientated in time,* but other modalities may also be affected.

Long-term memories are relatively well preserved. The patient may provide plausible but incorrect answers to questions that he cannot answer – *confabulation.* There is also an apathy or air of blandness and lack of concern about the failure to answer the questions correctly. Other aspects of cognitive functioning are preserved and the patient does not show clouding of consciousness. Peripheral neuropathy occurs commonly with these disorders.

NEUROPATHOLOGY

Symmetrical lesions are found in the walls of the third ventricle, the periaqueductal region, and the floor of the fourth ventricle; also the medial dorsal nuclei of the thalamus and the mamillary bodies. There is proliferation of blood vessels and glia, with petechial haemorrhages. Ocular signs are related to lesions in the third and sixth cranial nuclei, nystagmus to lesions in the vestibular nuclei, and ataxia to lesions in the vestibular nuclei and the vermis of the cerebellum.

Most cases are due to thiamine deficiency, but rarer causes of damage to this part of the brain are: bilateral temporal lobectomy, tumours of the third ventricle, anoxic brain damage, subarachnoid haemorrhage, tuberculous meningitis, and viral encephalitis.

DIFFERENTIAL DIAGNOSIS

Acute brain syndrome of other causes. The history of alcoholism is helpful but in Wernicke's encephalopathy the neurological signs confirm the diagnosis, while in Korsakow's syndrome there will be absence of clouding. The neurological signs also help to distinguish the condition from delirium tremens, another acute brain syndrome resulting from alcoholism, which is four times more common than Wernicke's encephalopathy.

Chronic brain syndrome. The specific nature of the memory defect is the principal differentiating feature. Chronic alcohol ingestion may lead to a chronic brain syndrome because of cerebral atrophy (see p. 163).

INVESTIGATIONS

Psychometric testing will identify the specific memory impairment necessary to make the diagnosis. Take blood for pyruvate assay as soon as possible, and before giving intravenous parenterovite. Only if the expected history of heavy drinking is not obtained need the other causes be considered.

A lumbar puncture, EEG, and CAT scan would then be helpful. Investigations to identify other damage resulting from alcohol are appropriate.

TREATMENT

Wernicke's encephalopathy requires urgent treatment with large doses of thiamine, with the intention of treating the acute symptoms and modifying the memory impairment. The vitamin is given together with other vitamins of the B group intravenously initially ('Parenterovite' contains 250 mg of thiamine in each ampoule), then intramuscularly. Other aspects of management are attention to infection, dehydration, and electrolyte balance. Bed rest is required initially. Sedation may be required and is similar to that used for delirium tremens.

COURSE AND PROGNOSIS

Sixth nerve palsies clear rapidly with prompt treatment, ataxia clears over a few months in many patients, but the neuropathy resolves slowly if at all.

The subacute brain syndrome sometimes clears rapidly without lasting amnesia. Otherwise it clears over one to two months, leaving the amnesia, which only shows any subsequent improvement in half of the patients. In this chronic state the retrograde amnesia is pronounced, there is apathy, but confabulation is rare.

Temporal lobe lesions

Lesions of the *dominant temporal lobe* produce sensory dysphasia together with alexia and agraphia if the lesion extends posteriorly towards the parietal lobe. *Non-dominant temporal lobe lesions* may be relatively asymptomatic though visuospatial difficulties may occur. *Bilateral lesions of the medial parts of the temporal lobes* are those which cause severe memory deficits in the absence of other intellectual impairment.

Of special interest to the psychiatrist are temporal lobe lesions which present with personality change, unpredictable aggressive behaviour, and 'symptomatic schizophrenias' associated with chronic lesions. These have been recognized principally in relation to temporal lobe epilepsy (see p. 148).

Frontal lobe syndrome

Frontal lobe tumours may present to the psychiatrist because of the predominance of behavioural and mood changes over neurological signs. Lateral lesions have been associated with disturbances of volition and psychomotor activity, whereas lesions in the medial and orbital areas affect the limbic system and reticular formation leading to disinhibition and mood changes.

The patient typically shows *lack of spontaneity* and initiative and a general diminution of motor activity, although when others provide the stimulus he may behave quite normally. The mood is one of rather inappropriate mild *euphoria* – sometimes described as a 'fatuous jocularity' – alternating with apathy, irritability, or even depression. *Over-familiarity* occurs sometimes progressing to sexual disinhibition. The patient seems unaware of his unsocial behaviour and irresponsible attitude. Judgement and foresight are impaired. Cognitive functions are largely unimpaired although specific tests for frontal lobe function are available. Neurological signs include combinations of optic atrophy and papilloedema if the lesion involves the optic nerves, or contralateral spastic paresis, grasp reflex, increased tendon reflexes, and a positive Babinski response if the lesion extends posteriorly on to the motor cortex.

Parietal lobe lesions

There are changes in the cognitive and visuospatial spheres: *agnosia* is a disturbance of recognition without sensory disturbance or intellectual impairment. *Apraxia* is the inability to carry out motor activity when motor and sensory systems are intact. Lesions of either parietal lobe produce visuospatial difficulties.

Right (non-dominant) hemisphere lesions produce:

1. Neglect of contralateral sensory field and anosagnosia (failure to recognize disabilities on that side).
2. Disturbance of body image.
3. Dressing apraxia.
4. Visuospatial agnosia (constructional apraxia).
5. Inability to follow a route on map ('topographagnosia').

Left (dominant) hemisphere lesions produce:

1. Motor aphasia (anterior lesions).
2. Sensory aphasia (posterior lesions).
3. Difficulty writing and drawing ('dysgraphia').
4. Difficulty reading ('dyslexia').
5. Right–left disorientation.

HEAD INJURY

The severity of brain damage

A patient who has sustained a closed head injury will report a loss of memory from some time before the injury to the time of the injury itself – called the *retrograde amnesia*, or *RA* – and a loss of memory from the time of the injury to some time afterwards when consecutive memory resumes – called the *post-traumatic amnesia*, or *PTA*. The RA is usually considerably shorter than the PTA, and does not in any case give a very reliable indication of brain damage. The two factors from the history which best correlate with the severity of organic damage are the *duration of unconsciousness* and the *duration of the post-traumatic amnesia*. Most of those who report a PTA of more than twenty-four hours will be fortunate if they recover without some degree of intellectual impairment.

The location of brain damage

The effects of location of brain injury on subsequent psychological dysfunction can be examined by studying soldiers who have suffered penetrating injuries to the brain. *Frontal lobe damage* causes severe effects on both mood and behaviour, with injuries to the orbital surface producing severe effects on the personality such as lack of perseverance, inability to maintain relationships, and disinhibition especially affecting sexual and aggressive impulses, while those on the convex lateral surface produce lack of drive, indifference, and incapacity for decisions.

Left hemisphere lesions are associated with global intellectual impairment as well as dysphasias and impaired memory, while injuries to the *right hemisphere* are followed by affective and behavioural disorders and by somatic complaints. Injury to the *parietal or temporal lobes* is associated with intellectual impairment and dysphasia.

Long-term psychological sequelae of closed head injury

Since there are many possible sequelae, we will organize our account by starting at the top of our hierarchy (see p. 50) and working downwards.

CHRONIC BRAIN SYNDROME

In very severe head injuries the chronic brain syndrome will be accompanied by dysphasias and quadriparesis, and the patient may be apathetic, slow, or even mute. Control of affect will be poor, and loss of libido is the rule. Such severe disabilities present formidable problems for rehabilitation, although assessment is usually straightforward. The main problems of assessment are presented by minor degrees of global damage involving minimal degrees of intellectual impairment and claims for compensation.

POST-TRAUMATIC EPILEPSY

This develops in about 5 per cent of closed head injuries and over 30 per cent of injuries involving penetration of the dura mater. After closed head injury, temporal lobe epilepsy (see p. 145) is the commonest form, and is the form most likely to be followed by psychiatric disability. Epilepsy developing in the year following injury is particularly likely to be associated with psychiatric disability.

PSYCHOTIC ILLNESS

A *post-traumatic psychosis* refers to a psychotic illness manifest as soon as consciousness is resumed after injury: these usually remit with treatment. There is an increased incidence of all types of psychotic illness after head injury, although the available evidence suggests that there is a constitutional predisposition in cases of schizophrenia and affective psychosis, so that the role of the head injury is to increase the likelihood of the disorder being manifested.

DEPRESSIVE ILLNESS

Symptoms of affective illness are very common after head injury, and all combinations of non-psychotic symptomatology occur. Indeed *suicide* accounts for 14 per cent of all deaths following head injury. A triad of persistent headache, dizziness, and irritability is sometimes described as a *post-concussional syndrome*, although the longer it lasts the more it tends to merge with non-specific patterns of psychiatric disorder, and the less likely are such symptoms to be a pure expression of brain damage. Abnormal illness behaviours, such as hypochondriacal symptoms (see p. 236) and hysterical symptoms (see p. 239), commonly accompany such illnesses. Obsessional neuroses (see p. 228) have also been shown to be more common after head injury.

One theoretically important study compared head-injured twins with their normal co-twins some ten years following the injury. Although the head-injured twin was found to be inferior to the normal co-twin on a variety of tests of intellectual function, such differences were subtle and unobtrusive in everyday life. The MZ twins were more concordant than the DZ twins for the 'post-concussional' symptoms described above; and those twins thought to have shown a 'change in personality' consisting of tension, fatiguability, and lessened ability to work were found to have co-twins with the same traits. Once more, it is clear that constitutional predisposition to such symptoms must play a major role, with the function of the head injury being to release the symptoms in the short term.

PERSONALITY DISORDER

The personality changes which go to make up the *frontal lobe syndrome* (see p. 171) have already been referred to, while another pattern consists of *explosive aggressive outbursts* on minor provocation. As you have seen from the twin study reported above, constitutional factors are likely to play a decisive role in the development of non-specific 'neurotic' symptoms.

FURTHER READING

Lishman, A. (1990) *Organic Psychiatry*. Oxford: Blackwell Scientific.

12 / SCHIZOPHRENIA AND ALLIED STATES

EPIDEMIOLOGY

Approximately 1 per cent of adults are diagnosed as schizophrenic at some time during their lives. The inception rate (new illnesses) is 15 to 20 per 100,000 in the UK, and the point prevalence is about 200 per 100,000. The large difference between these figures implies a mean duration of illness of approximately fifteen years; schizophrenia is often a chronic condition, but the course of the illness may vary greatly.

Recent studies have demonstrated that the incidence of schizophrenia is similar in countries all over the world but tends to run a less chronic course in the developing countries. The peak incidence occurs between twenty-five and thirty years of age and there is another smaller peak in the over sixty-five age group.

Although higher rates of schizophrenia are found in lower social classes and in central zones of large cities, these findings are the result of the illness rather than its cause. The social class distribution of fathers of patients with schizophrenia approximates to that of the general population and the downward social drift is accounted for by the many handicaps that accompany schizophrenia. These also result in people with chronic schizophrenia living alone in the cheap hotels and lodging houses that are found in the centres of large cities.

CLINICAL FEATURES

Schizophrenia is a term used to describe a syndrome of abnormalities in the history and mental state. This does not imply a particular cause or course of the symptoms, which may be quite variable. There is frequently a *prodromal stage* in which non-specific symptoms such as loss of interest, neglect of personal hygiene, and mild affective symptoms precede frank psychotic phenomena. The psychotic symptoms occur in several spheres and are divided into *positive* and *negative* symptoms.

Positive symptoms
(sometimes called type 1 schizophrenic symptoms)

These are made worse by *over-arousal* and respond to medication with *neuroleptics.*

1. **Contact with reality** is reduced. The normal mental processes which allow clear differentiation between subjective experiences and the outside world break down. The patient may state that his thoughts are known to others or are not his own, that is, caused by others (**disorders of thought possession**). His own movements, or his own feelings and impulses, may be experienced as being generated by, or under the control of, other people or forces (**passivity phenomena**). In **thought withdrawal** the patient feels that his thoughts are being actively removed from his head ('*My thoughts are removed by a phrenological vacuum extractor*'). These phenomena are sometimes described as **disintegrative delusions** (see p. 49).

2. **Hallucinations** are common, usually of the auditory type. Thus the person with schizophrenia may experience his own thoughts as coming from the outside world spoken aloud (**thought echo**). Another typical form is for the patient to hear himself referred to as 'he' or 'him' (**third-person auditory hallucinations**). (Other auditory hallucinations which are common in schizophrenia are voices which make obscene, threatening, or highly critical comments: *but these occur in other conditions as well.*)

3. **Thinking** may become disturbed so that the patient's speech shows unusual logic, idiosyncratic use of words or made-up words, called **neologisms** (see p. 27). Associations between concepts becomes loosened, so the usual flow of logical ideas is replaced by passages of speech which are difficult to follow ('knight's move' in thought, or 'derailment'). In **schizophrenic thought disorder** the patient's speech contains thoughts which do not directly follow from one another (see p. 27).

4. **Delusions** of various types may occur. Delusions which cannot be derived from some other abnormality are called **primary delusions.** (see p. 31). A form of primary delusional experience which is diagnostic of schizophrenia is called **delusional perception** (see p. 31). Such experiences usually have a vivid quality, and are well remembered by the patient. (As a result of abnormal experiences such as hallucinations, the patient may develop **secondary delusions,** so that X-rays, computers, bugging devices, witchcraft, or hypnosis may be blamed for the occurrence of these phenomena. These should be thought of as the patient's attempts to make sense of his puzzling experiences, and *they are of no diagnostic significance in their own right.*)

5. The normal **control of emotions may be disturbed**, with outbursts of laughter or anger without any appropriate stimulus (**incongruous affect**). This may occur spontaneously but may also reflect the patient's psychotic experiences – threatening hallucinations, or the experience of being controlled by others – and may cause resentment or hostility in the patient.

Negative symptoms

(sometimes called type 2 schizophrenic symptoms)

These symptoms are exacerbated by living in an *under-stimulating environment* and contribute to the features of *institutionalization*; in some patients they are associated with enlarged cerebral ventricles on CAT scan and 'soft' neurological signs.

1. **Poverty of speech.** The patient has little to say for himself, and tends to give empty or laconic replies to questions. The patient's thinking has lost richness and complexity, and this is reflected in his speech.

2. **Slowness of thought and movement** also contribute to the picture of an unresponsive person and clear psychomotor retardation may occur.

3. **Emotional flatness** tends to accompany slowness and poverty of speech, and refers to the absence of normal modulation of mood, with lack of facial expressiveness and emotional responsiveness.

4. **Loss of volition** indicates that the patient seems unable to motivate himself to work satisfactorily or, in severe forms, even to be able to care for himself on a day-to-day basis. Movements and speech become slow. This lack of drive leads to under-activity and social withdrawal – symptoms which are greatly exacerbated if the patient lives in an under-stimulating environment.

Many other psychotic phenomena may occur (see Chapter 3) but these are not characteristic of schizophrenia and may occur with any psychotic illness. In addition, patients with schizophrenia may complain of depression, anxiety, irritability, and somatic symptoms of tension. However, in the presence of schizophrenic phenomena symptoms from lower down the diagnostic hierarchy (see p. 49) do not alter the diagnosis.

Classification of schizophrenic disorders

Schizophrenia is best regarded as a group of disorders, rather than a single entity. Because it is stigmatizing to be diagnosed as a 'schizophrenic', and acute transient illnesses with schizophrenia-like symptoms but full recovery are fairly common, patients who have had illnesses lasting for less than a month are said to have **'schizophrenia-like disorders'** rather than schizophrenia. The main groupings of the established illness were originally described by Emil Kraepelin as **paranoid, hebephrenic, and catatonic**. This classification is still used, although in England the last two are now seen only rarely. After a number of years these groups tend to merge into one another anyway, and patients with persisting illnesses from all groups show the same features: **residual or chronic schizophrenia.**

Acute schizophrenia-like disorder

An acute psychotic disorder in which hallucinations, delusions, and perceptual disturbances may be present, and in which emotional turmoil – ecstasy, irritability, or anxiety – is frequent. Typical schizophrenic symptoms may also be present, but the most characteristic feature of the disorder is an *unstable, changing clinical picture which will typically have had an acute onset, and will resolve rapidly.* (If schizophrenic symptoms persist for more than a month the patient will then fulfil requirements for a diagnosis of schizophrenia.) In a proportion of these patients there is clear precipitating stress.

Paranoid schizophrenia (F20.0)

This is the commonest form of schizophrenia, characterized by stable, often persecutory delusions which are usually accompanied by auditory hallucinations and other perceptual distortions such as sexual and other bodily sensations. Hallucinations of taste, smell, and vision may also occur.

Disturbances of volition, affect, and speech are not prominent, there is relatively little deterioration of personality, and the patient may be able to live independently in the community.

Hebephrenic schizophrenia (F20.1)

Disturbances of affect and volition are common, and thought disorder is usually prominent. Delusions and hallucinations are fleeting and fragmentary, the mood is shallow or inappropriate with silly behaviour, giggling, grimaces, and mannerisms. Thought is disorganized, speech rambling and incoherent. The illness usually starts between the ages of fifteen and twenty-five and has the worst prognosis, with rapid development of negative ('type 2') symptoms.

Catatonic schizophrenia (F20.2)

Prominent psychomotor symptoms are essential to the diagnosis with features such as stupor, excitement, posturing, negativism, catatonic rigidity, waxy flexibility, and command automatisms (see p. 336). The patient alternates between extremes such as stupor and excitement; negativism and automatic obedience. There may be dream-like states with vivid visual scenic hallucinations. This state is now rarely seen in the United Kingdom, but still occurs in the developing world.

Residual ('chronic') schizophrenia (F20.5)

Chronic schizophrenia is characterized by a protracted course and the gradual development of pronounced negative symptoms, leading to pronounced disability. This state must be differentiated from **post-schizophrenic depression** (F20.4), which may follow an acute episode with positive symptoms.

DIAGNOSTIC CRITERIA

Because schizophrenic forms of experience can occur for other reasons, the diagnosis 'schizophrenia' is only made after excluding other conditions.

In the absence of epilepsy, mania, intoxication, or other evidence of gross cerebral damage, the presence of ONE OR MORE of the following symptoms for a period longer than one month indicates a likely diagnosis of schizophrenia:

1. **Disorders of thought possession:**
   - Thought insertion.
   - Thought withdrawal.
   - Thought broadcasting.

2. **Auditory hallucinations in which the person hears:**
   - His own thoughts echoed out aloud ('thought echo').
   - Two or more people discussing or arguing about him in the third person ('He's a silly old man, isn't he?').
   - Voices that form a running commentary on his behaviour ('Now he's drinking his tea').

3. **Passivity experiences:**
   - Feeling that one's movements, thoughts, impulses, or sensations are under some outside control.

4. **Persistent delusions, and delusional perception:**
   - Persistent delusions that are culturally inappropriate and completely impossible (being able to control the weather; being Jesus Christ; being in communication with extra-terrestrial beings).
   - Delusional perception (see p. 31).

The diagnosis should also be considered if the patient has TWO OR MORE of the following:

5. Persistent hallucinations in any modality.
6. Incoherent or irrelevant speech; mannerisms or neologisms.
7. Any catatonic phenomena (see above).
8. Negative symptoms (see above).

Schizophrenia or mania?

Recent studies have demonstrated that typically schizophrenic forms of experience can occur in mania. The differentiation between these two conditions rests on two sets of criteria:

The first regards the **mental state** of the patient; the presence of pronounced elation of mood characterizes **mania**, together with the other features of that condition (see p. 203).

The second regards the **course** of the illness. Repeated episodes of illness occur in both mania and schizophrenia but the latter is more likely to result in a gradual accumulation of negative symptoms, while the former is associated with episodes of depression, and complete recovery between episodes of illness.

DIFFERENTIAL DIAGNOSIS

Symptomatic schizophrenia

Sometimes psychoses resembling schizophrenia occur secondarily to known organic diseases (F06.2) or disorders due to psychoactive substances (F1x.50, where 'x' is a code for the particular substance).

Examples of *organic diseases* include:

1. Temporal lobe epilepsy.
2. Huntington's chorea.
3. Neoplasms of the cerebral cortex.

The psychoses secondary to temporal lobe epilepsy (see p. 145) usually follow some three to five years after the fits, while those secondary to Huntington's chorea usually (but not always) follow the onset of the choreic movements.

Diagnosis of schizophrenia-like illnesses caused by cortical neoplasms depends on eliciting other neurological signs: it means that *every patient with an apparently schizophrenic illness must have a thorough neurological examination.*

Examples of *psychoactive substances* include:

1. Amphetamine.
2. Other stimulant psychoactive substances such as cannabis.

The psychosis secondary to intoxication with amphetamine (or other sympathomimetic amines) can appear identical to paranoid schizophrenia. Since the patient does not always admit to taking drugs, a urine specimen should always be sent for amphetamines in any young person with an unexplained psychotic illness. (If the drug is withdrawn, these psychoses should remit completely within ten days.)

A number of 'hallucinogenic' drugs – such as mescaline, lysergic acid, and psilocylin (the 'magic mushroom') – can produce toxic psychoses which are superficially similar to schizophrenia. However, they are usually readily distinguishable because of the disturbances in time perception and in both colour and shape constancy.

Alcoholic hallucinosis (F10.52) (see p. 212)

Here the primary abnormality is an auditory hallucinosis, and any delusions are secondary.

Delusional disorder (F22)

This is an illness with persecutory or other delusions but without other evidence of schizophrenia. Such patients do not have an increased genetic loading for schizophrenia, but the illness often represents a development of a previous sensitive, suspicious, and rigid personality. The delusions may form a complex and logically elaborated system which leaves other areas of the personality intact. Morbid jealousy and erotomania are specific examples of this syndrome, also convictions that some part of one's body is misshapen, or that one is giving off a bad smell.

Schizoaffective disorder (F25)

This is an episodic disorder in which both affective and schizophrenic symptoms are prominent *within the same episode of illness,* either simultaneously or within a few days of each other. (Patients with separate episodes of schizoaffective episodes and typical episodes of depression or mania should be regarded as having variants of manic-depressive illness – see p. 203.)

NEUROCHEMISTRY

The most influential biological theory of schizophrenia has been the '**dopamine hypothesis**'. This hypothesis assumes a functional abnormality in the mesolimbic and mesocortical dopaminergic neuronal systems of the brain. This theory is based on the effects of drugs: those leading to a stimulation of central dopamine receptors (L-Dopa, amphetamine) can cause 'schizophrenia-like' states; and the most effective drugs in the treatment of schizophrenia, neuroleptics, are potent blockers of central dopamine receptors. Dopamine receptors can be divided into two functional subtypes, D_1 and D_2 receptors. The strongest evidence for the dopamine hypothesis has been the correlation between the ability of anti-psychotics to block central D_2 receptors and their clinically effective dose.

However, some currently available atypical anti-psychotics (for example, clozapine) do not show this relationship, indicating that actions on other receptors are also likely to be important. Attempts to investigate dopamine receptor function in the brain of schizophrenic patients (post mortem or using *in vivo* imaging techniques) have yielded conflicting results. It is clear that anti-psychotic medication increases the number of D_2 receptors in the brain but whether drug-naive schizophrenics have a pre-existing abnormality of brain dopaminergic function remains controversial. Some authors claim that dopamine levels are increased in areas of the limbic system and that the increased numbers of D_2 receptors in the basal ganglia cannot be entirely accounted for by previous anti-psychotic treatment. It is generally agreed, however, that schizophrenia is not caused by simple 'dopamine excess'.

Other neurotransmitters are implicated in schizophrenia, in particular the excitatory amino-acid transmitter **glutamate** (which has functional interactions with dopamine systems). In post-mortem schizophrenic brains an increase in markers for glutamate nerve endings and glutamate receptors has been found in pre-frontal cortical areas, while the opposite, a decrease in both measures, occurs in the medial temporal lobe. This suggests that there may be an abnormality in connections between frontal and temporal areas (both of which have been implicated in schizophrenia) involving glutamate pathways, and it is interesting that phencyclidine, a drug acting on glutamate receptors, has been reported to cause a schizophrenia-like psychosis in normal subjects.

It is clear from the above that it is not possible to hold a simple neurochemical theory of schizophrenia and that a complex interplay between structure and function underlies the illness.

AETIOLOGY

The aetiology of schizophrenia can be considered under several headings. The theories regarding aetiology are not mutually exclusive and evidence for each should be sought in examining each individual case.

Genetic causes

These have been repeatedly demonstrated. Whereas the lifetime risk for schizophrenia in the general population is approximately 1 per cent, that for a person who has a sibling or one parent suffering from the illness is about 12 per cent, and for the child of two parents with schizophrenia it is approximately 40 per cent. The concordance rate for dizygotic twins has been found to be roughly that of siblings whereas the concordance rate for monozygotic twins is much higher: 40–60 per cent. This holds even for those twins who have been reared apart, which overcomes the criticism that the high concordance rates might reflect environmental rather than genetic effects. Adoption studies have confirmed the importance of genetic factors, as children of schizophrenic mothers adopted by families which are free of the disease show a similar chance of developing schizophrenia to those brought up by their own mothers.

No single genetic model can account for these findings, and certain subgroups of schizophrenia may have particularly strong genetic components in their aetiology.

A well-recognized predisposing factor is a pre-morbid *schizoid personality* (see p. 62). There is an increased incidence of schizoid personalities in the first-degree relatives of schizophrenic probands. Such people show a marked degree of shyness and reserve, they may be socially phobic, have few or no friends, and behave in an eccentric fashion. They are at higher risk for schizophrenic illness, and when one develops it has a worse prognosis.

Environmental factors

The importance of environmental events in the genesis of schizophrenia is inferred from:

1. The lack of 100 per cent concordance for schizophrenia in monozygotic twins.
2. The excess of winter births in schizophrenic patients, suggesting a possible viral factor.
3. The increased incidence of birth complications.

As a group schizophrenic patients have enlargement of ventricular size on CT and magnetic resonance imaging (MRI) brain scans. There is some evidence that schizophrenic patients without a family history of schizophrenia ('sporadic' cases) are more likely to have been born in winter, to have a history of perinatal trauma, and to have enlarged cerebral ventricles than those with a family history ('familial' cases). The implication of these findings is that vulnerability to schizophrenia may arise from a structural brain abnormality as a result of an environmental insult, through a genetic factor not related to obvious structural damage, or through a combination of both (see also 'Neurodevelopmental theories' below).

Neurological theories

These are stimulated by the fact that schizophrenic symptoms may be caused by organic brain disease. Of particular relevance is the fact that long-standing temporal lobe epilepsy may lead to the development of schizophrenic symptoms.

Neurodevelopmental theories

Neurodevelopmental theories propose that a combination of genetic and early environmental factors (the relative importance of which are disputed – see also 'Environmental factors' above) lead to defective development and maturation of the brain (particularly the medial temporal lobe). They have arisen from the following findings:

1. Enlargement of cerebral ventricular size antedates the development of schizophrenia and is not progressive in the majority of cases.
2. Boys who go on to develop schizophrenia exhibit more abnormalities in pre-morbid personality, intelligence, and social adjustment than their peers.
3. Structural brain abnormalities (particularly a reduction in temporal lobe and hippocampal size) are not associated with gliosis, which would be expected if destructive or degenenerative processes were at work.

A version of this theory involving an abnormality in the development of **cerebral laterality** has been proposed to explain certain structural findings and the sex differences in age of onset and clinical picture. (As a group males show more structural abnormalities, have more pre-morbid difficulties, have an earlier age of onset of schizophrenia, and show a more typical and chronic course than females.)

Psychological theories

Schizophrenic patients have been shown to be in an abnormal state of arousal which has been related to social withdrawal. This may be the necessary response if a schizophrenic is faced with an overwhelming number of conflicting stimuli which he is unable to sort out. A reduction of arousal is brought about by drug therapy and this leads to improvement and protects against relapse.

Abnormalities in parenting and disordered family communication (for example, according to the **double bind** theory there may be conflict between the overt verbal message and the tone or manner in which the message is given) may occur in families with a schizophrenic member, but a causal role remains to be proved. It now seems likely that this is often a consequence of the illness rather than a cause.

Sensory impairment

Impaired sensory input such as *deafness and blindness* predisposes individuals (especially the elderly in whom such handicaps may be multiple) to develop persecutory states.

Precipitating factors

An acute episode of a schizophrenic illness may be precipitated in a predisposed individual by environmental stress. Stressful life events in the three weeks before the onset of psychotic symptoms are more frequent than would be expected by chance. This includes desirable (such as promotion) as well as undesirable events (such as redundancy), the common ingredient being some form of increased tension.

An increased chance of relapse of schizophrenia has been shown to occur if the patient lives in an environment where he receives much criticism. The relapse rate has been shown to be nearly four times increased if the patient returns from hospital to a family in which there is a high level of hostile or critical *'expressed emotion'*. Tape-recordings of conversation in such families reveal frequently expressed critical comments directed towards the patient. The chance of relapse in such a situation can be reduced by the use of neuroleptic medication and by ensuring that the patient spends less time in face-to-face contact with emotionally arousing relatives. It has been shown that certain forms of family therapy can effectively reduce the expression of hostility in the family, with a consequent reduction in the relapse rate.

COURSE

Schizophrenia is generally considered to be an illness which has a characteristic chronic course and leads to the person becoming progressively disabled. The exception to this lies in the recognition of acute schizophrenia with positive symptoms, from which the patient may make a complete recovery. Overall figures for the outcome of schizophrenia are as follows:

- 10% show rapid and permanent deterioration,
- 35% show mild and persistent symptoms which require continuing care either in a hostel or in the patient's home,
- 35% appear 'cured' for long periods of time but have relapses of their illness, and
- 20% are apparently 'cured' and stable.

Repeated episodes of psychosis together with hospitalization lead to a set of **secondary handicaps** in addition to the negative symptoms of the illness itself. The patient's job will be disrupted by repeated absences through illness; and the onset of psychotic symptoms at the place of work will again increase the chance that he may lose his job and find further employment difficult to obtain. Similarly, personal friendships may be severed and relatives may reject the patient if they have been involved in his delusions or affected by difficult behaviour during his illness. The patient may experience prejudice against him in his attempts to find independent housing or to arrange his finances. Increasing inability to work leads to a decline in skills which often leads to a slow movement down the social scale.

INVESTIGATIONS

Investigations are aimed at confirming the diagnosis, and at elucidating aetiological and prognostic factors.

Physical

1. Drug screen for amphetamines.
2. Tests for organic illness if clinically indicated: e.g. EEG, lumbar puncture, CAT scan.

Psychosocial

1. History from relatives and other informants to confirm history of illness, assess presence of precipitating life events, and supplement information about genetic factors.
2. Social worker or other team member to assess home environment concerning attitudes of the family, and their level of 'expressed emotion'.

TREATMENT

Although in the past many patients with schizophrenia were treated as long-term in-patients, the emphasis today is on brief hospital treatment for the acute episode followed by sustained treatment in the community. The aim of the latter is to prevent relapse and reduce the chances of negative symptoms and secondary handicaps developing.

Acute phase

MEDICATION

Treatment in the *acute phase* usually involves admission to the in-patient unit or day-hospital for all the appropriate investigations to be performed and medication to be increased rapidly to therapeutic levels.

Oral neuroleptic medication is started in a dose that suppresses the psychotic phenomena and accompanying disturbances of behaviour and affect but without causing undue sedation (often chlorpromazine, in the range 300–900 mg per day).

NURSING

Nursing at this time is aimed at keeping the patient in an environment which is reasonably free of stressful situations and conflict while maintaining as normal a daily routine as his clinical condition permits. If the patient holds ideas which render him a danger to himself or others it may be necessary to detain him in hospital compulsorily (see pp. 331–3). Rehabilitation should start early. The patient is seen and assessed by the *occupational therapist* as soon as is practicable.

Long-term treatment

MEDICATION

Medication is usually changed to long-acting injections (flupenthixol or fluphenazine) which need only be given every two to four weeks. The drug is dissolved in an oily solution from which it is gradually absorbed into tissue fluid. The drug passes straight into the blood stream without passing through the liver (where phenothiazines are metabolized); the absorption is such that a small quantity leads to a constant plasma level. This form of administration of neuroleptic drug is usually started by a psychiatrist, rather than the GP, because it is only one aspect of specialist continuing care for schizophrenic patients in the community (see below). The depot injections are usually commenced at the second or subsequent episode, or where there are indications during the first illness that the patient is likely to relapse. The advantages of depot injections include the fact that the patient does not have to take oral medication (unless they require concurrent anti-Parkinsonian medication) and compliance with medication is greatly improved. The medication is given two–four-weekly, usually by a community psychiatric nurse, who can regularly review the patient's mental state and check for side-effects of medication at each visit.

Anti-Parkinsonian medication should only be given if extra-pyramidal symptoms are present and it is not practicable to reduce the dose of the neuroleptic. A few patients who do not respond to the usual neuroleptic drugs may improve dramatically with clozapine (see p. 87). This is an expensive treatment but the clinical benefits may be so considerable that a previously hospitalized patient may be able to live independently in the community, in which case the cost savings greatly outweigh the cost of the drug.

ACCOMMODATION

The patient should live in suitable accommodation, where relationships are smooth and the patient will be encouraged to lead a normal, active life. If this is to be his own home, a member of the team should help the other members of the family to understand the patient's illness and cooperate with his gradual return to a normal life style, which should include a good level of self-care, social activity, and occupation. If no such home environment exists and the illness is severe the patient may be best placed in a hostel where his daily routine and independence may be preserved. It is useful to be able to offer care in a *day-hospital* or in a *day-centre* operated by local social services to help provide some useful structure to the patient's day, to reduce contact with emotionally arousing relatives, and to cover relapses which do not necessitate admission to the in-patient unit. *Voluntary organizations* such as the National Schizophrenia Fellowship may offer considerable support to the patient's family.

PROGNOSIS

Poor prognostic factors are:

Pre-morbid

1. Family history of schizophrenia.
2. Schizoid personality.
3. High expressed emotion home environment.
4. Poor previous work record.

Illness

1. Gradual onset without clear precipitating cause.
2. Absence of prominent affective or catatonic symptoms.
3. Pronounced negative symptoms.

A MODEL FOR SCHIZOPHRENIA

Many students or doctors other than psychiatrists view the diagnosis and treatment of schizophrenia as an exercise quite different from the rest of medicine. In fact the similarities with **diabetes** are numerous and the routine care of the schizophrenic patient in the community has many similarities with that of diabetics.

Both conditions are **diagnosed** by precise criteria (blood glucose level or the presence of first-rank symptoms) which have been chosen to correspond most closely with the other clinical characteristics of the condition. The **aetiology** of each condition includes genetic predisposition and environmental stressors. In either disease, the genetic predisposition may be clear early in life, with an early onset, pronounced symptomatology, and numerous complications (negative symptoms in schizophrenia). A later onset may be associated with environmental factors, such as obesity in diabetes, or sensory or cognitive impairment in the elderly person who develops schizophrenia. In either disease acute symptoms may be **precipitated** by stress – a glucose load or stressful life event.

The **treatment** of both conditions is similarly divided into acute and long-term. Both conditions require very large doses of drugs in the acute phase but smaller maintenance doses.

The routine assessments in the maintenance phase of treatment are as follows:

1. Good control of the illness (glucose level and absence of psychotic symptoms).
2. Prevention of complications: maintenance on adequate doses of the drug, leading as normal a life as possible, avoiding severe stress (dietary restrictions/low expressed emotion environment).
3. Encourage a normal life: encourage interest and motivation for self-care and education about the illness and its treatment.

It is the role of the specialist nurse (community psychiatric nurse for schizophrenia) to administer and monitor the depot medication, and to arrange for other members of the psychiatric team to be involved as necessary. The psychiatrist periodically reviews the patient's mental state, including negative symptoms, and may alter the dose of medication accordingly. From time to time the patient may benefit from a period of more intensive treatment in a rehabilitation unit or other day-care facility. The occupational therapist may offer increased activities at home and the social worker can help with accommodation, housing, or financial problems. Without such assistance these problems may become severely neglected in this group of patients, whose disabilities may greatly limit their capacity to cope with life in the community.

The general practitioner will see the schizophrenic patient from time to time in the surgery, often with unrelated health problems, but should not miss the opportunity to check that this framework of support and periodic review is in place and operating satisfactorily. Good communication between GP, social services, and psychiatric services is essential for adequate community care for patients with chronic schizophrenia living in the community.

FURTHER READING

Warner, R. (1985) *Recovery from Schizophrenia: Psychiatry and the Political Economy.* London: Routledge & Kegan Paul.
Wing, J.K. (1978) *Schizophrenia: Towards a New Synthesis.* London: Academic Press.

13 / AFFECTIVE DISORDERS

An affective disorder is a disorder of mood. **Anxiety, depression**, and **elation** are all associated with clinically important syndromes, although only the first two are common in general medical settings. In the interests of clarity we will describe anxiety states and depressive disorders separately, but it should be grasped from the outset that combinations of the two syndromes are very common both in general hospital and in general practice settings.

Affective illnesses occur in both psychotic and non-psychotic forms: we will first of all describe the common, non-psychotic form of illness (anxiety-related disorders and depressive illness), and then describe the severe, psychotic forms of illness, psychotic depression, and mania.

ANXIETY STATES AND RELATED DISORDERS

Epidemiology

Symptoms of anxiety and worry are among the commonest psychological symptoms encountered in the normal population: however, most worried people do not have enough other symptoms related to anxiety to justify a diagnosis of anxiety state. The prevalence of anxiety states has been estimated at between 2 per cent and 4 per cent for men, and between 3 per cent and 4.5 per cent for women in three recent surveys of the normal population. There have been no reliable estimates of inception rate. However, one study of inceptions of illnesses seen in general practice settings showed anxiety disorders to constitute about 10 per cent of all new illness onsets, and to account for about one-third of all those with a diagnosable psychiatric disorder. There are therefore grounds for supposing that the prevalence of anxiety states is considerably higher in medical settings than in the general population.

Most acute anxiety reactions are of relatively short duration, but in contrast phobic illnesses last longer and affect about 3 per cent of men and 6 per cent of women.

Neurochemistry

The syndrome of anxiety is characterized by increased arousal, increased sympathetic activity (mydriasis, tachycardia, perspiration), and unpleasant subjective sensations of fear and apprehension. It is believed that both ascending **noradrenaline and 5-hydroxy-tryptamine containing neuronal pathways**, innervating the limbic lobe and neocortex, play important roles in mediating the symptoms of anxiety. Increased activity of nor-adrenergic neurones appear to be involved in symptoms and signs of heightened arousal, while increased activity of 5-hydroxytryptaminergic neurones enhance responses to aversive stimuli, so that blocking the effects of 5-hydroxytryptamine with antagonist drugs makes animals more likely to brave an aversive stimulus in order to gain a reward, suggesting that they are less anxious or at least less inhibited than normal. Antagonists at $5-HT_2$ receptors have been shown to be anxiolytic in humans and the anxiolytic effect of anti-depressant drugs may be mediated by their ability to decrease the sensitivity of $5-HT_2$ receptors. As discussed elsewhere (see p. 196), changes in the functioning of noradrenergic and 5-hydroxytryptaminergic neurones are also implicated in the aetiology of depressive illness and it is believed that different but related neural pathways using different receptor subtypes are involved, which is consistent with the clinical overlap seen between the two disorders.

Neurones containing **gamma-amino butyric acid (GABA)** provide the principal inhib-itory system in the brain and act to decrease the activity of other neurones including those containing monoamines. Drugs which increase GABA function such as barbiturates and benzodiazepines are potent anxiolytics. Benzodiazepines act via receptors which are found in the limbic lobe and neocortex and are associated with, and modulate, post-synaptic $GABA_A$ receptors (the $GABA_A$-benziodiazepine receptor complex). Benzo-diazepines increase the effect of GABA whereas there are a group of compounds known as '**inverse agonists**' which bind to benzodiazepine receptors but have the opposite effect and act to decrease the effects of GABA. As might be predicted these compounds are anxiogenic. There are a number of candidates for endogenous compounds which bind to benzodiazepine receptors and could theoretically contribute to pathological anxiety states.

Other neurotransmitters may be important in mediating anxiety. Cholecystokinin and related peptide neurotransmitters cause symptoms of panic when infused into humans.

Symptoms

ANXIOUS RUMINATIONS

These often come about because the patient anxiously broods about the significance of the somatic symptoms (do the palpitations mean a heart attack, does the tiredness mean cancer?); or because he is afraid that others notice symptoms such as tremor. Such thoughts exacerbate the original anxiety, and in turn the somatic symptoms are magnified. Anxiety states are especially common in medical settings, for reasons that were explained in Chapter 10, p. 136. Patients who present with a single somatic symptom of anxiety such as tachycardia or tremor may present a diagnostic problem until it is appreciated that other psychological and somatic symptoms of anxiety are present.

In addition to subjective feelings of tension and worry, the symptoms of anxiety states can conveniently be thought of in three groups:

autonomic symptoms of anxiety include	symptoms relating to motor tone include	symptoms of hyper-vigilance include
palpitations	shakiness	irritability
tachycardia	tremor onset	insomnia
cold, clammy hands	muscular aches	trouble staying asleep
sweating	lump in throat	easily startled
blepharospasm	distractibility	poor concentration
paraesthesiae	restlessness	feeling keyed up
dizziness	easily tired	
hot and cold spells	trouble swallowing	
frequency of micturition		
diarrhoea		
nausea		

PANIC ATTACKS

Sometimes patients experience episodes of severe, uncontrollable anxiety called **panic attacks**. These usually take the form of intense anxiety of sudden onset with both cognitive and somatic accompaniments. The patient thinks some misfortune will befall him: death by heart attack, madness, or just a nameless dread; typically accompanied by one or more symptoms such as sweating, tremor, palpitations, and paraesthesiae due to overbreathing. The attacks last from anything between a few minutes and some hours, and often present in the casualty department.

Patients whose only symptoms are panic attacks are said to suffer from **panic disorder (F41.0)** if they are experiencing several severe attacks each month. In practice, there is a strong overlap between panic attacks and other disorders described in this chapter, notably agoraphobia.

PHOBIC ILLNESSES (F40)

Patients with **phobic illnesses** become anxious only in particular situations and have no trouble providing that they avoid the object or situation that arouses their anxiety. However, their avoidance behaviour may become extreme.

Objects about which people develop specific phobias include spiders, snakes, dogs, rats, and moths; while **situations** include high places (**acrophobia**), enclosed spaces (claustrophobia), air-travel (air phobia; all F40.2), and social gatherings (social phobias: F40.1).

Agoraphobia (F40.0) commonly develops in women between the ages of eighteen and thirty-five, and anxiety symptoms are only experienced in situations which share certain characteristics: being a long way from home; in crowded places such as public transport, department stores, or cinemas; in shops where one must queue to pay before leaving; or in any situation which is difficult to leave quickly. The anxiety may be reduced or be quite tolerable if a trusted person is with the patient: some women can manage even with a small child, others need an adult or cannot face the feared situation at all. The patient may feel quite safe in her car, but is in real trouble if the car breaks down when she is on her own.

As time goes on the symptoms tend to progress and to generalize: panic attacks may occur even at the thought of going out, and eventually without obvious provocation. By this time the patient is likely not to be going out at all, and is then said to be 'house-bound'.

Patients often develop depressive symptoms as well, but these will be described in the next section, and are not central to the agoraphobic symptom-complex.

Diagnosis

There is no natural dividing line between normal people and those with **anxiety states** that would enable us to lay down firm criteria for diagnosis. In this respect anxiety disorders resemble conditions like hypertension and anaemia in general medicine. There are various research criteria for the diagnosis, but they are arbitrary. In practical terms, any patient whose pronounced symptoms of anxiety are accompanied by three or more of the other symptoms given above can usefully be thought of as satisfying the requirements for diagnosis, while with increasing numbers of symptoms there is increasing certainty that such a disorder is present.

Panic disorder should only be diagnosed if an individual describes recurrent panic attacks, and does not satisfy the criteria for either anxiety state or depression (see below).

Phobias refer to a persistent, irrational fear with a compelling desire to avoid the objects or situations described above. The disorder should cause the patient significant distress, and the patient should regard his fear as excessive or unreasonable.

Agoraphobia should be diagnosed when there is marked fear in the situations described above and there is increased constriction of normal activities until fears or avoidance behaviour dominate the patient's life.

Post-traumatic stress disorder (F43.1) refers to a syndrome which follows exposure to unusual stress – such as a battle; or being attacked or raped; or a natural disaster like a fire or flood. The patients 'relive' the distressing experience with intrusive flashbacks or vivid memories; and may start to avoid circumstances which remind them of the original trauma. For example, a woman who has been raped in a car-park may start to avoid all car-parks. The symptoms begin within a few months of the original stressor, and typically occur in settings of other symptoms of anxiety.

Differential diagnosis

OTHER PSYCHIATRIC ILLNESSES

Symptoms of anxiety commonly accompany more differentiated kinds of psychiatric disorders. Easily the commonest of these is **depression**; but such symptoms also occur in any **psychotic illness** (that is, above anxiety state in the diagnostic hierarchy). Anxiety is also an integral part of an **obsessional state** (see pp. 228–9). So, make sure that you have elicited all the patient's symptoms, and that those that you have elicited can be accounted for by morbid anxiety.

THYROTOXICOSIS (see p. 138)

Look for symptoms suggestive of hyperthyroidism. Atrial fibrillation, exophthalmos, or a thyroid bruit make thyroid function tests mandatory.

DRUG INTOXICATION

Think of stimulants such as caffeine and methyl phenidate; also sympathomimetic agents such as bronchodilators.

DRUG WITHDRAWAL (see pp. 210, 217, 219)

Sometimes anxiety symptoms are caused by the patient running out of sedatives – whether these be benzodiazepines, alcohol, or barbiturates. Diagnostic difficulties arise when the patient wishes to conceal his drug use, but wants help for the anxiety symptoms. (If drugs are obtained illicitly, and the patient thinks the doctor may prescribe a sedative as a treatment, he may be unwilling to give an honest history.)

PHAEOCHROMOCYTOMA

Thought of by every medical student, but in fact very rare indeed! The history of flushing attacks accompanied by diarrhoea alerts one to the possibility.

Investigations

It is not necessary to carry out tests for thyrotoxicosis or phaeochromocytoma unless they are indicated by the results of the history and physical examination.

Aetiology

It is convenient to distinguish between long-term factors that predispose to symptoms of anxiety, and factors that release a particular episode.

PREDISPOSING FACTORS

Twin studies have shown that there is an undoubted genetic component in the propensity to anxiety state: however, it only accounts for rather a small proportion of the variance, and it seems probable that a polygenic mechanism is responsible. Adults with anxiety states consistently report childhoods that were more traumatic than do controls, with inconsistent support from parents and higher rates of parental divorce. Sexual abuse during childhood is associated with higher levels of both depressive and anxious symptoms during adult life.

The pre-morbid personalities of patients with anxiety states are heterogeneous, so that although the states occur more easily in those with anxious temperaments, they can also occur in obsessional, dependent, and even schizoid personalities. However, it seems likely that those individuals who score highly on questionnaires measuring neuroticism or 'trait anxiety' are more vulnerable to symptoms of anxiety than those with a more phlegmatic disposition.

Those with chronic social adversity are at greater risk, and this adversity may take the form of difficult interpersonal problems or unfavourable living conditions.

PRECIPITATING FACTORS

Anxiety states are usually in some understandable relationship to stressful life events. In general medical settings anxiety symptoms are often related to worries about physical health, and it is therefore essential to allow patients to express their own fears about the nature of their illness before the doctor provides information from the medical viewpoint. Anxious ruminations are especially difficult to handle if the patient has no one in whom to confide, or is unable to find reassurance from people in his immediate social field.

However, in other cases the anxiety will not be related to physical health, but will be found to be a somatic expression of some interpersonal problem. It will often be the case that the patient has not connected the psychological problem with the physical symptom for which help is sought, so that taking a proper history not only helps us to understand the aetiology of the disorder, but is also an indispensable first step in treatment.

Treatment

GENERAL MEDICAL CARE

Taking a history, physical examination, and carrying out any essential physical investigations are all part of treatment, provided that they are done properly. The history must be taken in such a way that the patient has had an opportunity to ventilate problems and has received reassurance about any irrational fears: both these procedures are therapeutic. The physical examination should if possible be done in such a way that it reassures the patient: for example, if the doctor knows that the patient is afraid that he might have a gastric cancer, it is helpful if the doctor says that no mass can be felt, nor are there other signs that suggest cancer. Finally, physical investigations can be therapeutic if they are carried out to produce final reassurance, but actively harmful if they signal to the patient that his doctors do not know what is wrong with him, but are prepared to go on and on because they can think of endless possibilities! Thus a patient who is told *'There isn't any evidence of cancer to account for this pain, but we'll put a tube in your tummy and look so that we can be quite certain'* is likely to be reassured by the subsequent investigation showing no abnormalities, while a patient who is given no explanation for an endless series of physical investigations will become more anxious as each normal finding is reported to him, because it looks as though the doctors are sure that there is something wrong, but do not know what it is!

ADVICE

All anxious people need advice, most don't actually want sedative drugs, and even fewer need such drugs. So what advice should they be given?

First, an explanation that their various symptoms make up a common syndrome with which the doctor is familiar, and that the symptoms do not indicate serious disease. Next, advice on what to do during an anxiety attack: sit down if possible, try to relax and breathe no more deeply than usual, and the symptoms will pass off by themselves. Finally, advice on the advisability of going to relaxation classes, to meditation, or to yoga, depending on the patient's interests.

In the course of taking the history the doctor will usually have heard about other related problems, and must use judgement to decide on whether the nature of these problems is such that help from others should be sought.

HELP FROM SOCIAL WORKERS

Patients with anxiety disorders often have social or interpersonal problems that can be helped greatly by a trained social worker. It should not be thought that only those with obviously soluble problems that can be 'talked out' should be referred: on the contrary, the social worker is often aware of resources that can be mobilized to help people with seemingly quite intractable problems, and should in any case be given the chance of making up her own mind about what might be done.

HELP FROM CLINICAL PSYCHOLOGISTS

People whose anxiety states do not remit with simple measures, or who are unable to learn relaxation from such local classes as are available, will sometimes succeed in learning relaxation in one-to-one treatment. If there is a pronounced element of anxious ruminations (see above) then one should also consider the possibility of an 'anxiety management package'. Patients with phobic illnesses should be treated with relaxation and graded *in vivo* exposure (see pp. 103–4).

Patients with post-traumatic stress disorder may benefit from a cognitive-behavioural approach (see p. 103) to their problems.

DRUG TREATMENT

This should be avoided except in the management of short-term situations: for example, a patient who is anxious about some medical procedure despite reassurance, or someone who is very anxious about the outcome of a child's surgical operation and asks for help in staying calm. It will sometimes be necessary to offer benzodiazepines for a course of a few weeks at most, but the prescription should not be renewed, since these drugs produce dependence (see p. 219).

Drug treatment of post-traumatic stress disorder should be with tricyclic anti-depressants in the first instance, with monoamine oxidase inhibitors being offered to those who do not respond.

Course and prognosis

Most acute anxiety states remit, which is an excellent reason for avoiding dependence-producing drugs. Many of those put on to benzodiazepines and then thought to have developed 'chronic anxiety states' are experiencing anxiety symptoms when their drugs are withdrawn, but such symptoms often improve dramatically after a week to ten days. Some patients with chronic anxiety will be found to have social problems, but such problems should attract social interventions. In fact, most patients with persistent anxiety symptoms will gradually develop depressive symptoms as well: these will be dealt with in the next section.

DEPRESSION

Most patients with persistent anxiety symptoms will eventually develop depressive symptoms as well. There is therefore a sense in which depressive symptoms represent a more differentiated form of psychological illness than anxiety states, and for this reason we described anxiety states first. Some depressed patients seem to develop both anxiety and depressive symptoms simultaneously, while others – as already mentioned – develop depressive symptoms only after experiencing anxiety symptoms for some time: it is possible that the longstanding anxiety symptoms increase their vulnerability to develop depressive symptoms under stress.

There has been a long controversy about the best way to classify depressive illnesses, and the non-psychiatrist is well advised to ignore it. The common form of depression encountered in general medical settings is described here as **depressive illness (F32.0)**. There is also a more severe form of illness, which we have called **depressive psychosis (F32.3)**. These two forms of illness have been described elsewhere as 'reactive/endogenous' or as 'neurotic/psychotic', but neither set of terms is really satisfactory. It is now known that both sorts of depression are equally likely to be secondary to stressful life events, so the term 'endogenous' is actively misleading. The term 'neurotic' is best avoided, since it implies that people who become depressed are neurotic, and this is far from being the case. It is true that people who score highly on 'neuroticism' scales are more vulnerable to develop depressive illnesses when under stress, but with sufficient adversity depressive illnesses can develop in stable, phlegmatic people.

Epidemiology

Although depressive symptoms are somewhat less common than anxiety symptoms, they are nonetheless to be found in between 10 per cent and 16 per cent of men, and between 20 per cent and 24 per cent of women in community surveys. Once more, people with **depressive illnesses** – that is to say, with more than a critical number of depressive symptoms – are very much less common, accounting for between 2.6 per cent and 4 per cent of men, and about 7 per cent to 8 per cent of women in surveys carried out in London, Canberra, and the United States. The annual inception rate in the community is not known, although it seems likely that it is over half the point prevalence.

The prevalence of depressive illness is very much higher in consulting populations. Depressive illnesses are the commonest diagnosis in a study of inceptions of illness in general practice, accounting for 12 per cent of all new illnesses and 45 per cent of all psychiatric diagnoses made in this setting. It is important to emphasize that most of these depressed patients were consulting their doctors either with somatic symptoms related to their depression, or with physical illnesses that they had in addition to their depression.

Neurochemistry

According to the **monoamine theory** of affective disorders, depressive illness is due to a functional impairment in central noradrenaline and/or 5-hydroxytryptamine-containing neurones.

This theory is based on the actions of drugs: reserpine, a drug which depletes central neurones' monoamine stores, causes depression, whereas drugs which increase central monoamine levels (monamine oxidase inhibitors, tricyclics, selective noradrenaline or 5-hydroxytryptamine re-uptake inhibitors) relieve the symptoms of depression. More modern versions of this theory concentrate on **adaptive changes** in monoamine neurones caused by long-term medication with anti-depressants to explain the two-week delay in the onset of therapeutic effect. In animal studies effective anti-depressants (including electroconvulsive treatment) cause a number of changes in neuronal function and monoamine receptors. There are multiple subtypes of receptors for monoamines (for example, noradrenaline receptors – a_1, a_2, b_1, b_2; 5-hydroxytryptamine receptors – $5\text{-HT}_{1\text{-like}}$, 5-HT_2, 5-HT_3, 5-HT_4) and many anti-depressants share common effects, for example, increasing neurotransmission mediated by 5-HT_1 receptors in the hippocampus and reducing the sensitivity ('**down-regulation**') of β-adrenoceptors. While it is possible that there is a single common action underlying the action of all anti-depressant treatments, it is more likely that the anti-depressant response is a result of a variety of effects on interrelated neurones.

There is evidence that depressed patients free of drug treatment have abnormalities in monamine neurotransmission. Some depressed patients have reduced levels of 5-hydroxyindoleacetic acid (5-HIAA) in the cerebrospinal fluid, possibly reflecting a reduced turnover of central 5-hydroxytryptamine, and this is consistent with the reduced ability of indirect 5-hydroxytryptamine agonists to stimulate prolactin secretion and with reduced levels of 5-hydroxytryptamine in the brains of some suicide victims (in whom a depressive illness could be inferred). In severe depression the α_2-adrenoceptor-stimulating drug, clonidine, has a reduced effectiveness in enhancing growth hormone output, suggesting a decreased sensitivity of central adrenoceptors.

Depressed patients have abnormal neuroendocrine regulation which may be a consequence of changes in monoamine function. Many have raised plasma concentrations of cortisol, which are believed to result from increased secretion of corticotrophin-releasing factor from the hypothalamus. This underlies the reduced effectiveness of dexamethasone to suppress cortisol secretion which has been proposed as a diagnostic 'test' for depressive illness (the *dexamethasone suppression test*). While up to two-thirds of severely depressed patients demonstrate this abnormality it is not specific enough for routine clinical use, as it occurs in other psychiatric disorders.

Symptoms

These will be described under four headings: **emotional changes**, **cognitive changes**, **motivational changes**, and **neurovegetative symptoms**. Symptoms of anxiety, restlessness, and agitation may also be present.

EMOTIONAL CHANGES

In the early stages of a depressive illness the patient may notice that he no longer derives pleasure from life: this **anhedonia** may precede experience of sadness or unhappiness. Sense of humour is often lost, so that although he may see the point of a joke, he doesn't find it funny. Eventually the mood becomes one of **sadness** and misery, with the content of the patient's thought accompanying his mood. Thus the past supplies evidence of failures and wrong decisions, what is dismal about the present is dwelt on inordinately, and the future is seen as threatening or **hopeless.** This sadness is often accompanied by **crying spells**, although some patients report that they feel like crying but are unable to do so. The patient may feel that life isn't worth living, and begins to think of ways of ending his life. Feelings of affection for those close to him are often reduced, and the patient may lose his religious faith.

COGNITIVE CHANGES

These include feelings of **self-dislike** with an exaggerated assessment of current life problems. Changed self-concept and **self-blame** should be assessed by asking how the patient compares himself with other people, and whether he blames himself for being as he is. Depressed women may complain that they are ugly, or find their bodies repulsive. **Ideas of reference** may occur in which the patient feels that others look critically at her or make disparaging remarks about her. Religious patients may feel that they are **wicked or sinful.** There may be **difficulties about making decisions**, either because of **lack of confidence** or because of subjective **difficulty in thinking**. In severe forms of depression ideas of **guilt and worthlessness** appear. **Suicidal ideas** are particularly serious in the presence of such other symptoms. **Nihilistic ideas** take the form of the patient's saying that he has no money, he has no feelings, he is already dead, or the world does not exist.

MOTIVATIONAL CHANGES

Low energy, fatigue, apathy, and **inability to concentrate** may occur secondarily to depressed mood, and are especially common in depressive states following infectious diseases such as glandular fever, infectious hepatitis, influenza, or brucellosis. Depressed patients tend to escape responsibility and to avoid demanding tasks. They may do this because their usual tasks seem boring or meaningless, or because they lack confidence to make the right decisions. Failure to complete tasks may reinforce ideas of self-blame or worthlessness. Patients are often said to be 'dependent' because they become willing to allow others to take over responsibility for giving them guidance.

NEUROVEGETATIVE SYMPTOMS

These include disturbances of **appetite, weight, sleep rhythm, libido, energy level,** and **posture.** Depressed mood may influence the way the patient speaks, walks, and sits. In minor depressive illnesses increased appetite with weight gain is almost as common as anorexia and weight loss, but the latter symptoms predominate in severe depression. There is diminution of sexual interest and performance. Sleep is hard to come by, light, and unrefreshing. Emotional energy no longer flows outwards to the world of people and events, and the patient becomes lost in miserable self-absorption with his discomforts. In this way the patient may present the doctor with **headache, backache,** or some other **regional pain,** and the doctor may be so distracted by these symptoms that the depressive syndrome of which they form a part goes unrecognized. In severe depression the patient may report **early waking,** and **diurnal variation of mood,** with his worst mood in the mornings.

Diagnosis (of depressive illnesses: F32)

As with anxiety states, there is no point of discontinuity between normality and depression, so the dividing line between the two must be arbitrary. One widely used criterion requires:

A. Depressed mood or inability to experience pleasure to be prominent and fairly persistent,

and to have had AT LEAST THREE of the following seven symptoms on each day for the previous two weeks:

B. 1. Poor or increased appetite/weight loss or gain.
    2. Insomnia or hypersomnia.
    3. Agitation or retardation.
    4. Loss of energy or fatigue.

have been shown to be associated with authoritarian styles of parenting as well as with indifferent and neglectful parenting.

PROVOKING FACTORS

Loss events, physical illness, and adverse social circumstances all favour the release of depressive phenomena:

Loss events may be bereavements, threatened future losses, as when a near relative develops a fatal illness, the loss of a relationship, or even a failure to be promoted. These are especially likely to precipitate depression in those with low self-esteem, in those without intimate confidants, and in those with some pre-existing conflict that is exacerbated by a stressful event. The loss may precede the episode of depression by as much as one year.

Physical illness commonly contributes to the genesis of depressive illnesses seen in general medical settings. The patient may have been mildly dysphoric before the onset of such illnesses, but experiences a marked exacerbation of depressive symptoms after the physical illness. Although the association between depression and infections like infectious hepatitis, influenza, and glandular fever has been recognized for many years, it should be appreciated that other infectious illnesses such as herpes zoster and urinary tract infections often seem to contribute to the development of depressive disorders. It has been shown that those with a lower self-esteem are at higher risk for developing depressive illnesses after episodes of infectious illness.

Stressful social circumstances are protean in their manifestations. Patients may have very little in the way of social support, or they may have lost what little they had. Unsatisfactory living conditions, chronic illness in close relatives, and poor interpersonal relationships are recurrent themes in individual case histories.

Treatment

There is good evidence that anti-depressant treatment shortens the course of depressive illness: the more severe the depression, the more likely are anti-depresssants to be helpful. Patients with lesser degrees of depression are more likely to remit spontaneously and are likely to be helped as much by non-specific aspects of therapy as by anti-depressant medication. However, in order to regain his normal adjustment the patient must be kept alive, so we will first deal with suicidal threats.

SUICIDAL THREATS (see also pp. 323–6)

One should establish the extent to which the patient has been preoccupied with ideas of suicide, and whether any concrete steps have been already carried out. Has the patient decided when, where, and how? A serious view should be taken of plans which involve a painful method such as hanging or swallowing disinfectant; or one which is likely to be successful, such as jumping from a high building. Have materials been especially obtained? If the patient intends to take an overdose, has he handled the bottle, or tipped the tablets out and looked at them? If it turns out that some of these events have occurred, then what has so far prevented the patient from carrying out his plans? If the patient is to be allowed to go home, one must consider the environment to which he will return. Has the patient anyone in whom he can confide? Will he be under surveillance from others? Has he a past history of self-injury or self-poisoning? Is he prepared to give an undertaking that he will not harm himself before his next appointment?

There is no evidence that asking about suicide increases the likelihood of an attempt: on the contrary, many patients report relief of feelings of anxiety and guilt after they have had such a discussion. It would be quite impracticable if all those who thought of suicide were to be referred to a psychiatrist, but it is reasonable to refer those where there is doubt, or where the risk to life is thought to be real. Patients with symptoms of psychotic depression should all be referred for specialist treatment: the risk of suicide is great, and so is their suffering.

SPECIFIC PHARMACOLOGICAL TREATMENT

Anti-depressants are dealt with on pp. 91–5. However, it is worth noting that if the decision to prescribe an anti-depressant is made, compliance will be very much greater if the doctor anticipates possible side-effects, predicts the likely duration of treatment, and explains that the drug will not produce dependence and that cessation of treatment will be an easy matter when the time comes. Will the patient give you an undertaking not to take an overdose of the anti-depressant? It is irresponsible to give tricyclic anti-depressants to patients who are likely to take an excessive dose, since they are cardiotoxic in overdose. Consider asking a spouse or parent to look after the tablets, and remember that tetracyclic anti-depressants are much less toxic, and only slightly less effective! If there is a real risk to life, the patient should be offered admission to hospital.

SPECIFIC PSYCHOLOGICAL TREATMENTS

It is usual to discover that depressive illnesses are in an understandable relationship to the patient's life situation and to the way in which he handles **interpersonal rela-tionships**. Rather than endlessly dwelling on his symptoms, provide the patient with an opportunity to tell you about these problems. Most depressive illnesses will remit on a combination of anti-depressants and kindness; if material arises which cannot be handled consider referral to a psychiatrist.

Cognitive therapy for depression (see pp. 106–7) is given by some clinical psychologists, and is useful for patients whose depressive illnesses have not responded to anti-depressants but in whom there is no risk to life, or are recurrent and accompanied by depressive ideas about the self. It has been claimed to reduce the relapse rate.

ELECTROCONVULSIVE TREATMENT

This is the treatment of choice for psychotic depression, as it produces improvement very rapidly. Severe depression is an appalling experience for the patient; any treatment which shortens it is a major benefit. It is described fully on pp. 98–101.

In drug trials of anti-depressants in primary care settings many patients improve on placebo medication. It is naive to suppose that all these patients would have got better without treatment, although many would probably have done so. *The doctor's confidence that he can help his patient* – whether based on his own personal qualities or on his faith in the content of his pills – *promotes hope*, and with it *an expectancy that improvement will occur.* By his offer of return visits he implicitly offers to monitor the patient's return to effective social functioning and makes the patient feel that he has a powerful ally, so that the way becomes clearer for the resolution of both hopelessness and helplessness. The doctor's power to remove both social and occupational obligations may allow the patient to *rest without a sense of failure;* and if *sleep* can be restored there is often a major improvement in how the patient feels.

Course and prognosis

There is much variation in outcome of depressive illnesses seen in general medical settings, and although many will become symptom free within four to six weeks, about a third are likely to follow a protracted course. Illnesses following severe loss events in those with stable pre-morbid personalities are likely to have a good outcome, while those associated with chronically adverse social and interpersonal circumstances are likely to have a poorer outcome. **Depressive illnesses** associated with abnormal personalities, especially those described as manipulative, unstable, or highly dependent, are likely to have a poor outcome, with hostile depressive outbursts accompanied by dramatic behaviour and impulsive suicidal attempts.

Depressive psychosis is highly responsive to treatment, but there is a high likelihood of recurrent episodes: when this happens the patient is thought of as having a variant of bipolar affective illness where the episodes have so far been of the same type, and are sometimes called 'unipolar' illnesses.

BIPOLAR AFFECTIVE DISORDER
(also known as MANIC-DEPRESSIVE PSYCHOSIS)

In this illness the patient typically has episodes of depression – often psychotic in intensity – and at other times has episodes of psychotic excitement. In severe degree this illness is called mania; in milder degree hypomania. The sections which follow on symptoms, pathophysiology, diagnosis, and differential diagnosis will be confined to excited episodes since depressive psychosis has already been covered; the sections on epidemiology, treatment, course, and prognosis will be concerned with bipolar affective disorder.

Epidemiology (of bipolar disorder)

The lifetime morbid risk for bipolar disorders is approximately 1 per cent, with an annual inception rate of about 10 in 100,000 for men, and 15 in 100,000 for women. This means that in a standard catchment area of 250,000 there will be approximately 30 inceptions a year.

Neurochemistry (of mania)

A corollary to the 'monoamine theory of affective disorders' states that the biological abnormality in mania is the opposite to that found in depression: while in depression there is a lowered activity in central monoaminergic neuronal systems, an **increased monoaminergic activity** could be found in mania. This hypothesis of mania is based partly on the clinical observations that the symptoms of the depressive and manic syndromes are often polar opposites, and partly on the ability of drugs which can induce increased levels of noradrenaline and/or 5-hydroxytryptamine to produce manic reactions. These drugs, however, do not have consistent effects; they include *L-Dopa, amphetamine, monoamine oxidase inhibitors, and tricyclic anti-depressants*. Dopamine has also been implicated in mania since the most effective anti-manic drugs are the neuroleptics which are potent dopamine receptor antagonists. Biochemical studies in manic patients have not produced consistent results: some studies show evidence of increased central noradrenaline turnover (increased urinary excretion of 3-methoxy-4-hydroxyphenylglycol (MHPG)); other studies, however, show normal values.

Symptoms (of mania)

The central features of mania are **elevation of mood, increased activity**, and **grandiose ideas.** The elevation of mood may take forms ranging from **euphoria** to **elation**, and in such patients there may be an infectious gaiety. Others are not so lucky. Some are **irritable** rather than euphoric and the irritability can easily turn to anger. As with depression there may be diurnal variation of mood, and there may be brief episodes of depressed mood between episodes of high spirits. The elevation of mood is part of a **disinhibition** which affects social, sexual, and financial behaviour.

Thus the patient may make tactless or rude remarks in social situations, may make inappropriate sexual advances to strangers and fail to take precautions against pregnancy, and expensive goods that are not needed may be ordered from shops.

Increased activity involves motor behaviour, speech, and appetite, with sleep being correspondingly reduced. In lesser degree the increased activity may be associated with getting more done, but as the patient restlessly moves from one activity to another they surround themselves with chaos. **Speech** is rapid and **thoughts are speeded**. Eventually the thoughts come faster than they can be uttered, and ideas become more loosely connected with **punning** and jumping from one topic to another using rhymes – or '**clang associations**'. Eventually speech may become completely unintelligible.

Appetite is increased and at first food is eaten greedily and with poor manners; eventually the patient becomes too over-active either to eat or to sleep.

These symptoms often cause patients to abandon good jobs and steady sexual partners: they may embark on hare-brained schemes and become progressively more **grandiose.**

The patient may believe that he has some special mission, is extremely rich, or has some special message for others. Such **delusion-like ideas** are congruent with the patient's mood, so that if the predominant mood is one of irritability and suspiciousness they can be persecutory, if of elation they are expansive and grandiose. Schneiderian **positive symptoms of schizophrenia** (see p. 175) can occur, including delusions of reference and passivity experiences. **Hallucinations** may also occur but once more are congruent with the prevailing mood, taking the form of voices giving advice or telling the patient of his special powers, and occasionally that of visions of an ecstatic or religious character. None of these symptoms tends to last long (hours rather than days): one is struck by a kaleidoscope of psychotic experiences which vary with the mood disorder. **Insight** is almost invariably impaired, with the patient seeing no need for treatment. However, others with whom he comes in contact rarely have doubts!

Diagnosis (of manic episode: F30)

A period of elevated or irritable mood lasting at least a week, severe enough to disrupt work and social activities completely, with AT LEAST THREE of the following:

1. Increased activity or restlessness.
2. Pressure of words.
3. Subjective increased speed of thought.
4. Increased self-esteem, or grandiose ideas.
5. Decreased need for sleep.
6. Abnormal distractibility.
7. Disinhibited behaviour (see above).

Hypomania refers to similar, milder disorders, in which work and social activities are not completely disrupted.

Differential diagnosis (of mania)

SYMPTOMATIC MANIA

A manic illness does not always indicate a bipolar illness, since mania can be produced by drugs such as sympathomimetic amines, steroids, isoniazid, or L-Dopa; or it may be secondary to metabolic disorders such as renal failure or thyrotoxicosis; or it may follow cerebral insult such as encephalitis or a cerebral neoplasm.

SCHIZOPHRENIA (see p. 178)

The differentiation can be very difficult, especially as manic phenomena may occur during the course of a schizophrenic illness. If allegedly 'schizophrenic' phenomena have only occurred at times of elation and over-activity, the patient should be diagnosed as manic.

SCHIZO-AFFECTIVE DISORDER (see p. 180)

This is a psychotic disorder in which affective and schizophrenic psychotic phenomena are prominent within the same episode of illness. Patients with complete recovery between episodes of illness should be regarded by non-psychiatrists as variants of manic-depressive illness.

CYCLOTHYMIA (see p. 200)

This is a persistent instability of mood where the individual recognizes variations in energy and outlook which appear like *formes frustes* of bipolar illness. The diagnostic criteria given above should assist in the differentiation.

Aetiology (of bipolar disorder)

GENETIC FACTORS

Family and twin data indicate that bipolar affective disorder is aetiologically distinct from most cases of unipolar depression. However, the genotype underlying bipolar illness may sometimes produce unipolar illness, and sometimes cyclothymic personality. While genetic factors are undoubtedly important, no specific mode of inheritance has been established. With bipolar probands (although not with probands with depressive illness), there is an increased incidence in sibs reared under unfavourable conditions. The genetic predisposition is very much greater in early onset cases.

PERSONALITY

People with cyclothymic or depressive traits are at greater risk of bipolar disorder (see earlier discussion, p. 200).

DRUGS

Some patients have their only episode of manic illness during treatment of a depressive episode with an anti-depressant. Some people tolerate vast doses of amphetamines without developing psychotic illnesses, while others develop a manic illness on relatively small doses: in both cases, we are probably dealing with an interplay between genetic factors and environmental releasing factors.

STRESSFUL LIFE EVENTS

First episodes of mania often follow the same sort of stressful life events as precipitate episodes of depression. Once more, the stressful event is probably a releasing factor responsible for the timing of the episode.

Treatment (of mania)

NEUROLEPTICS

Haloperidol (pp. 85–7) and chlorpromazine (pp. 85–6) are drugs of choice for the symptoms of excitement and for suppressing any hallucinations.

LITHIUM CARBONATE (see p. 96)

Lithium is used both to make attacks less frequent and to lessen the severity of attacks. It also has some value in the treatment of mania, although it is not a drug of first choice.

ELECTROCONVULSIVE TREATMENT (see p. 98)

This is not usually necessary, but can be helpful in cases that do not respond to drug therapy.

ADMISSION TO HOSPITAL

This will often be necessary to contain episodes of mania which are very difficult to manage without specialized nursing care. It must not be forgotten that there is an increased risk of depression during mania: especially after the more excited symptoms have responded to treatment, while the patient is still active and disinhibited but during the brief episodes of depressed mood that have already been described.

Treatment (of recurrent illnesses)

Prophylactic lithium (see p. 96) is recommended for both bipolar (manic-depressive) illnesses and recurrent, unipolar psychotic depressions (see below). **Carbamazepine** (see p. 82) can be tried for 'rapid cycling' illnesses.

Course and prognosis

The natural history of bipolar illness is for the patient to have episodes of increasing frequency and duration over the course of his lifetime. However, lithium treatment has made a great impact on the course of the disorder, and there is good evidence that it reduces both the intensity and frequency of attacks. However, even without lithium there were always some people who recovered from a single attack of either mania or depressive psychosis and never had a recurrence: so lithium should only be offered after it is clear that a pattern of recurrence has been established.

FURTHER READING

Ashton, H. (1992) *Brain Function and Psychotropic Drugs*. Oxford: Oxford University Press.

Brown, G. and Harris, T. (1990) *The Social Origins of Depression*. London: Routledge.

Goldberg, D. and Huxley, P. (1991) *Common Mental Disorders – a bio-social model*. London: Routledge.

Paykel, E. (1992) *A Handbook of the Affective Disorders*. Edinburgh: Churchill Livingstone.

Williams, J. (1992) *The Psychological Treatment of Depression: A Guide to the Theory and Practice of Cognitive Behaviour Therapy*. London: Routledge.

14 / MALADAPTIVE BEHAVIOURS

The apparently heterogeneous conditions described in this chapter have a number of features in common:

1. Each of the behaviours considered represents an *exaggeration of normal behaviour:* consumption of alcohol, the taking of drugs, dieting, and overeating are normal behaviours, and obsessional traits are common in normal people. They are **maladaptive** in the sense that they cause the individual to suffer, and usually place him at a biological disadvantage: there is a *morbidity* associated with all of the conditions described in this chapter, and many also have an increased *mortality*.

2. *Response to anxiety:* each behaviour tends to become worse with increased anxiety and there is a component of each which is associated with reduction of anxiety. The consumption of alcohol or drugs relieves anxiety, and washing the hands relieves the anxiety that results from the obsessional idea that they may be contaminated. In each case this reduction in anxiety is only short-lived and in the longer term further anxiety is generated, which leads to the repetition of the behaviour, causing a vicious circle. Thus the alcoholic feels better after a few drinks but is left in a more anxious (withdrawn) state the next morning. This leads to further anxiety and further drinking.

3. A sense of subjective *compulsion* is experienced by the patient in most of these conditions. However hard he tries to resist, the person feels compelled to drink, starve, binge, or perform a certain act. The doctor must understand this so that he doesn't simply expect the patient readily to stop the behaviour.

ALCOHOL DEPENDENCE AND ALCOHOL-RELATED DISABILITIES

The concepts of dependence and alcohol-related disabilities are first defined.

Alcohol dependence (F10.2)

Alcohol becomes a drug of dependence when there is a compulsion to take it on a continuous or a periodic basis. The concept of dependence has three components:

1. Subjective awareness of a **compulsion to drink**.
2. **Increased tolerance**.
3. **Withdrawal symptoms**.

Awareness of a **compulsion to drink** is reported by the person, so that the first drink after a period of abstinence inevitably leads to a return to the previous level of consumption. The desire for a further drink is seen as irrational, the desire is resisted, yet the further drink is taken. If he tries to abstain, he may experience cravings for alcohol.

Increased tolerance develops so that large amounts of alcohol can be consumed without inebriation. The patient may have derived confidence from this, when in fact it indicates that dependence is beginning.

Withdrawal symptoms occur when there is an abrupt drop in the blood alcohol in someone who has maintained a high intake over a prolonged period of time. These typically occur in the morning, since this is the time when blood alcohol is at its lowest. They consist of shaking of the hands ('morning shakes'), nausea, sweating, and agitation. They are relieved by taking an alcoholic drink. More severe withdrawal symptoms include illusions, a sense of dread, and jumbled auditory hallucinations. *Generalized epileptic seizures* may occur, and after some forty-eight hours *delirium tremens* (see p. 157).

After a while, drinking begins to take priority over everything else: work, family life, social life, and even health. The drinking repertoire is restricted to a stereotyped pattern each day and drinking acquires salience over other activities. The concept of dependence leads to the discussion of whether someone is 'an alcoholic' or not. This is seldom a useful discussion. *It is better to ask whether a dependent individual has developed any related disabilities.*

Alcohol-related disabilities

These include physical, psychological, and social problems that result from persistent heavy drinking. Since alcohol-related disabilities may occur in the absence of dependence, this term includes many who come into contact with the medical services but would not be regard as alcoholics.

Epidemiology

Problem drinkers are greatly over-represented among medical in-patients. Eight per cent of women and 29 per cent of men in general medical and orthopaedic wards have been found to be problem drinkers. Higher figures will be found in casualty departments because accidents often involve those with a high blood alcohol, and in gastro-intestinal clinics, since these deal with many of the physical complications of alcohol. Yet most alcohol abusers in the general hospital go undetected. Twenty per cent of psychiatric admissions are associated with alcohol dependence.

General population surveys of alcohol abusers are notoriously difficult but also demonstrate that many problem drinkers are not known to any form of helping agency. However, it is probable that the prevalence of alcohol dependence is between 0.9 per cent and 1.4 per cent in England, while perhaps as many as 5 per cent of the adult population drink to excess. Figures for alcohol abuse are consistently higher among men than among women. Highest rates are found in those twenty to thirty years old but patients hospitalized for alcohol-related illness tend to be in their forties. Lowest rates are found in the middle classes. The upper social classes have a pattern of prolonged heavy drinking, while the lower classes drink extremely heavily at weekends.

Clinical features

PHYSICAL DISABILITIES

Cirrhosis of the liver is the best-recognized complication. Deaths from cirrhosis have risen in the UK recently because of the marked increase in alcohol consumption. For men the risk of cirrhosis increases as a result of drinking four pints of beer a day (or a quarter of a bottle of spirits or one bottle of wine); for women two pints of beer or equivalent is sufficient. Persistent heavy drinking is most likely to lead to cirrhosis, which will occur in 80 per cent of those who drink ten or more pints a day for fifteen years.

Hepatitis is also common among heavy drinkers and may lead on to cirrhosis. **Hepatic encephalopathy** occurs in liver failure.

Half the cases of **chronic pancreatitis** occur in heavy drinkers, especially chronic calcifying pancreatitis. **Acute gastritis** is common among heavy drinkers and peptic ulcers are three times more common than in non-drinkers. These illnesses together with **oesophageal varices** and **oesophagitis** mean that a problem drinker may present with abdominal pain, with a haematemesis, or with an iron-deficient anaemia. **Macrocytosis without anaemia** occurs as a result of folate deficiency. **Megaloblastic anaemia** may result from folate or vitamin B_{12} deficiency or as a direct toxic effect of alcohol. **Haemolytic anaemia** or **thrombocytopenia** may arise from cirrhosis.

The risk of **ischaemic heart disease** and **cerebrovascular accidents** is increased with alcohol abuse. **Cardiomyopathy** is more specifically linked to alcohol, which is associated with 50 per cent of cases of primary degeneration of the heart muscle.

Peripheral neuropathy occurs in 10 per cent of dependent drinkers and affects both sensory and motor systems, especially in the lower limbs. It is due to thiamine deficiency but rarely responds to treatment. **Cerebellar degeneration, myopathy,** and **Wernicke's encephalopathy** (see p. 168) occur. The alcoholic is at greater risk of **subdural haematoma** and **traumatic neuropathy,** as well as injuries of all kinds due to accidents at home and at work, to road traffic accidents, and to episodes of violence.

Many of these physical disabilities are due to, or made worse by, dietary deficiencies and general poor health which predispose the alcohol-dependent patient to develop infection.

PSYCHOLOGICAL DISABILITIES

Depression is common among alcohol abusers. Three patterns may be discerned:

1. Alcohol has a *direct depressant effect* and the alcohol abuser may have a persistently depressed mood that responds to abstinence.
2. Alcohol abuse leads to *social problems,* such as unemployment, divorce, and debts, and these lead to the person becoming depressed.
3. Depression, occurring for some other reason, may be *relieved temporarily* by drinking. This is one way in which heavy drinking starts, with an eventual worsening of the depression.

The depression may lead to deliberate self-harm. Nearly half of the males who take overdoses are dependent upon alcohol. The risk of **suicide** is increased many times among the population of alcohol abusers admitted for treatment.

Anxiety is related to alcohol abuse in a similar way to depression. In addition, anxiety is marked during alcohol withdrawal.

Alcoholic hallucinosis is a rare condition separate from the acute effects of withdrawal. In the setting of clear consciousness, auditory hallucinations occur which are generally in the second person and may be derogatory. They are often in the form of a conversation about the patient. The phenomenon usually occurs when prolonged heavy drinking ceases or is considerably reduced. It generally clears within a few days. If not, a state similar to schizophrenia develops. In this case it is likely that latent schizophrenia is released by the heavy alcohol intake.

Dissocial personality (see p. 63) may lead to alcoholism, but a normal personality may be evident before persistent heavy drinking leads to mood changes, inability to hold a job, and disruption of personal relationships.

MEMORY IMPAIRMENT

1. This occurs during acute intoxication with alcohol. Although the person may function quite normally during an evening of heavy drinking, on waking the next day there will be a dense amnesia for those hours (**alcoholic amnesia**, or 'palimpsest', or alcoholic 'blackout').
2. A specific memory impairment occurs, **Korsakow's syndrome** (see p. 168).
3. **Alcoholic dementia**, which may resolve if the person stops drinking.

SOCIAL DISABILITIES

Marital problems occur because the alcohol abuser is late coming home, and may be abusive or violent while drunk, incur debts, lose his job, and become impotent. The spouse may be disgusted by her drunk husband and embarrassed by his social behaviour.

She may therefore become depressed and anxious herself, or even take an overdose, and the astute general practitioner may detect alcohol abuse in this indirect way. Effects on the children may predominate if it is the wife who is abusing alcohol.

Work problems develop if the person attends late, is drunk and argumentative at work, and fails to perform at his former standard. Alcoholics miss much time from work and lose their jobs more frequently than their sober colleagues.

Alcoholics often come into contact with the **police** because of antisocial behaviour while intoxicated, either being disorderly or committing a petty crime.

Vagrancy has many causes but alcohol abuse often combines with other factors to lead to this state. Such people may present very considerable problems to the health services because of their multiple physical illnesses, their poor living conditions, and their insistence on continued drinking.

The detection of alcohol-related disabilities

Doctors do not detect alcohol abuse in general medical practice because they fail to ask the appropriate questions.

WHEN TO SUSPECT A PROBLEM MAY BE PRESENT

1. When any of the physical problems mentioned on p. 211 present (do not be satisfied with diagnosing a peptic ulcer: ask yourself whether alcohol could be responsible).
2. When the patient seems evasive or unclear while describing his complaint (this might represent concealment of heavy drinking or indicate a memory impairment).
3. When the patient is in a high-risk occupation (barman, publican, wine merchant, or brewer carries a high risk; well above average are company directors, commercial travellers, the armed forces, journalists, entertainers, and doctors).
4. When another family member has alcohol-related problems.
5. When investigations provide evidence of pathology which may be due to alcohol (for example, an unexpected elevation of the γ-GT).

THE CAGE

In any of these circumstances, you may find that the CAGE questions are useful (see the Card).

C. Have you ever felt you ought to CUT down on your drinking?

A. Have people ANNOYED you by criticizing your drinking?

G. Have you ever felt bad or GUILTY about your drinking?

E. Have you ever had a drink first thing in the morning to steady your nerves or get rid of a hangover (EYE OPENER)?

If you get positive replies to any TWO of these questions, it is worth taking a proper 'drinking history'. (Probability of being a case if score is 2 or > 2 = 45 per cent; probability of being a non-case if score is 0 or 1 = 97 per cent.)

TAKING A DRINKING HISTORY

Start by asking the patient (and later an informant) to describe a **typical drinking day**. One starts with the morning and proceeds through the day establishing what is drunk and when:

1. Establish if the first drink of the day is taken to combat withdrawal symptoms.
2. Does the patient drink throughout the day without getting drunk, or in bouts – usually at lunchtime and the evening?
3. How much is drunk at each session?
4. Does a single drink always lead to many more, and the person generally become drunk? If so, has this led to blackouts or falls?
5. Establish whether drinking takes place alone, and whether the person drinks only in response to certain moods or situations.

In this way the doctor and patient together estimate how much is being spent on drink each week. This is compared to the patient's previous estimate of expenditure per week and is often an eye opener (!) for the patient.

Having established the current drinking pattern one then tries to ascertain the **development of heavy drinking** over the years. There are often key points in the patient's life, such as working in the armed forces or in the wine trade, where a great increase in drinking occurred. The patient may recall his daily drinking pattern at times when he lost a particular job or when his marriage broke up. Contacts with the police may also be dated. In this way the doctor establishes the duration of heavy drinking and which of the related disabilities have developed.

Aetiology

GENETIC FACTORS

The prevalence of alcoholism amongst parents and siblings of alcoholics is two-and-a-half times that of the general population. This is not solely an environmental effect as sons of alcoholic fathers adopted away are just as likely to become alcoholics as those who remain in the original parental home.

PSYCHOLOGICAL FACTORS

Prospective studies have shown that although neurotic traits in childhood do not relate to the later development of alcoholism, children who were impulsive, aggressive, and hyperactive are more likely to become alcoholic as adults.

However, alcohol is a potent anxiolytic and agoraphobics, social phobics, and other neurotic personalities are likely to use alcohol in this way. In some this will lead on to clear dependence upon alcohol. The relief of tension or distress by alcohol can be viewed as a reward in behavioural terms. If this happens repeatedly the consumption of alcohol becomes a self-perpetuating habit. Any difficulties that arise from heavy drinking, including withdrawal symptoms, increase anxiety which can once again be relieved by the ingestion of alcohol. Thus a vicious circle with increasing consumption is set up.

SOCIAL FACTORS

Several *occupations* have more alcoholics than would be expected, and these have been listed above. Predisposing effects of these occupations include availability of cheap or free alcohol, strong peer pressure to drink, lack of supervision at work, and estrangement from the stabilizing influences of home life.

Cultural factors are important as the taboos against drinking among Muslims and Mormons, and against drunkenness among Jews, lead to very low rates of alcoholism compared to cultures where drinking is equated with masculinity.

Availability of alcohol is being increasingly recognized as a factor. There is evidence for a direct relationship between per capita consumption in a population and the number of people with alcohol-related problems. The former is determined by the real price of alcoholic beverages and as this is reduced the mortality rate from cirrhosis increases.

Investigations

TO ESTABLISH THE DIAGNOSIS

Physical – test blood or urinary alcohol to detect alcohol in the patient's blood stream when he denies having drunk; or abnormal liver function in someone who denies drinking very much.

Social – interviewing an informant to establish the patient's true drinking pattern and extent of related disabilities when these are not clear from the patient. Assessment of family relationships, financial position, and job situation will reveal the true extent of social disabilities, which are often more serious than the patient has led the doctor to believe.

A knowledge of these social factors may allow the doctor to understand the aetiology of the person's heavy drinking (this may be years previously) but also allow him to assess the factors which reinforce his current consumption.

TO ESTABLISH THE EXTENT OF ALCOHOL-RELATED DAMAGE

Physical – test liver function, especially γ-glutamyl transpeptidase (γ-GT), which is raised in 75 per cent of dependent drinkers.
Blood film for macrocytosis in the absence of anaemia.
Thereafter test to detect the physical sequelae of heavy drinking listed above.

Psychological – test for memory impairment (see p. 72).

Treatment

PHYSICAL

Drug treatment, to be given only in hospital, is required for withdrawal symptoms. *Diazepam* or *chlormethiazole* for nine days is usually sufficient (typical daily doses of chlormethiazole would be 6 g for three days, 4 g for three days and 3 g for three days). Treatment for delirium tremens is described on p. 157.

Parenterovite injections are given if there is any possibility that the person might be thiamine deficient.

Serious depression or anxiety occasionally requires drug treatment but usually depression improves as the person is detoxified.

Any accompanying physical illnesses must be treated.

Disulfiram (Antabuse) can be given daily and will help the impulsive drinker, who knows that he will become acutely ill if he drinks during the subsequent twenty-four hours. The patient must be motivated to take the tablet each day for this to be a useful adjunct to other treatment. It is only likely to be effective if given by a third person.

PSYCHOLOGICAL

Supportive psychotherapy is essential. This alone may be the appropriate treatment for mild alcohol abuse in general practice or the general medical clinic. Often the assessment procedures described above may enable the patient to realize that his drinking is causing physical or social damage. If this motivates him to reduce his drinking he is asked to keep a *daily diary* of his consumption. A gradual reduction will avoid withdrawal symptoms and drug treatment will be unnecessary. The major complaint is likely to be of insomnia but hypnotics can be avoided if the patient is warned of this beforehand and encouraged to do without. The doctor should ask the *patient's spouse* to encourage and help the patient especially at times of wanting a drink.

SOCIAL

Involvement of the family to understand the nature of the problem, provide support for the patient, and to help them cope.
Activities other than going to the pub or mixing with drinking friends should be encouraged.

The doctor must use his judgement as to whether total abstinence or controlled social drinking should be the aim of treatment. If alcohol-related problems are severe, or the patient has relapsed after previous periods of abstinence, total abstinence should be the goal.

With more serious cases *admission to a psychiatric ward or alcohol treatment unit* is recommended so that the commencement of psychological treatments occurs together with the detoxification.

Group therapy is useful to help the person to be honest about the nature of the problem and find ways of coping without alcohol.

Alcoholics Anonymous is very helpful for many patients. It advocates a strict abstinence policy and provides a social structure to replace drinking. Support is available at all times and often from ex-alcoholics with whom the patient can identify.

DRUG DEPENDENCE (F1x.2; where x refers to the particular drug)

Most of what has been written about alcohol-related problems applies to drug-related problems, so only a few points will be highlighted in this section.

Opiate dependence (F11.2)

Opiates in the UK come from three sources: legal prescriptions, theft from chemists, and smuggled oriental heroin.

The addict takes the drug by mouth ('dropping'), inhales the fumes of burning heroin ('chasing the dragon'), nasally inhales it ('snorting'), injects it intramuscularly (a 'fix'), or subcutaneously ('skin pop'), or intravenously ('main-lining'). Initially the drug taker experiences a 'rush, thrill, buzz or flash' following intravenous heroin. This is described like a rather superior sexual orgasm and is the reason for taking heroin at first. Appetite and sexual desire are decreased, and constipation is common.

As tolerance develops larger doses are required, dysphoria and somatic side-effects are experienced, and the person takes the drug increasingly to avoid withdrawal symptoms.

WITHDRAWAL SYMPTOMS

The latter start eight to ten hours after the last dose with **rhinorrhoea, lacrimation, yawning, sweating,** and **craving. Nausea, vomiting, diarrhoea, abdominal cramps,** and **muscle pains** develop.

Central nervous system *rebound excitability* is shown by **mydriasis, tachycardia, hypertension, flushing,** and **involuntary movements.**

These symptoms ('cold turkey') are much feared by addicts because they are so unpleasant, but in fact recede after seventy-two hours and do not carry the same risk to life as delirium tremens.

MORTALITY AND MORBIDITY

Mortality among opiate addicts is almost *fifteen times* that of the non-drug-taking population.

This is accounted for by the *morbidity* associated with opiate dependence, itself mainly related to:

1. *Dirty injection technique* leading to **sepsis, hepatitis, endocarditis, tuberculosis** and **nephrotic syndrome**. (See also p. 141 on HIV and AIDS.)
2. *Drug overdosage* which may cause **respiratory failure**.
3. Feelings of *desperation and depression* which often lead to **suicide**.

Morbidity and mortality of injecting drug abuse is set to rise significantly as some of this group become affected by *HIV infection and AIDS*. Injecting drug abusers contract this infection usually by sharing dirty injecting equipment and they are also one of the main sources of spread of HIV and AIDS into the general heterosexual population by sexual contact. HIV infection rates in drug abusers vary widely in different parts of the UK.

CLINICAL FEATURES

During withdrawal, the patient will have widely dilated pupils, tachycardia, and pilo-erection as well as the symptoms listed above. Look for thrombosed veins, and other complications of dirty injections.

TREATMENT

As with alcohol-related problems this is largely concerned with helping the individual to develop a new life style free of the drug. This may involve changing the social group in which the person mixes if this includes other drug abusers. Financial and family problems and involvement with the law will all require social help.

It is often the general practitioner, casualty officer, or general physician who is initially faced with an addict claiming to be in withdrawal. *It is illegal to prescribe certain narcotics (heroin and diconal) to those who are dependent upon them unless you have been approved by the Home Office.*

When deciding whether to prescribe **methadone** – this drug is used because it can be given orally, it prevents withdrawal symptoms, but does not produce the pleasurable 'buzz' of heroin – it is best to err on the side of caution; there are some heroin takers ('chippers') who only take the drug occasionally and are not dependent.

In the GP surgery and casualty department it is generally better not to prescribe in the absence of clear withdrawal symptoms or without the patient signing a *treatment contract*. This defines a withdrawal regime of reducing doses over a two to three week period and states conditions which the patient must fulfil (for example, abstinence from additional drug-taking checked by urine samples each visit) if the doctor is to continue prescribing. Without such precautions the doctor may find himself becoming obliged to continue prescribing.

For serious cases of dependence, admission to a *specialist treatment unit* is advisable so that rapid detoxification may take place with minimal withdrawal symptoms, and a long-term treatment plan commenced. This includes social treatment, rehabilitation, and, very occasionally, longer-term prescribing of methadone.

A minority of patients have developed dependence on opiates as a result of prescriptions from a doctor ('iatrogenic drug dependence'). In the case of terminally ill patients this does not matter. For the remainder opiates have usually been prescribed for a painful condition, so alternative methods of controlling the pain must be sought before the opiate can be withdrawn gradually.

Barbiturate dependence (F13.2)

Barbiturates are now very little used (see p. 79), but there are still some young multiple drug-abusers who manage to obtain these drugs through medical channels.

Barbiturate abusers may develop *tolerance* but the risk of **respiratory depression** increases with large doses and these may be fatal. Drug-dependent individuals are particularly likely to take an overdose of barbiturates. A *withdrawal syndrome* similar to that of alcohol is recognized, and **epileptic fits** and **delirium** are common.

CLINICAL FEATURES

The younger barbiturate addict may have injected these highly irritant drugs in aqueous solution, and so produced phlebitis, indolent abscesses, and sloughing ulcers. He may be unkempt, dirty, and malnourished. He may appear drunk, with slurred speech and incoherence, or be sleepy. Nystagmus is usually present, and depression is a common complication.

TREATMENT

Replacement with a short-acting barbiturate (for example, pentobarbitone) is recommended for those dependent upon high doses, with 10 per cent reduction of dosage per day and possible concurrent cover with an anticonvulsant. Subsequently prolonged difficulty with sleep occurs and **nightmares** result from REM rebound.

Benzodiazepine dependence (F13.2)

Benzodiazepines are widely prescribed drugs that are increasingly recognized as causing dependence. They cease to be effective anxiolytics once the user is habituated to them, yet severe symptoms of anxiety will be experienced if withdrawal is attempted. The withdrawal *symptoms* also include **giddiness**, **trembling**, **faintness**, **insomnia**, and **hypersensitivity**. These can be minimized by using a long-acting drug, such as diazepam, and withdrawing it very slowly. Irritability and insomnia are severe in the first two weeks after withdrawal, but have virtually disappeared three months later. Large numbers of people have become dependent on these drugs as a result of their widespread therapeutic use. In addition, young multiple drug-abusers often use them (especially Temazepam) in extremely high doses in combination with other drugs, as an alternative to barbiturates, which are less readily available.

The following drugs do not cause physical dependence but are of importance to psychiatry because of the abnormal mental states that they produce. They are often used alongside other drugs, and they may precipitate psychotic illness.

Amphetamines

These drugs are still occasionally prescribed for hyperkinetic children and adults with narcolepsy. (Amphetamine abusers sometimes claim to suffer from the latter condition.) Most street usage is of a very impure powdered preparation ('speed' or 'whizz').

They are taken to produce a state of increased awareness, energy, and concentration, together with reduced hunger and fatigue. Taken intravenously they may produce a short-lived 'flush' and are used in this way by opiate addicts. These effects are followed by depression, anxiety, irritability, and anergia. Barbiturates may also be taken to combat the insomnia produced.

CLINICAL FEATURES

The patient will be talkative and over-active if intoxicated, sleepy or depressed if withdrawn. He may be malnourished because of the anorexia, and lick his lips because of the dry mouth. The pupils are dilated, there may be sweating, tachycardia, high blood pressure, or arrhythmias, and there is usually a generalized hyperreflexia.

Amphetamines may produce a **symptomatic schizophrenia** (see p. 179) in otherwise normal people, with persecutory delusions, accompanied by visual, tactile, and auditory hallucinations in a state of clear consciousness. They will also exacerbate schizophrenic symptoms in those vulnerable to the disorder. In other patients a **symptomatic mania** can be precipitated. The mental state usually returns to normal over five to seven days as the drug is excreted, but occasionally a persistent psychosis requires treatment with phenothiazines.

Cocaine

Cocaine may be 'snorted' into the nostril and absorbed through the nasal mucosa, injected, or smoked (the 'crack' preparation of the drug is used in this way). It is a central nervous stimulant with effects similar to amphetamine but said to be less sharp and more subtle. It may produce disorientation and depression. It resembles amphetamine in its ability to produce a symptomatic psychosis.

CLINICAL FEATURES

The intoxicated patient may be excited, with dilated pupils and tremulousness. He may report a feeling of insects crawling under his skin ('formication'). At later stages, dizziness, convulsions, and cardiac arrhythmias occur. Death may be from cardiac arrest.

Hallucinogens

Mescalin, lysergic acid diethylamide (LSD, or 'acid'), dimethyltryptamine ('angel dust'), and psilocybin ('the magic mushroom') are hallucinogens. At the time of writing LSD and psilocybin are most commonly used in the UK.

CLINICAL FEATURES

Taken orally LSD causes perceptual changes within forty minutes. Sensation in all modalities is heightened and distorted and may be translated from one modality to another so sounds may be seen and colour smelled: *synaesthesia*. The body image may be terrifyingly distorted; the patient may regard himself as able to fly or to walk on water. Numerous deaths have occurred in this way. Extreme emotional changes may occur, which result in anxiety and terror of imminent insanity: these are described as a 'bad trip'. Such states are best managed by someone 'talking down' the patient, emphasizing that the alarming experiences are due to the drug.

· The acute effects die down over twenty-four hours, but perceptual changes may last longer. A more prolonged psychosis may result as with amphetamines, although it may be that the drug has merely released the psychosis in a vulnerable personality.

Sometimes *flash-back experiences* occur some months later when, under stress or the effect of another drug, the person relives part of the perceptual distortion that occurred during an LSD trip.

Cannabis

Cannabis is widely abused by young people, notably students and members of some ethnic groups. 'Grass' refers to the dried plant, *Cannabis sativa*, while 'resin' is secreted by the female parts of the flowering plant. The effects largely depend on the circumstances in which the drug is taken, and it is generally used as a social drug. There is no withdrawal syndrome, nor is there evidence of tolerance.

Feelings of well-being, relaxation, and tranquillity are induced within minutes of inhalation but prevailing moods of anger or depression may be aggravated. Perceptual disturbances of time, sight, and sound may occur but the person generally retains insight throughout.

Acute schizophrenia-like episodes can occur with high doses, and these may last up to forty-eight hours. Cannabis use is a risk factor for schizophrenia.

Solvent sniffing

Euphoria may result from the sniffing of solvents which contain toluene and acetone, but continued inhalation leads to stupor and loss of consciousness as these toxic substances are powerful CNS depressants and may cause neuronal destruction. Psychological dependence occurs and this causes concern because it involves children, especially those from a deprived background. The mortality is considerable; about 50 per cent due to direct toxic effects of the solvent, the remainder mainly due to asphyxia from the plastic bag from which the solvent was inhaled, or from inhalation of gastric contents.

CLINICAL FEATURES

Look for glue on the hands, face, or clothes, and the glue sniffer's rash over the mouth and nasal area. The patient is usually a child or adolescent, and males outnumber females by thirteen to one. The glue may be smelled. There are rapid variations in the level of consciousness; disorientation; sometimes slurred speech and an ataxic gait.

Non-opiate analgesics

Those who regularly take large doses of aspirin, phenacetin, and paracetamol may do so secretively, against medical advice, and with serious physical consequences.

Psychological dependence occurs, and women with chronic depressive illness or personality disturbance are particularly prone to use these drugs in this way. The principal physical related problem is *analgesic nephropathy*.

Multiple drug abuse seems to be the norm rather than the exception, especially if alcohol is included as a drug. Therefore a drug-dependent person who has taken an overdose may have done so with several drugs. An opiate-dependent person denied his normal dose will turn to other drugs.

ANOREXIA NERVOSA (F50.0)

This condition predominantly affects adolescent girls, and takes the form of **self-induced loss of weight**, so that body weight is at least 15 per cent below standard weight (the body-mass index, that is, weight in kg /(height in metres)^2, is 17.5 or less), accompanied by an intense wish to be thin. The patient has an intense **fear of fatness**, and this takes the form of an *over-valued idea* (see p. 31) that she is fat, although aware that others regard her as thin – this feature distinguishes anorexia nervosa from all other causes of either weight loss or anorexia. There is a widespread endocrine disorder involving the hypothalamic–pituitary–gonadal axis, manifested in females by **amenorrhoea**, and in males by **loss of sexual interest and potency**. If onset is pre-pubertal, the sequence of pubertal events is delayed or arrested.

The patient may successfully conceal abnormal eating habits, and sometimes even be under intense medical investigation for somatic complaints such as diarrhoea, metabolic disorder, or amenorrhoea before the diagnosis is recognized.

Epidemiology

In Scotland, the prevalence has been estimated at 10.8 per 100,000 for females in the fifteen to thirty-four age group. Over 90 per cent of patients with anorexia nervosa are female. Surveys in England have indicated that between 1 per cent and 2 per cent of adolescent females are affected, with highest rates for the age group between thirteen and twenty, and with a few cases starting either before puberty or during adult life.

Clinical features

Emaciation with a weight of 35–40 kg is common. If the weight has dropped as low as 30–35 kg the patient may present with fainting. She may wear heavy clothes to mask the thinness. This weight loss results from calorie restriction and selective exclusion of carbohydrate from the diet, but protein deficiency can develop in the chronic state, which may present as swelling of the ankles. *Abuse of diuretics* leads to dehydration and *purgative abuse* leads to diarrhoea and hypokalaemia in severe cases.

The patient's apparent unconcern about her condition may be balanced by her parents being distraught; whereas she may cook for the rest of the family she starves herself. *Preoccupation with calorie counting, avoidance of all carbohydrate, vomiting after meals, vigorously exercising, and taking laxatives* are common behaviours. The patient may deceive those around her into thinking that she is eating adequately and often does so in the medical ward.

The anorexia may be interspersed with bulimic episodes when binge eating is followed by vomiting and guilt. The underlying panic in relation to weight gain becomes obvious at such times. The patient may show signs of depression or obsessionality, especially in relation to food preparation and consumption.

The body shows evidence of chronic starvation with:

1. Cold, blue extremities.
2. Fine, downy hair – 'lanugo' – on back and face.
3. Slow pulse: 40–60 per minute.
4. Low blood pressure: 90/60.
5. Low body temperature.
6. Reduction of LH and FSH with amenorrhoea.

The amenorrhoea is usually secondary to the loss of weight, but occasionally precedes it.

Differential diagnosis

Dieting is to be distinguished from anorexia by the absence of amenorrhoea and over-valued ideas about being fat.

Weight loss may also result from psychological or physical illnesses: *hyperthyroidism* and *diabetes* are examples of the latter that occur at this age. Organic causes of diarrhoea, such as *idiopathic steatorrhea* or *inflammatory bowel disease,* may need to be considered.

Amenorrhoea may result from *ovarian or pituitary disease*, following use of the *contraceptive pill* or from *psychological stress*.

Depressive and obsessional features may suggest these illnesses, and occasionally *psychotic illnesses* can present with avoidance of food, but the central fear of weight gain and distorted body image generally indicate the true diagnosis.

Aetiology

Eating disorders tend to run in families so obesity and alcoholism among older relatives are common. Episodes of anorexia during the teenage years of female relatives may have occurred though not necessarily reached medical treatment.

The anorexic patient is often obese during her younger childhood years and may have been teased for being so. An early menarche and rapid growth increase pubertal fatness. The subsequent dieting may start as a reasonable behaviour but get out of control in relation to a precipitating event. More commonly there is a background of disturbed family relationships with a dependent and immature patient. There may be competition with other sibs for parental attention, or conflicts about leaving home with an avoidance of mature responsibilities. This avoidance often involves sexual behaviour.

Maintaining factors are sometimes very important in prolonging what might otherwise have been a brief episode of dieting. For example, there may be some crisis within the family, such as the parents' marriage breaking up, or psychiatric illness in one of the parents, or a family situation which the daughter seems to be able to control with her anorexia.

Investigations

Physical investigations may be necessary to exclude other conditions listed in the differential diagnosis. More important is the need to assess the extent of malnutrition and electrolyte disturbance due to vomiting. *Confirmation of the diagnosis comes from the patient directly expressing her fear of weight gain* to the doctor. The doctor must allow the patient to develop enough trust for this to occur, preferably at the first interview. The patient may also indicate to a sympathetic doctor that she has other fears about growing up even if she is not prepared to describe these in detail at an early stage.

Assessment of body image in a standardized way by a psychologist is possible but often unnecessary, as experience over a short time generally provides evidence that the patient is afraid of gaining weight and does not do so even when she has initially promised to do so.

Luteinizing hormone levels have been shown to be low, and to show an impaired response to LH-releasing factor. Even when weight is restored, cyclical LH activity may not resume – suggesting an abnormality of the hypothalamo-pituitary axis. There may be raised levels of growth hormone and cortisol and abnormalities of insulin secretion.

Social investigations – a member of the team attempts to identify any problems in the parental or other family relationships which might cause or exacerbate the anorexia of the patient. The possibility of family therapy or support for the parents is investigated.

Treatment

Treatment is aimed first at restoration of normal body weight, and then assistance with maturation and establishment of independence appropriate to the patient's age.

RESTORATION OF BODY WEIGHT

Out-patient treatment may be appropriate: sometimes separation of the patient from her parents leads to weight gain – so moving to another house or hostel may help to avoid hospital admission.

In-patient treatment may be required from the outset if the patient's weight is very low and secondary physical problems are severe. Rarely the emaciation is extreme and the patient refuses voluntary treatment so admission under section 3 of the Mental Health Act (see p. 332) has to be considered. Restoration of body weight in hospital can be achieved in various ways, but perhaps the simplest has regard to three points:

1. Bed rest.
2. Supervision during meals and for at least half an hour afterwards.
3. Controlled diet, avoiding excessive weight gain. Aim at increasing by 3–4 lb per week.

Drug treatment is sometimes helpful. *Chlorpromazine* reduces anxiety and stimulates appetite, but occasionally leads to epileptic fits. *Anti-depressants* are used if there is evidence of a concurrent depressive illness, which sometimes occurs in older patients. Correction of *hypokalaemia* may be urgent if vomiting has been a pronounced feature, and of severe dehydration if diuretics have been abused. Other dietary deficiencies may need attention.

Behaviour therapy may be used as an adjunct to restoration of body weight. A target weight is set, and the weight to be gained is divided into steps with a clearly stated reward for each intermediate target weight. The gaining of rewards must be very strictly related to weight gains. The patient is initially confined to bed and denied visitors, only earning privileges such as getting dressed, going out, and having time at home once she puts on weight. One must guard against patients gaining weight quickly so that they can be discharged and then lose it again.

Psychotherapy

A relationship of trust with the patient from the first interview is essential. It is likely that the patient will attend the first interview eager to discover whether the doctor will side with the parents' wish for increased weight or the patient's desire to stay thin. In fact the doctor makes it clear from the outset that weight gain is essential for a full recovery, but that he or she understands the patient's fears of weight gain.

MATURATION AND ESTABLISHMENT OF INDEPENDENCE

Treatment in the longer term is principally by **psychotherapy** with the patient and/or her family. Once trust has been established the aim of psychotherapy is to encourage the patient to discuss those powerful inner feelings which she has been unable to express previously and which have led to the anorexia.

Course and prognosis

The disorder usually lasts for at least two years. Weight gain in the short term is usually satisfactory in most cases. This is maintained in approximately 60 per cent and normal menstruation is restored in a similar proportion. Eating habits can only be regarded as returning to normal in 40–50 per cent and some patients present later with obesity. Psychiatric illness occurs in approximately one-third; this is usually depressive illness, obsessional illness, anxiety, or phobias.

Approximately 15 per cent of cases become chronic, that is, continuing over five years or more, and the chance of recovery in these cases is poor. The condition carries a mortality rate of up to 10 per cent; death occurs through emaciation or suicide. Factors that indicate a *good prognosis* are an onset very soon after puberty, a brief illness with brisk response to treatment, and satisfactory family relationships. A poor prognosis is indicated by the presence of vomiting, purgative abuse, and bulimic episodes with extreme weight loss and development of a chronic illness.

BULIMIA NERVOSA (F50.2)

This is a form of eating disorder where the abnormality is of uncontrolled and excessive eating ('**binge-eating**'). During the eating binges – which tend to last less than two hours – there is a feeling of loss of control of the eating behaviour, and the binge is followed either by *self-induced vomiting*, by the use of *laxatives*, or by *rigorous dieting* to counteract the effects of the binge. The patient typically eats high-calorie foods on their own, and reports a relief from tension during the binge.

Binge-eating occurs in both anorexia nervosa and obesity, and can also be a mild intermittent behaviour that cannot be regarded as pathological. It is always preceded by attempts to diet. Occasionally it occurs with sufficient frequency to be regarded as an eating disorder.

Diagnostic criteria

1. Recurrent episodes of binge-eating.
2. A feeling of lack of control during binges.
3. Self-induced vomiting, purgation, or severe dieting afterwards.
4. At least two binges per week for at least three months.

The patients presenting with bulimia tend to be older than those with anorexia nervosa, but often report a previous episode of anorexia that may have gone undetected. Virtually all are women, and the psychopathology overlaps with that described in anorexia nervosa. However, body weight is often normal, menstrual disorders occur in only about a half of the cases, and most readily agree that they have an eating disorder even though the bingeing may always have been done in secret. They may complain about their preoccupation with food and weight changes. Mood disturbances are common. Again, the eating disorder tends to mask other psychological problems and a binge may be a repeated way of relieving distress.

Complications

These can occur due to vomiting and purgation which result in potassium deficiency with weakness, cardiac arrhythmias, and renal damage; teeth may become pitted by gastric acid.

Treatment

This differs from that in anorexia because the patient's weight is normal. A *behavioural assessment* is employed to examine the circumstances in which bingeing occurs. This is usually when the person is under stress, which triggers negative thoughts about herself. Alternative strategies to over-eating are then put into practice at such moments. *Psychotherapy* is aimed first at getting the patient to express verbally her underlying conflicts and problems, and secondly at finding ways of coming to terms with these.

OBESITY (ICD-10: E66)

Obesity refers to an **abnormally high proportion of body fat**, and can best be estimated by comparing body weight with height (the body-mass index is greater than 25). About one-third of adults in Britain and the USA are obese by this definition.

Aetiology

The aetiology is partly constitutional, partly social – a combination of over-eating and under-exercise. In some obese people an additional contribution comes from *abnormal eating patterns* such as eating to deal with stress, comfort eating, night-eating, continuous snacking, and binge-eating. Those who were **overweight in childhood** are a special group with a greater tendency for abnormal eating patterns, and a greater likelihood of self-loathing and disparagement of their own body image.

Community studies have demonstrated that there is no direct link between obesity and neurotic illness. However, obese patients seen in medical clinics who find it impossible to lose weight may be an unrepresentative sample, and thus at greater risk for mental disorders like anxiety and depression. The excess in weight may enable the patient to deny problems in the personal and sexual spheres. If weight loss is successfully achieved these problems may become prominent and disrupt personal relationships whose precarious stability seems to have depended on the patient being obese. It is not uncommon for such patients to have a history of anorexia when younger, which may not have reached medical attention, when similar sexual or interpersonal problems were evident.

Treatment

All obese patients should be given advice on *diet and exercise*, and many benefit from self-help groups although relapse is frequent.

One should consider patients with abnormal eating patterns, low self-esteem, and a negative attitude towards their body image for a cognitive-behavioural approach. *Such an offer of treatment will be made only to a small minority*, since most moderately obese patients do not over-eat, are not unduly sensitive to food cues, and their eating style is no different from that of other people.

Appetite-suppressant drugs have no place in the treatment of obesity: they produce dependence and such effect as they may have on body weight is likely to be short-lived.

Good results have been reported by surgical procedures in the treatment of severe obesity (body-mass index > 40). Both *gastric resection* and *jejuno-ileal bypass* are followed by weight reduction as a result of decreased food intake, and there may be psychological benefits including increased self-confidence, elevation of mood, and decrease in negative self-image. The former operation is technically difficult, but associated with fewer post-operative complications.

OBSESSIVE COMPULSIVE DISORDER (F42)

An obsessional illness is a state in which the outstanding symptom is a sense of subjective compulsion, which the patient feels must be resisted, to carry out some action, dwell on an idea, recall an experience, or ruminate upon some abstract topic. The obsessional urge or idea is seen to be senseless but recognized as arising from within oneself, rather than being imposed from outside. Attempts to dispel the inner thought, or to resist the compulsion to carry out some act, usually lead to anxiety. (See definitions of both *obsessions* and *compulsions* in the Glossary.)

Obsessional phenomena include:

1. **Thoughts** of an unpleasant or obscene nature.
2. **Images** in the form of disgusting but vividly imagined scenes.
3. **Impulses** to perform acts of a violent or embarrassing nature.
4. **Rituals** such as hand-washing or elaborate ways of dressing or cleaning oneself.
5. **Ruminations** (see p. 30) about the pros and cons of everyday actions.
6. **Doubts** concerning whether or not actions involving safety (locking doors, turning off gas-taps and switches) have been completed.

Diagnostic criteria

An obsessional illness refers to symptoms as described above, in the absence of symptoms higher in the hierarchy (such as organic states, schizophrenia, or depression), when they cause significant distress and interfere with the individual's social or occupational functioning. Related phenomena include *slowness* and *depersonalization* (see p. 336).

Approximately two-thirds of patients who develop obsessional illness show *obsessional personality traits* (see p. 66). Indeed, those with such traits often experience some obsessional symptoms, but if they are able to function socially and occupationally they are not said to be *ill*. Such patients often experience a great increase in such symptoms if they develop a depressive illness, but in that case they are described as having depressive illnesses – since depression is higher in the hierarchy, and the obsessional symptoms will remit with treatment of depression.

Epidemiology

Estimates vary between 0.1 and 2 per 1,000 per year. Obsessional illnesses do occur without depressive symptoms, but they are comparatively rare. Obsessional illness accounts for only 2 per cent of the illness seen by psychiatrists.

Differential diagnosis

Obsessional symptoms may occur secondary to depression, schizophrenia, or organic brain disease – in which case treatment is usually directed at the precipitating condition.

Treatment

Behaviour therapy is the treatment of choice and consists of **response prevention** (see p. 106) for compulsive rituals and **thought-stopping** for obsessional thoughts. In the latter treatment the patient is helped to substitute neutral or pleasant thoughts for the distressing thought.

Tricyclic anti-depressants, especially clomipramine, may be helpful even in the absence of marked depression. Anxiolytic drugs provide only temporary relief from the worst anxiety. Supportive, rather than interpretive, psychotherapy is helpful at times when the symptoms are worst.

FURTHER READING

Beech, H.R. and Vaughan, M. (1978) *Behavioural Treatment of Obsessional States.* Chichester: John Wiley.

Edwards, G. (1987) *The Treatment of Drinking Problems: A Guide for the Helping Professions.* Oxford: Blackwell Scientific.

Hore, B. (1976) *Alcohol Dependence.* Oxford: Butterworth.

Kessel, N. and Walton, H. (1986) *Alcoholism.* Harmondsworth: Penguin.

15 / ABNORMAL ILLNESS BEHAVIOUR

NORMAL ILLNESS BEHAVIOUR

Illness behaviour has been defined as *the ways in which given symptoms may be differentially perceived, evaluated, and acted (or not acted) upon*. For example, two healthy people run for a bus and both notice palpitation. One assumes that it is a normal experience, the symptom is transient and soon forgotten. The other, whose spouse recently died of a myocardial infarct, notices it more, worries that she has heart disease, and consults her general practitioner.

The definition is extremely broad and includes all aspects of thinking, emotion, and behaviour related to the symptoms of illness, whether or not these are associated with objective evidence of physical or mental disorders. The more important aspects of illness behaviour are listed in *Table 15.1*.

The term 'illness behaviour' does not imply that the behaviours are necessarily pathological. Illness behaviours that are appropriate are adaptive. They facilitate recovery in those with disease, for example, by consultation, compliance with treatment, and rest when indicated. They also allow those with trivial symptoms to function well by recognizing them as such and avoiding unnecessary invalidism.

For individuals, illness behaviour includes both *traits* (the lifelong tendency to have a low or high threshold for being aware of and worrying about symptoms and consulting doctors) and *state* (the behaviour at a particular time). There is evidence that such traits are acquired during childhood, by learning the patterns of illness behaviour that are characteristic of the culture or family. The majority of consultations, particularly in general practice, are determined to a considerable extent by current social and psychological factors, including recent life events, the extent of social support, and distress – this is illustrated by the example of palipitation described above. Thus many of the behaviours related to illness are not directly determined by disease processes but by the psychological and social state of the patient.

Table 15.1 *Different aspects of illness behaviour*

Symptom perception	quality, distribution, intensity, frequency, duration, number
Symptom evaluation	beliefs about significance and morbid risk; ability of symptoms to be controlled by self or others
Actions	
Communication	
verbal	complaint behaviour; sighs, groans
non-verbal	posture, gait, use of aids
Consultation	medical, non-medical, number consulted, total consultations
Treatment	number of medications and other treatments received, treatment adherence, self-treatment
Disability	maintenance of customary roles: self-care, family, social, recreational activities
Mood states	may include anxiety, depression, anger; denial of negative mood states

ABNORMAL ILLNESS BEHAVIOUR

The term **'abnormal illness behaviour'** is used to refer to illness behaviours which are regarded as inappropriate or maladaptive, that is, they are motivated by goals other than maintaining function or recovery from disease. The rest of this chapter describes the different aspects of abnormal illness behaviour and these are summarized in *Figure 15.1*.

There are two major aspects of abnormal illness behaviour, which have been described as **'illness denial'** and **'illness affirmation'**.

Illness denial is a term used to describe the behaviour of people with significant physical or mental disorders who use denial (see p. 59) to avoid the stigma of a physical disorder such as heart disease, or a mental disorder such as manic-depressive illness. They avoid appropriate consultations and there are also likely to be problems with treatment adherence, for example, failure to follow advice about exercise, diet, or taking lithium.

Illness affirmation is a term used to describe the behaviour of those who inappropriately affirm illness although they are well or have only minor disorders. They present symptoms or are disabled to an extent which is disproportionate to any objective evidence of physical or mental disorder. All of the disorders which are described in the rest of this chapter have in common the fact that they are forms of abnormal illness affirmation.

The development of invalidism can be of benefit (whatever our state of health or disease) because it allows us to avoid unpleasant obligations or predicaments: for example, abdominal pain preventing a child from going to school when he has not done his homework or expects to be bullied; or headaches preventing a man who has recently been made redundant from seeking work, despite his limited skills.

Figure 15.1 *Processes involved in abnormal illness behaviour, showing examples of common diagnoses in italics.*

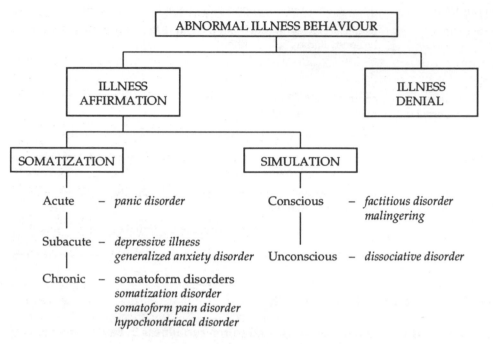

If successful this leads to **'primary gain'**, that is, relief from stress, due to avoidance of the underlying predicament. (An example is described in the section on dissociative disorders, p. 241.) Following the onset of invalidism, there may be other tangible benefits (referred to as **'secondary gain'**), such as increased care and concern from family, friends, and medical services, as well as financial gains such as disability benefits, pensions, and compensation payments. If successful, such mechanisms are more likely to be used in the future. Invalidism can benefit others too – this process has been referred to as **'tertiary gain'**.

A man who has been made redundant develops 'tension headaches'. His wife has devoted her life to bringing up their children, who have left home, and her life is now empty. She responds to his headaches with increasing care, so that she satisfies her own thwarted need to care for others, and consequently he does less for himself, worries about the significance of his headaches, and becomes disabled.

Similarly, some doctors are able to resolve uncomfortable feelings of uncertainty by diagnosing non-existent illnesses or offering inappropriate treatments. This also illustrates the way in which abnormal illness behaviour is commonly facilitated by doctors – that is, it is partly *iatrogenic*.

Usually, patients and others who are involved do not consciously plan to benefit from invalidism, that is, these are **unconscious defence mechanisms** (the exception is 'malingering' – see p. 238).

SOMATIZATION

Somatization is an aspect of abnormal illness affirmation (see *Figure 15.1*) and can be defined as *the expression of personal and social distress in an idiom of bodily complaints with medical help-seeking.*

The terminology is potentially confusing. *Figure 15.1* should help to illustrate that 'somatization' is the term used for the *process* we have just defined; the 'somatoform disorders' are a *group of diagnoses*; and 'somatization disorder' is the term used for one *diagnosis* in this group.

The majority of patients with somatization are also experiencing symptoms of depression and anxiety, but they do not present these symptoms to the doctor or recognize their connection with current psychosocial problems. Instead, they complain of pains and other somatic symptoms, and they do not consider themselves psychiatrically unwell. They may have physical disease as well; or it may not be possible to demonstrate any physical disease.

Acute somatization tends to be associated with sudden brief fear or panic, as when someone develops palpitation before an examination or worries about having a 'heart attack', but then probably recognizes the true nature of the experience as soon as their anxiety, and its cause, subside. The psychological disorders will probably be viewed as **adjustment disorders (F43.2)**. *Subacute somatization* is more prolonged, lasting for weeks or several months, and is more commonly related to anxiety states and depressive disorders. *Chronic somatization* is best regarded as lasting for six months or more and is particularly associated with somatoform disorder diagnoses (see *Figure 15.1* and below).

Epidemiology

Community-based surveys indicate that the most severe and chronic forms of somatization are found in about 0.5 per cent of the general adult population and that about 10 per cent are suffering from less severe disorders. In primary care almost 20 per cent of patients presenting to their doctors with new episodes of illness can be shown to satisfy criteria for acute or subacute somatization because, in addition to the features described above, a research diagnosis of a depressive illness or an anxiety state can be made, treatment of which would ameliorate the patient's presenting somatic symptoms. A physical disease will be demonstrable in about 70 per cent of such somatizing patients, but it will not by itself account for the patient's symptoms. Most surveys have shown that between 20 per cent and 40 per cent of patients admitted to medical wards have a psychiatric illness. However, only a small minority of these see themselves as psychiatrically ill: most will satisfy criteria for somatization.

Clinical features of abnormal illness behaviour and somatization

It is important to recognize that both abnormal illness behaviour and somatization are *not diagnoses but processes*, with related behaviours, which can occur in the setting of any physical or mental disorder.

In most settings the majority of somatizers have **depressive or anxiety disorders** (often with mixed symptoms) and others have **adjustment disorders**. An important minority have **alcohol- and drug-related disorders**. In addition there is a group of psychiatric disorders which are particularly characterized by abnormal illness behaviour and somatization, that is, these constitute the core of the symptoms and signs. They include the **somatoform disorders – somatization disorder, somatoform pain disorder,** and **hypochondriacal disorder** (see *Figure 15.1* and below).

Aetiology of somatization

We must now understand why these patients choose to focus upon somatic symptoms to the relative neglect of their affective symptoms and psychosocial problems:

1. The patient does not connect his affective symptoms with his physical symptom, e.g. pain, and concentrates on the pain **because it hurts**.

2. The patient is afraid that the pain may indicate some **serious physical disease**, so he gives it increasing attention, leading to further exacerbation of the pain.

3. The patient may feel that his emotional problems are his own affair, but excluding physical causes for pains is very much his doctor's job. Some doctors share this view, feel unfamiliar with or intolerant of their patients' emotional problems, and may respond with greater interest to physical symptoms than they do to psychological symptoms. This is **differential reinforcement** by the doctor. Doctors may investigate physical symptoms repeatedly despite negative findings, give misleading and conflicting diagnoses, and give physical treatments for non-existent disorders. This encourages their patients' inappropriate worry about a physical disorder. So somatization is often at least partly *iatrogenic*, that is, caused by doctors.

4. Somatization tends to run in families. One reason is that the patterns of behaviour are copied (or 'modelled'). Another is that key people in the patient's family may be more sympathetic to physical symptoms than they are to psychological problems: this is **differential reinforcement by relatives**.

5. The patient may feel that there is some **social stigma** attached to emotional illness: societies vary in the extent to which they stigmatize such illnesses, but in the UK it is more acceptable to be thought to have a physical illness.

6. The last reason is a development of the same point: a somatizing patient who fails to recognize that he is emotionally unwell does not have to ask himself awkward questions about his own personal contribution to the life predicament that he is in, particularly if it can be blamed on physical illness. To have a physical illness is a misfortune, but in most cases one does not need to feel responsible for it. A somatizing patient **need not blame himself,** examine the life problem in which he is enmeshed, or accept some responsibility for resolving it. Thus **somatization acts as a defence mechanism**.

Recent research into somatization in primary care settings has indicated that adult somatizers are more likely to have experienced lack of care from parents during their childhood, serious physical illness before the age of seventeen, and serious physical illness in one or both parents. The more of these experiences there have been, the more likely they are to develop chronic somatization. It has also been shown that, when compared with patients in primary care who present psychological complaints, somatizers are less depressed, report lower levels of social dissatisfaction and stress, have a less sympathetic attitude towards mental illness, are less likely to consult doctors about psychological symptoms, and have received more medical in-patient care for previous complaints.

SOMATOFORM DISORDERS (F45)
(somatization disorder, persistent somatoform pain disorder, and hypochondriacal disorder)

These three syndromes are all forms of **chronic somatization**, characterized by repeated physical complaints, concern about health, requests for medical examinations, investigations, and treatments (often from many different doctors), and failure to be reassured by negative findings and explanations. Although there may be some evidence of a physical disorder, this cannot account for either the complaints or the associated disability, which is sometimes severe so that the patient may become chair- or bed-bound. Somatization is a predominant feature: anxiety and depressed mood may be present (and there may be an associated diagnosis of an affective disorder – see above), but this may be denied. Precipitation and maintenance of the physical complaints are often closely related to distressing life events but the patient tends to resist any exploration of possible psychological causes. Although the following disorders are described, in practice there is often some overlap and it is uncertain to what extent they are separate conditions.

Somatization disorder (F45.1)

This is a form of chronic somatization in which the patient has many different symptoms which fluctuate and recur over many years. Very few complaints will have adequate physical explanation. It is much more common in women than men, starts in early adult life or even childhood, and tends to run in families. Symptoms may be referred to any system of the body and are particularly likely to include various aches and pains, and gastro-intestinal, sexual, and menstrual complaints.

Patients are likely to have visited numerous hospital departments (for example, the neurology department for headaches, cardiology for palpitation and breathlessness, gastroenterology for abdominal distension and flatulence, gynaecology for dysmenorrhoea and menorrhagia) where they receive multiple inappropriate diagnoses and accumulate thick medical records. Doctors feel frustrated by these patients, as attempts to relieve their symptoms are unsuccessful. Often they claim that their symptoms have been caused by treatments, particularly surgery, given by previous doctors. A description of a patient with typical somatization disorder is provided in a formulation at the end of Chapter 9.

DIAGNOSIS

The following are ALL required:

1. At least two years of multiple and variable physical symptoms for which no adequate physical explanation has been found.
2. Persistent refusal to accept reassurance from doctors that there is no physical explanation.
3. Impairment in social function associated with the symptoms.

Persistent somatoform pain disorder (F45.4)

In this form of chronic somatization the essential feature is pain which persists, for at least some months and often for many years, and cannot be adequately explained by any identifiable organic pathology or physiological process, despite appropriate examination and investigation. The disorder is diagnosed more often in women than men and can start at any age. The pain may be felt at a single site, or at multiple sites, or may be diffuse, and may affect different sites at different times. Its distribution is usually incompatible with any recognizable pain representation of the central or peripheral nervous systems, for example, a dermatome or peripheral nerve distribution. On examination, clinical signs are either absent or inconsistent with any known organic syndrome. Patients with this disorder often have additional physical complaints, and preoccupation with ill health and 'missed' diagnoses, so that they tend to see many different doctors in their search for a 'cure' and cannot be reassured by negative findings.

Although there is often evidence of current or past organic disorders which have contributed to the symptoms, this is never sufficient to account for the severity or distribution of the pain or the associated disability, which may be profound. In some cases the pain is initiated by trauma, for example following a road traffic accident, but fails to improve as expected, and this pattern is seen particularly in those seeking compensation.

Often there is evidence of social and psychological predisposing factors (such as childhood physical or psychological neglect or abuse), precipitating factors (such as negative life events), and gain resulting from the symptoms. These are not always obvious from the history because the patient tends to present an idealized picture of a 'perfect' life.

Hypochondriacal disorder (F45.2)

The essential characteristic of this form of chronic somatization is persistent preoccupation with the possibility of having a serious physical disorder (for example, heart disease or cancer) or an abnormality in physical appearance (for example, nose or breasts too small or too large), despite appropriate medical examination, explanation, and reassurance about the lack of physical abnormality. The beliefs take the form of **over-valued ideas** (see p. 31) – they are not delusions – and their content and strength are liable to vary from time to time. The physical symptoms which the patient presents to support his case can often be recognized as elaborations of normal bodily sensations (for example, heart beat or gut peristalsis), to which the patient pays excessive attention and attributes inappropriate significance. The patient may present specific diagnoses but often will be quite vague, saying 'I'm not the doctor but I know something has been missed'. The prevalence is similar in men and women, usually starts before the age of fifty, and tends to run a chronic course.

The term **dysmorphophobia** has been used to describe the idea that the body is deformed in some way; particularly the nose, but sometimes other parts of the body such as face, hair, breasts, or genitalia. Patients with such beliefs commonly and repeatedly consult plastic surgeons but are unlikely to be helped by surgery. These ideas are included in the syndrome of hypochondriacal disorder if they take the form of over-valued ideas but not if they are delusions, in which case they indicate the presence of a psychosis (usually schizophrenia).

DIAGNOSIS

The following are BOTH required:

1. Persistent belief in serious physical illness underlying the presenting symptoms, although repeated examinations and investigations have not revealed any adequate physical explanation; or persistent preoccupation with presumed deformity.

2. Persistent refusal to accept medical advice and reassurance that there is no physical disorder or abnormality.

SIMULATED DISORDERS

Finally, there are three forms of abnormal illness behaviour in which organic disorders are simulated by the patient: factitious disorder, malingering, and dissociative disorders.

In **factitious disorder** the patient is aware of the simulation but not the gain; the **malingerer** is aware of both simulation and gain. In **dissociative disorders** it is thought that the patient lacks insight into the fact that symptoms are simulated and also into the gain derived from them; the simulation is at an unconscious level. However, it is possible for them to overlap, as in the case of a patient with a dissociative disorder who gradually acquires insight and then consciously maintains his symptoms in order to 'save face'. It can therefore sometimes be extremely difficult to differentiate between them.

Factitious disorder (F68.1)

Some patients consciously feign the symptoms and signs of disease, by self-injury or other subterfuge, in order to deceive doctors ('factitious' means artificial). They may present with many different signs, including rashes – **'dermatitis artefacta'**; infections, for example, of the urinary tract or septic arthritis, due to the introduction of infected material; 'pyrexia of unknown origin' which results, for example, from putting the thermometer in a cup of tea; or lapses of consciousness due to the injection of insulin. Usually the patients are well aware of the deception but may have little or no insight into the motives for their behaviour. In this respect they differ from malingerers. Their motives in general are to maintain themselves in the role of invalidism, from which they derive comfort and care: they either fail to receive these normal human requirements from the more usual sources, or they are dependent personalities with excessive needs. Formal psychiatric assessment rarely leads to any diagnosis other than personality disorder.

MUNCHAUSEN SYNDROME

This is a form of factitious disorder. Baron Munchausen was an eighteenth-century Hanoverian cavalry officer who was famous for his inventive story-telling. His name has therefore been given to this form of factitious illness, sometimes referred to as 'hospital addiction'. Patients may present to any department but particularly to surgical units, usually as an emergency, for example, with signs of an 'acute abdomen' or with haematemesis, complete with blood-stained vomitus. The patient may give a polished but totally invented history, which can include a false name and past medical history, and this often has the desired result of major surgery. Characteristically, the patient bears the scars of many previous episodes. If the suspicions of staff are raised and the patient's history is checked by contacting other hospitals, he is often found to have mysteriously left the ward and is never seen again. Such patients tend to roam the country, from one hospital to the next, using different names at each admission. They rarely wait to be seen by psychiatrists but if assessed appear to have grossly disturbed personalities or may be seeking narcotic analgesics.

MUNCHAUSEN SYNDROME BY PROXY (MEADOW'S SYNDROME) (ICD-10: T74.8)

'Munchausen syndrome by proxy' consists of factitious disorder presenting in children, caused by a parent, almost always the mother. *It should be thought of as a form of child abuse.* Apart from demonstrating the abnormal needs of the mother, it often results in serious physical and psychological abuse of the child. It is thought to be relatively common and sometimes results in the child's death, for example, due to hypoxia caused by smothering, hypoglycaemia due to insulin, or poisoning with other medication. These are caused either directly by the mother, or by doctors who are induced by the mother to give inappropriate treatments. The range of presentations is as broad as those resulting from factitious disorder in adults. It is important to be aware of this if you work on a paediatric unit.

Malingering (ICD-10: Z76.5)

Malingering is a form of feigned illness in which the subject is conscious both that he is simulating the symptoms of disease and also of the purpose (the nature of the gain): for example, this may be to get time off work, to avoid responsibility for some criminal action, or to obtain financial compensation for an alleged injury. The presentations are similar to those of dissociative and factitious disorders. In practice it can be extremely difficult to differentiate between them.

Dissociative disorders (conversion disorders) (F44)

These disorders are a form of abnormal illness behaviour in which the patient develops an often dramatic symptom of physical or mental illness, usually with an acute onset. Thus the patients may present with paralysis, pseudo-seizures, anaesthesia, amnesia, dysphonia, or blindness – but there are many others. These symptoms all involve unconscious simulation of the symptoms of illness. In addition, the physical symptoms, such as paralysis and blindness, involve somatization.

However, all these symptoms are thought to share an additional underlying psychological mechanism – the defence mechanism of **dissociation** (**conversion** is another similar mechanism: see p. 60). Our normal function is based on our ability to exert some degree of conscious control over our memories, sensations selected for attention, and choice of movements. It is thought that in the dissociative disorders this ability is partly or completely lost and this can result in impairment of many different functions. The symptoms are believed to be entirely psychological in origin, due to the unconscious mechanisms which have been described in the section on somatization (above).

EPIDEMIOLOGY

The prevalence of dissociative disorders in the community is uncertain as the nature of the disorder may go unrecognized. However, it is thought to have become less common in recent years, although it remains a common presentation in developing countries. Hospital surveys show that between 1 per cent and 5 per cent of all referrals have this disorder, which is more common in women than men. The onset may be at any age but the majority start before age thirty, and it is likely that transient symptoms may be quite common in children. Of patients who have been referred to hospital, about 70 per cent recover during the first year, 80 per cent in five years, and few of the remainder recover subsequently.

Dissociative symptoms are liable to show **epidemic spread** (referred to as '**mass hysteria**') particularly amongst adolescents and young adults who are in close proximity. There are generally several accounts of outbreaks, which can affect hundreds of people, for example in schools or at 'pop' concerts, reported in the national press each year, sometimes masquerading as some new or mysterious disease. One interesting facet is the widespread vulnerability of the general population to the development of dissociative symptoms by suggestion, given 'favourable' conditions; they are by no means limited to a few 'weak' or abnormal personalities.

SYMPTOMS

Dissociative symptoms have two distinguishing characteristics:

1. They mimic the phenomena of neurological and psychiatric disorders but *reflect the patient's concept of how such disorders present*. Thus a dissociative paralysis will not show the range of features of a typical upper or lower motor neurone lesion. A dissociative anaesthesia will fail to show the distribution of either a central or peripheral sensory loss: for example, it may be of 'glove' or 'stocking' distribution on perhaps a single limb, rather than conforming to the distribution of a dermatome, a peripheral nerve, or the symmetrical distribution of a peripheral neuropathy.

2. The function that appears to be lost *can often be demonstrated to be intact* in conditions which the patient does not associate with the symptom. For example, a leg which is 'paralysed' when the patient attempts to walk may show normal tone and reflexes in the relevant muscle groups and may be raised against gravity from the examination couch. Similarly a patient with hysterical dysphonia may phonate normally if coughing or laughing, and the vocal cords are seen to be normal on laryngoscopy. It is often possible to remove dissociative symptoms by hypnotic suggestion and this may be helpful diagnostically.

An important difference between hypochondriacal disorder and dissociative symptoms is that patients with the former show excessive concern about their health, but the latter present with clinical signs. Because of their value, dissociative symptoms often result in a surprising lack of distress and the patient may pay little more than lip service to the wish to overcome his disorder. French physicians have referred to this bland lack of concern as **'la belle indifférence'**.

Generally, dissociative symptoms tend to have a sudden onset, following a major stress, seemingly insoluble predicament, or interpersonal problem. This may not be evident from the history provided by the patient and information from other informants is essential. The patient clearly believes that the symptoms are organic and will usually reject any suggestion that they are psychological in origin.

A complicating factor is that symptoms which are themselves dissociative may be released by other mental disorders – particularly organic brain disorders, functional psychoses, and affective disorders – which are all higher in the diagnostic hierarchy. For this reason, in the presence of symptoms suggestive of one of these other disorders, the dissociative symptoms have no diagnostic value and are ignored. The preferred diagnosis is the one highest in the diagnostic hierarchy for which characteristic symptoms are present.

Dissociative symptoms can also occur in the setting of somatization disorder. The latter diagnosis is made rather than dissociative disorder if there have been many different symptoms over a number of years.

AETIOLOGY

The predisposing factors and unconscious mechanisms involved are those described for abnormal illness behaviour and somatization (see above). Primary gain is thought to play a particularly important role, but secondary and tertiary gain may also contribute. It should be possible to demonstrate that the symptoms have some adaptive value for the patient. For example, anxiety is at least partly relieved when the development of a symptom removes the patient from conflict.

A student who feared he might fail his exams developed a paralysis of his arm which prevented him from completing his course and sitting the exams.

DIAGNOSIS

1. The main requirement is a symptom or impairment of sensory or motor function suggestive of disease of the central nervous system, which is inconsistent in form with the characteristics of such disease, and in the absence of any objective evidence of organic pathology that can account for it. It follows that dissociative symptoms cannot be identified correctly unless you are thoroughly familiar with the symptoms of organic disorders.
2. There should be no evidence of other major psychiatric disorders – this point is explained above.
3. There should be some evidence of psychological causes, based on the onset following stress, and of gain, although this may not be evident from the patient's history.

A NOTE ON 'HYSTERIA'

The terms 'hysteria' and 'hysterical' originated in ancient Greek medicine and, like many other long-established concepts, have acquired a wide range of different and ambiguous meanings. In order to avoid confusion, we have abandoned the use of these terms (but not the concepts), in line with the major classifications of mental disorder. We advise you to do the same. Because these terms are likely to continue in medical usage for some time to come, we include a summary of the commonest ways in which they have recently been used:

1. 'Hysterical' has been used by lay people as a pejorative term to describe **dramatic** or **histrionic behaviour**: these latter terms are more appropriate.
2. 'Hysterical personality' is an old-fashioned term for **histrionic personality** (see p. 65).
3. 'Hysterical symptoms' are now referred to as **dissociative symptoms** (or **conversion symptoms**).
4. 'Hysteria' and 'hysterical neurosis' have now been replaced by **dissociative disorder**.

These usages have nothing to commend them and they should be avoided. We are left with 'mass hysteria' (see p. 239), for which the only synonym is epidemic hysteria. Fortunately, it is rare.

DIFFERENTIAL DIAGNOSES OF ABNORMAL ILLNESS BEHAVIOUR

The following must be considered:

1. **Physical disorders**. Patients suffering from somatization disorder have the same risk of developing a new physical disorder as others, but it is unusual to discover an organic cause for long-standing multiple symptoms which have previously been adequately investigated with negative results. Organic disorders are particularly likely to be missed in patients who present their symptoms in dramatic ways. Also, dissociative symptoms are liable to be misidentified as due to physical disease.

2. **Affective disorders**. If the presentation satisfies the criteria for somatization disorder then it should be diagnosed as such but there may also be grounds for an additional diagnosis (see p. 50) of a mood disorder. Because patients with these disorders tend to confirm that they have symptoms that are suggested to them, it is important to base diagnoses of the affective disorders on objective changes (for example, observed sleep disturbance and measured weight loss) rather than rely entirely on the patient's own account.

   Some patients focus on symptoms which are limited to the autonomic nervous system and appear to represent physiological responses to anxiety, for example, sweating, palpitation, hyperventilation, and 'tension' headaches. The diagnosis will depend on the other clinical features: they may justify an anxiety disorder diagnosis, or that of a somatoform disorder.

3. **Other somatoform disorders**, dissociative disorder, factitious disorder, and malingering. In practice, patients may satisfy criteria for more than one of these diagnoses. The preferred diagnosis should be the one that fits the syndrome best.

4. **Dementias**, particularly in the elderly, who sometimes have multiple complaints related to a combination of physical and mental disorders. Also, remember that dissociative symptoms may be released by organic brain disorders.

5. **Substance abuse**. Alcohol abuse may cause multiple physical complaints due to physical pathology, as well as an associated mood disorder. There is also some evidence that alcohol abuse may predate the onset of somatoform disorders. Alcohol and drug abuse may result from the patient's or doctor's attempts to achieve symptomatic relief. Substance abuse must therefore be considered as part of the differential diagnosis and also as an additional diagnosis.

6. **Schizophrenia** and **depressive psychosis** must both be considered in the differential diagnosis of hypochondriacal disorder, because in these disorders there may be **delusions with hypochondriacal content** or of **distorted body image** – in these the beliefs take the form of absolute conviction and the patient cannot be argued out of them. These can occur in any of the **organic and functional psychoses**. In schizophrenia, delusions about disease or changes in the shape of one's body may be grotesque; for example, a young man thought his face was changing into that of a pig, developing a snout and bristles. In depressive psychosis, delusions tend to be 'mood congruent', that is, in keeping with depressive cognitions of hope-

lessness, and may take the form of impending and certain death due to cancer. In extreme cases the patient may believe that he is already dead: this would be an example of a nihilistic delusion.

7. **Personality disorders** are commonly found in patients who develop somatoform disorders, dissociative disorders, and factitious disorder. They should therefore be diagnosed in addition.

THE MANAGEMENT OF ABNORMAL ILLNESS BEHAVIOUR AND SOMATIZATION

Management can be divided into prevention; general measures, which can be applied in any medical setting; and specialized psychological approaches particularly for the more severe and persistent disorders – these will be considered briefly.

The prevention of somatizing disorders

Doctors make a major contribution to the development and chronicity of abnormal illness behaviour and somatization by responding to them inappropriately. It is important to avoid this by recognizing these problems and learning more appropriate ways of responding. We have already described how to avoid differential reinforcement of somatic complaints by acknowledging mood disorders and psychosocial problems. In addition:

1. Always provide clear information about negative clinical findings when you examine patients, and about negative investigations, otherwise they may assume the worst.
2. Avoid giving patients speculative or spurious diagnoses. Medical records are full of these, and the patient always remembers these diagnoses rather than the subsequent retractions.
3. Avoid treating disorders that the patient does not have – it is not unusual to find that patients who are told 'There's nothing wrong with your heart' have been offered medication commonly used for heart disease, without adequate explanation. Obviously, the patient will believe he is seriously ill.
4. Avoid carrying out and repeating investigations unless you think they are indicated, based on objective clinical findings. If you think they are indicated it is important to inform the patient of both the purpose and the result.
5. Avoid arranging consultations and referrals unless you think they are indicated. Always explain why.

The management of somatic presentations of mood disorders

In cases where either no physical disease is demonstrable, or the physical disease which is present does not account for the patient's symptoms, it is essential to help the patient to see his symptoms in a different way. The **worst thing you can do** is to indicate by your words or actions that: *'Our investigations are normal, so there's nothing wrong with you.'* The patient knows that isn't correct since his pain is real enough. The patient will usually be complaining of numerous other psychiatric symptoms, but he will not have connected them with the pain. You will have to help him.

Let us suppose that a patient with severe epigastric pain has reported numerous symptoms of a depressive illness, and you have been asked to tell him that the results of all investigations, including a gastroscopy, are quite normal. You should now go through the following steps:

1. **Provide clear information about negative physical findings while acknowledging the reality of the physical symptoms**

   I'm glad to be able to tell you that you haven't got an ulcer or a tumour causing this pain, and all our investigations have been completely normal. Nevertheless, you have had a lot of pain, haven't you, and it has gone well beyond your usual indigestion pain?

   (Having acknowledged the reality of the pain, pause for agreement.)

2. **Specify the relevant mood state and associated symptoms and refer to the psychosocial factors that were previously noticed** (this is called 'changing the agenda' – from the somatic complaints to the possible psychosocial causes):

   When you came into hospital you told me how depressed you have been feeling since you didn't manage to get promoted at work. You mentioned that you have lost over a stone in weight and tended to wake early in the morning brooding about the things that you feel you've made a mess of in your life.

   (Mention about three of the more striking symptoms, always including the mood disorder. Be prepared to remind your patient about the others if necessary.)

3. **Explain about the relationship of mood and pain:**

   We think that you are undoubtedly depressed, and that your depression has made your pain very much worse than it would have been otherwise. It's one of the things that depression does, I'm afraid.

   (Pause for patient's response; be prepared to repeat that you know that the pain is real, but depression can cause real pain.)

4. **Emphasize the positive aspects of treatment and provide reassurance, based on a realistic idea of outcome:**

   We think that it is very important to give you some treatment for your depression. Most people get over this sort of illness completely but it is likely to take some time. I would now like to discuss some of the ways we might help you.

   If you have got this far, you have done well. From now on the management is as described earlier in Chapter 13 (p. 201), but with one advantage. The patient's pain will act as a key symptom to indicate your success – or lack of it! – in dealing with the problem.

The management of more persistent disorders

All of the points covered in the preceding sections on treatment are relevant. If the problems continue, this is how to proceed:

1. Remember that anyone may have a physical disease, however obviously they show features of abnormal illness behaviour or an abnormal mental state. Frequently both physical and mental disorders occur in the same patient, so always look for evidence of both. All patients must be physically examined and investigated if they have a new episode of illness or new symptoms.

2. Few physical diagnoses are made as a result of further investigations more than six months after the initial presentation. Apart from the iatrogenic effects, repeated and inappropriate investigations also result in delay in initiating the appropriate psychiatric management.

3. At this stage it is essential to have a full psychiatric assessment and the purpose should be explained to the patient and his cooperation sought. The first step is to look for evidence of affective disorder (described above) or other treatable mental disorders, and to treat them.

4. Review the past medical records, particularly if they are voluminous, because it may become evident that far from being a new disorder the present symptoms are part of a chronic or recurrent pattern of somatization.

5. Arrange to see a key relative yourself in order to find out more about the psychological and social background of the disorder, to assess their knowledge and beliefs about the patient's symptoms (usually they have not been seen previously by a doctor and will probably share the patient's views that he has undiagnosed physical illness), and to explain the nature of the disorder.

6. Ask the medical social worker to help by carrying out a home visit, by seeing other relatives on your behalf, or by providing some tangible social help for the family.

7. It is essential for all doctors involved to work closely together and to take a consistent approach towards psychiatric management.

8. The cause of these disorders is primarily psychological and therefore the management should be psychological. However, the specific causes of a patient's illness will rarely be evident from the initial history: the effect of somatization and of gain is that usually the patient is unaware of underlying problems and relates all his difficulties to physical disease. Other factors will usually only come to light after taking detailed histories from the patient and others.

9. Insight-orientated psychotherapy can help the patient to face underlying problems and find more constructive ways to adjust to them. Behavioural psychotherapy can help the patient to give up inappropriate disability, by using a structured rehabilitation programme and rewarding achievement. Cognitive therapy is used to reduce inappropriate focus on and beliefs about symptoms, and to encourage positive attitudes and approaches to coping.

10. Often inappropriate attitudes and behaviours are reinforced by family members who are over-solicitous. They must therefore be included in the treatment plan to modify the effect they have on the patient. Sometimes they have a particular need to care for an invalid and are unable to tolerate the patient's recovery. They may then need help to find new ways of adjusting to their own problems.

11. Somatoform and dissociative disorders are often resistant to treatment, perhaps because they are rarely seen by psychiatrists in the early stages, and due to poor compliance by patients and/or their families. Those that fail to improve within the first year or two often run a chronic course subsequently.

FURTHER READING

Bass, C. and Benjamin, S. (1993) The management of chronic somatization. *British Journal of Psychiatry* 162: 472–80.

Benjamin, S. and Eminson, D.M. (1992) Abnormal illness behaviour: childhood experiences and long-term consequences. *International Review of Psychiatry* 4: 55–70.

Creed, F. and Guthrie, E. (1993) Techniques for interviewing the somatizing patient. *British Journal of Psychiatry* 162: 467–71.

Ford, C.V. (1983) *The Somatizing Disorders: Illness as a Way of Life*. New York: Elsevier.

Smith, G.R. (1991) *Somatization Disorder in the Medical Setting*. Washington, DC: American Psychiatric Press.

PART 3
DISORDERS RELATED TO STAGES OF THE LIFE CYCLE

16 / DISORDERS OF EARLY LIFE: MENTAL RETARDATION

TERMINOLOGY

A distinction has always been made between disorders of mental functioning which are developmental and those which are acquired. A developmental disorder is one which is usually first evident in infancy, childhood, or adolescence, and leads to permanent impairment of function. **Mental retardation** is the term used internationally for a developmental disorder affecting intelligence which leads to impairment of social functioning. In the United Kingdom the Department of Health has introduced the term **learning disability**, and most services use this term. We shall therefore use it in the remainder of this chapter.

Many terms have been used in the past: natural fool, idiot, imbecile, and moron were current in the English language long before they were given technical definitions. Some terms such as 'mongol' were introduced by the medical profession with the intention of being non-pejorative and objective. Others have been introduced by educationists or by legislators (for example, educational subnormality, mental subnormality, mental impairment).

The main reason for the changes in terminology is that this kind of disability is undesirable and associated with socially disapproved behaviour, therefore words describing it become insults. This presents a challenge to doctors, because it is necessary to be able to discuss disability with patients and their families. Unfamiliar, technical words become insults more rapidly than ordinary English, and it is unhelpful to use euphemisms. You should use terms that describe the disability accurately, such as 'slow to learn'. For this reason, the term 'learning disability' is helpful, and is likely to remain in use.

EPIDEMIOLOGY

Intellectual ability and social competence are continuously distributed variables; there is no clear cut-off between normality and disability, nor between the various degrees of disability.

It became possible to examine the distribution of intelligence in a population when psychologists developed methods for measuring cognitive performance in the first half of the twentieth century. Intelligence approximates to a Gaussian ('normal') distribution. The frequency distribution of a Gaussian curve may be described completely by the mean and standard deviation: about 95 per cent of the population falls within two standard deviations of the mean. IQ ('intelligence quotient') scores are adjusted so that the population mean is 100 and the standard deviation is 15. An IQ of less than 70 (that is, 2 standard deviations below the mean) is called subnormal. About 2.5 per cent of the population might be expected to have an IQ below 70. In practice the distribution of intelligence in a population depends on factors such as education and welfare provision.

The prevalence of **severe intellectual impairment** (IQ less than 50) is between 0.3 per cent and 0.4 per cent, and is similar wherever it has been measured. It changes a little from time to time, because of changes in the rates of onset and of survival (of both children and adults). For example, there has been a reduction in the proportion of pregnancies occurring in the second half of the childbearing age; this has led to a fall in the rate of Down's syndrome births. Factors such as cardiac surgery, treatment of childhood infections, and improvements in social care have led to increased survival in Down's syndrome. Also, families with disabled members have different patterns of migration to the rest of the population, and tend not to move from inner cities which are otherwise becoming depopulated, so rates there are higher than rural rates in the UK.

The inception rate is difficult to measure, because the identification of new cases does not occur at a single point in time. **Down's syndrome** (trisomy 21, or mongolism) is usually recognized at the time of birth, but most other causes are not. The prevalence at birth of Down's syndrome in England in the late 1970s was estimated at between 0.65 and 1.06 per 1,000 live births.

Most studies show a male preponderance. Mild and moderate disability are associated with low social class, probably because of their association with social and educational deprivation. Early studies of severe disability showed no association with social class, but recent studies show a weak association.

CLINICAL FEATURES

There are three main features:

1. Impairment of intelligence (or other cognitive function).
2. Impaired social functioning.
3. Onset before adulthood.

'Cognitive function' is the psychological term for information processing. Intelligence is not easy to define; it is concerned with the speed of understanding and the ability to learn from experience. This is an aspect of cognitive function, along with focusing attention (concentrating), registering, retaining and recalling information, and thinking. In a clinical setting, impairment of intelligence is often detected by attending to the complexity of language that a patient uses and understands. In childhood, parents or teachers may notice that a child is slower at attaining developmental milestones than their siblings or age-peers.

A person with intellectual impairment also has significant impairment of social functioning if they are unable to live independently (or, in the case of a child, have special educational needs). There are five areas of skills which are required for independence: *self-care, domestic activity, communication, social skills,* and *coping with stress.* Mental retardation may also affect academic skills such as reading, writing, numeracy, etc.; but these latter skills do not generally make the difference between dependence and independence.

There are, of course, many aspects of psychological development that may be impaired and cause difficulties in adult life, such as sexuality and emotional development. These do not generally cause severe educational problems, nor do they make people permanently dependent on others, and so they are not usually causes of learning disability. However, there are also some disorders which may affect cognitive development, notably autism and hyperkinetic syndrome, and several forms of specific learning disabilities, which may cause a person to need special education and support from learning disability services.

DIAGNOSTIC CRITERIA

The present legal definition is given in the Mental Health (Amendment) Act 1981 as 'a state of arrested or incomplete development of mind, including significant impairment of intelligence and social functioning'. This definition reflects the three defining characteristics of mental retardation but is conceptually flawed, because development can never be wholly arrested nor wholly complete.

IQ figures have limited reliability, and an incomplete correlation with practical and social competence. The criteria below are clinical guidelines, not rigid rules. The age at which mental development is regarded as stable is arbitrary; international classifications use the age of eighteen, but in clinical practice, leaving school is the dividing line.

Mild learning disability (F70) accounts for 2–3 per cent of the population, and 75 per cent of all people with learning disability. They are able to cope with self-care and domestic activity independently most of the time, but *have problems when faced with new or complex situations,* as executive speech problems interfere with independence. They are most likely to present to services such as GPs if they are faced with stress (for example, minor illness) and are unable to cope. They are usually able to learn occupational skills, but may have problems with the social skills required for employment. Common problems include budgeting, planning a healthy menu, and using the health service to best effect. Psychometric assessment usually shows an IQ in the range 50–69. Associated conditions include autism, epilepsy, conduct disorders, and physical disabilities.

Moderate learning disability (F71) is a term that is used differently in different publications; in the UK it usually means the lower end of mild learning disability (IQ 50–60), but in ICD-10 it means the higher end of severe learning disability (IQ 35–49). People with moderate learning disability *need supervision or assistance with complex activities, such as cooking, but the level of support needed is usually within the resources and abilities of families with no special training.* They can usually participate in simple conversations and can communicate their basic needs, although some never learn to use language. An organic aetiology can be identified in a majority. They will require specialist services if they have some additional problem or if they have no family support.

Severe learning disability (F72) accounts for about 25 per cent of all people with learning disabilities, usually associated with an IQ below 50: in ICD-10, below 34. They are *unable to cope independently because they need supervision or assistance with some skills required for independence (self-care, domestic, social, communication, and coping with stress).* Most will require supervision by a responsible person on a daily basis; they are very likely to be detected at school as having special educational needs. The great majority come to the attention of specialist services at some time, as they usually have a marked degree of motor impairment or other deficits indicating maldevelopment of the CNS.

Profound learning disability (F73) accounts for less than 0.1 per cent of the population, and 5 per cent of all people with learning disabilities. IQ testing is unreliable at this level of ability, where the person's development of language and other skills is equivalent to a normal child of two years or less. Comprehension of language is limited, at best, to understanding simple commands. An organic aetiology can usually be identified; severe neurological and physical disability is common. They require *assistance with all areas of life, including some skills required for basic survival (for example, feeding, clothing).*

AETIOLOGY

There are more than two thousand disorders recognized which can lead to learning disability, and there is little point in trying to remember them all. Instead, it is better to have a framework for understanding aetiology, which will enable you to conduct a rational investigation of any particular patient, based on the relative frequency of each category of disorder. The onset of the cause of disability may be prenatal, perinatal, postnatal, or unknown. The relative frequencies of each of these in Western Europe are shown in *Table 16.1.*

Figures are not available for developing countries, but it is known that **maternal malnutrition**, **dietary insufficiency of iodine**, and **inadequate perinatal care** are major causes of disability. In Western Europe, 'birth trauma' is an uncommon cause, and 'vaccine damage' extremely rare, despite the many people who believe the opposite.

The commonest single cause of severe mental retardation, which accounts for nearly all of the chromosomal causes of severe and profound disability, is **Down's syndrome**. This is due to trisomy 21, and the incidence increases with maternal age. It is often

Table 16.1 *Relative frequencies of causes of mental retardation in Western Europe*

aetiology	severe and profound mental retardation (%)		mild and moderate mental retardation (%)	
Prenatal	60		35	
(Chromosomal)		(35)		(15)
(Single gene)		(5)		(1)
(Alcohol)		(0)		(8)
(Infection)		(7)		(0)
(Other)		(13)		(9)
Perinatal	15		18	
Postnatal	10		2	
Unknown	15		55	

recognized at birth because of dysmorphic features, and the diagnosis may be confirmed by examining the chromosomes of cultured leucocytes.

Fragile-X syndrome is now known to be the second commonest cause. It accounts for 6 per cent of severe mental retardation and 10 per cent of mild mental retardation in boys, and a small proportion in girls. It is a familial condition associated with a gene whose length increases with successive generations, and with a 'fragile' site on the X-chromosome, detectable by examining chromosomes in leucocytes cultured under special conditions. The length of the gene is correlated with the degree of intellectual impairment. There are also dysmorphic features, including macro-orchidism.

Details about conditions which cause mental retardation should be obtained from a paediatric text. Conditions which are important because they are treatable if detected early are **hypothyroidism, phenylketonuria, metabolic disorders** (for example, hypernatraemia due to incorrectly formulated feeds), and **infections**. Doctors treating pregnant women should be aware of the risks caused by **alcohol, drugs** (especially anticonvulsants), **radiation** (including diagnostic radiography), **maternal phenyl-ketonuria**, and **metabolic disorders**.

Most people with severe mental retardation are disabled as a result of a biological impairment, but no biological impairment can be detected in about half of people with mild mental retardation. Mild mental retardation is associated with indicators of **social deprivation** and **poverty**, and also with low social class.

DIFFERENTIAL DIAGNOSIS

1. **Developmental disorders without impaired intelligence**
   - **Communication problems**. Any disorder that impairs communication may lead you to underestimate the person's intelligence; this includes sensory

impairments (deafness, blindness), motor impairments (cerebral palsy), other speech impairments (deformities of the mouth such as cleft palate), and other disorders that affect cognitive function (autism, hyperkinetic syndrome, and specific learning disabilities).

- **Emotional dependency.** People who are more dependent than expected for their chronological age may have the skills they require, yet fail to use them for some reason. If this is developmental, rather than acquired, it is usually part of a dependent personality disorder.

2. **Acquired impairment of intelligence**

- **Dementia** may occur at any age, and dementia before the age of eighteen leads to learning disability. There are some rare progressive disorders in childhood, such as Batten's disease and subacute sclerosing pan-encephalitis, which generally lead to death in childhood. Non-progressive dementia is caused by injury to the brain: traumatic, toxic (for example, heavy metals, alcohol), infective (for example, herpes encephalitis), anoxic, etc.

3. **Acquired disorders without impairment of intelligence**
Severe psychiatric illness may cause impairment of social functioning, and in some cases the person may have slowing or inhibition of cognitive function, or appear to have intellectual impairment because of poor concentration or lack of cooperation with testing. This non-specific phenomenon occurs with schizophrenia and depression more than with other diagnoses.

4. **Impaired social functioning, but no disorder**

- **Lack of education** may mean that a person has not acquired the skills required for independence, especially if their intelligence is at the lower end of the normal range.

- **Lack of opportunity to practise skills** due to living in a very restricted environment (such as prison or an institution) may have the same effect.

- **'Functional behaviour'** – in other words, behaviour which serves a purpose (whether or not the person is aware of it) – may sometimes convey the impression of learning disability. This is uncommon, and occurs mainly when a person is strongly motivated to avoid unwelcome responsibilities or demands; for example, a person charged with murder who wishes the charge to be reduced to manslaughter.

INVESTIGATIONS

Assessment of social and practical competence

In ordinary clinical practice, the method of assessing competence is to ask the individual, and to seek confirmation and elaboration by an informant, about the person's 'typical day'. The activities include rising, washing, choosing clothes, dressing, preparing breakfast, eating, clearing up, going out, using transport and roads, attending a place of occupation or education, shopping and using money, eating away from home, returning home, cooking, leisure, and recreation. For each activity, the degree of independence may be:

1. Unsupervised.
2. Checked after the event.
3. Prompted and checked.
4. Physically prompted or helped.
5. Done for the person by another.

Try to distinguish between activities that the person cannot do despite having the opportunity, and those that they never have the opportunity to try. Don't assume that a person is incapable, just because they are never allowed to do something.

Specialist services use standardized assessments which yield a profile of the person's abilities, and which indicate the areas to focus on for further training.

Developmental history

The parents, especially the mother, are the best informants about the rate of development of their child's abilities. Unfortunately, memory is unreliable, and it is vital to obtain and record this information at the earliest opportunity. Paediatric and community child health records are invaluable, and developmental records of disabled children should be preserved. Ask about problems during pregnancy, delivery, and the neonatal period, then ask about the age of reaching developmental milestones (see *Table 16.2*).

Psychometric assessments (measurement of cognitive ability)

Tests of performance of standardized tasks are necessary for epidemiological research, but are only useful in a few clinical situations. Psychometric assessment allows one to examine the component psychological functions underlying the skills which a person acquires. It is important to ask a clinical psychologist to do this if there appears to be a substantial variation between one aspect of a person's ability and another. It is also useful

Table 16.2 *Developmental milestones (adapted from the Denver developmental screening test)*

	6 months	12 months	24 months
posture and large movements	pulls to sit with no head lag	walks to the side holding furniture	kicks ball forwards
vision and fine movements	watches adult move, reaches for toy	grasps with thumb and finger	scribbles spontaneously
hearing and language	vocalizes with two syllables	imitates speech sounds	points to one named body part
social behaviour and play	smiles spontaneously	initially shy with strangers	uses spoon, spilling little

if the person's cognitive ability appears to be declining, as it assists one to diagnose and predict the course of dementia.

Special investigations

An attempt should always be made to diagnose the cause of the disability. In childhood, the cause may be remediable, and in adulthood may have significance for the onset of illness. It may also have significance for other family members planning to have children. Most diagnosable disorders are recognized on the basis of their clinical features (see Further Reading, p. 258).

A strategy for planning investigations should be based on the relative frequency of aetiologies, as listed above. For a person with severe mental retardation, these would include chromosome examination, urine and blood examination for in-born errors of metabolism, and investigations for intra-uterine infection (toxoplasmosis, rubella, cytomegalovirus, herpes simplex virus, syphilis).

TREATMENT

When developmental delay is first detected, it is important that the news is broken to parents in a sensitive way. This means telling them the facts at a speed and in a language that they can understand, and in a way that helps them to cope with it. As a rule, parents should be told jointly, in private, at the earliest opportunity after a problem is suspected. This will usually be done by a paediatrician, although it might be done by a GP. Non-technical language should be used, and it is important to realize that people retain only a very small amount of information when they first hear unwelcome news. There must be a follow-up interview soon, and preferably a written report for the parents. If a heritable condition is detected, families should be offered referral to a clinical genetics service.

A few conditions leading to learning disability are susceptible to medical treatment during childhood. People with learning disabilities also need diagnosis and treatment of any illness they may acquire, and are entitled to the same standard of medical care as the rest of the population. They have higher rates of some illnesses, yet use medical services proportionally less than the rest of the population. They need an active programme of health surveillance and screening, akin to the community child health programme.

Associated health problems may be considered under three headings:

1. **Specific associations. Down's syndrome** is common, and it is worth learning its associations, which include cardiac defects, obesity, respiratory tract infections, conductive deafness, skin problems (acne), chronic lymphatic leukaemia, Alzheimer's disease (leading to dementia, epilepsy, and early death), and, most importantly, hypothyroidism. Other examples include **rubella syndrome** associated with deafness, blindness, and cardiac defects; **hypothyroidism** associated with deafness; and **autism** associated with epilepsy.

2. **Shared aetiologies**. Learning disability usually indicates that the brain is not functioning normally, and this may be manifested in other ways, including epilepsy, sensory impairment, motor impairment (cerebral palsy), autism, and hyperkinetic syndrome. There is also an increased risk of mental illness, partly because of impaired brain function.

3. **Increased susceptibility**. People with learning disability are more likely than the rest of the population to live in social circumstances which carry risks to health. Even now in urban Britain, they may live in poverty, subject to crime, exploitation, and cruelty, and are likely to be unemployed and unmarried. Some still live in large institutions, where there are still risks of TB and hepatitis, and even malnutrition. Even where people receive good general care, they may have an inappropriate programme which makes too many demands of them. Behaviour problems and mental illness are common, partly related to these factors.

For most of the needs of most people with learning disabilities, the help they need is not treatment, but some other service. In addition to health care, there are some needs that everyone has:

1. *Housing*. A person with a disability may need supported housing, such as a substitute family or a staffed house, or a house with support from a neighbour or a warden.

2. *Education*. People with learning disabilities have special educational needs and should be able to receive appropriate primary, secondary, and continuing education.

3. *Occupation*. There are various ways of supporting disabled workers in the workplace, or in sheltered sections of the workplace, or in wholly sheltered workshops.

4. *Leisure and recreation*. Sports and social activities also offer opportunities for personal and social development.

In addition, there are some needs that are specific to disability which demand special attention, including:

1. Prevention of primary and secondary disability.

2. Specialized interventions to address sensory, motor, communication, and behavioural problems.

3. Advocacy.

4. Family support, respite care, holidays, and family advocacy.

There are several ways of meeting each need. A person could:

1. Have something done for them.

2. Be taught how to do it.

3. Be put into a situation where it did not matter whether the thing was done or not.

Services are provided by social service and education departments of local authorities, and by community support teams for people with learning disabilities (sometimes called community mental handicap teams). General practitioners are responsible for a person's primary health care, and may refer to consultants in psychiatry of mental handicap, or to child psychiatrists or neurologists as appropriate. Some parts of the UK also have mental handicap hospitals run by the National Health Service.

COURSE AND PROGNOSIS

The course of a learning disability depends on the interaction between the impairment causing the disability, and the education, training, and care the person receives. Most developmental disorders are stable in adult life with a tendency to progressive improvement. Behavioural problems are much less common after the age of twenty-five to thirty and autism also becomes less noticeable. People who receive suitable education, training, and care, and who receive treatment of intercurrent illness, gradually become more independent. Nevertheless, life expectancy is still reduced, because of the health problems listed above.

FURTHER READING

Hall, D.M.B. (1984) *The Child with a Handicap*. Oxford: Blackwell Scientific.

Office of Health Economics/MENCAP (1986) *Mental Handicap – Partnership in the Community?* London: Office of Health Economics/MENCAP.

Russell, O. (1985) *Mental Handicap*. 'Current Reviews in Psychiatry' vol. 1. Edinburgh: Churchill Livingstone.

Smith, D.W. (1982) *Recognisable Patterns of Human Malformation*. Philadelphia: W.B. Saunders.

17 / CHILDHOOD AND ADOLESCENCE

This chapter is concerned with the emotional and behaviour disorders of childhood and adolescence. Many of these disorders are an extreme form of everyday behaviour. Indeed, most young children go through patches of difficult behaviour at some time. It is only when a child's difficulties cause suffering, affect learning or relationships with others, or seriously interfere with development that we need to look further at the problem.

ASSESSMENT

There are six main stages in the assessment of psychiatric disorders in children:

1. The **family interview**.
2. The **parental interview**.
3. The **interview with the child**.
4. Obtaining **other sources of information**.
5. The **aetiological formulation**.
6. Making a **multi-axial diagnosis**.

THE FAMILY INTERVIEW

It is often helpful to see all of the family together at the start of the assessment. Conjoint interviews provide a way of observing interactions between family members. For example, they can be used to determine how the parents respond to the child's communications (for example, sympathetically, critically, etc.), whether the parents have difficulties in their own relationship, or whether one family member tends to be scapegoated or ignored. The interviewer needs to avoid exclusive questioning of individuals, but should set up opportunities for interactions between family members. This can be achieved by setting the family a task, such as drawing the family tree, or by asking questions that encourage such interactions. This is also a good time to establish the process of referral to the clinic and for finding out who has been experiencing the problem most acutely.

THE PARENTAL INTERVIEW

Like all interviews, the interview with the parents should start with **open questions** and minimal cross-examination to obtain the history of the presenting complaint. Try to clarify precisely what the parent means by terms such as 'naughty' or 'depressed'. Is the situation getting better or worse? What effects have the child's problems had on school-work, peer relationships, and the family? How long has there been a problem?

It is next necessary to cover systematically the child's **recent health and behaviour** (but bear in mind that parents do not have direct knowledge of the child's mental state, and may be unaware of important symptoms such as suicidal ideation). Direct enquiry should be made about each of the following areas: *emotional symptoms* (anxiety, fears, depression, suicidality); *behavioural problems* (stealing, aggression, disobedience, fighting, truancy, running away); *attention and concentration; motor skills* (activity level, clumsiness); *fits or faints; abnormal movements; school performance* (attendance, bullying, relationships with teachers); *peer and sibling relationships; bladder and bowel control; physical health* (appetite, weight, sleep, major illnesses); *recent adversity* (for example, bereavement or separations).

The **family history** should then be obtained, in much the same way as with adult patients. It is especially important to know about mental illness or personality problems in the parents. Find out about the parents' relationship, including marital problems. If the parents have separated, obtain details. Does the child have continuing contact with the other parent? To whom is the child closest?

The child's **family life and relationships** should be enquired about next. Key areas here include disciplinary practices, family activities that involve the child, and the child's role in the family.

Ask next about the child's **personal history**. Where was the child born? Any problems during the pregnancy or delivery? Birth weight? Neonatal problems? Immunizations? Early separations or 'bonding' difficulties? Motor and language milestones? Major illnesses? Schools attended?

Finally, ask about the child's **temperamental characteristics**. Have they always been a regular sleeper and eater? How well does the child adapt to new situations? Do they usually show emotions strongly? Is the child habitually sociable, or inhibited and slow to warm up?

THE INTERVIEW WITH THE CHILD

The examination that follows is based on one developed at the Park Hospital, Oxford. It may be possible with older children to follow something like the same procedure as used to examine an adult's mental state, but in young children formal examination of the mental state is often impossible. Every opportunity should be taken to observe the child's behaviour and this should be recorded systematically and objectively. Avoid global clinical impressions. Do not forget to obtain the child's view of the situation, including his likes, dislikes, and hopes for the future. Establishing a useful conversation with the child requires you to show warmth, interest, and respect for the child. Approach emotive topics gradually and carefully and use language that is appropriate (including use of play material for younger children).

When you require the child's cooperation, ask for it directly. Do not ask *'Would you like to . . . ?'*, because if the child would not like to, you are sunk.

THE MENTAL STATE

General behaviour

Dress and appearance.
(Is the child appropriately and cleanly clad?)
Parent–child interaction and separation.
(Do the parents seem able and willing to manage the child; was there a tantrum on separation?)
Emotional responsiveness and relationship with the doctor.
(Describe your own feelings about the quality of your interaction with the child.)
Habitual mannerisms.
(Does the child have tics, or recurrent speech or stereotypic mannerisms?)
Description of the course of the interview.
(What went on: drawing, play, tears, temper?)

Anxiety and mood

Signs of tension and sadness.
(include facial expression, apprehension, tearfulness)
Whether preoccupied by fears, worries, depressing thoughts.
Whether restless, disinhibited, assertive, aggressive.
Whether apathetic, withdrawn, or shy.

Talk (form)

Spontaneity, flow.
(Is speech painfully difficult to elicit or does it flow ceaselessly; or is the flow and exchange of talk normal?)

Defects of prosody, articulation, or sentence structure.
Coherence.
(Can you follow what is being said, or does it lose its point?)

Talk (content)

Attention or persistence.
(Whether easily distracted; whether interrupted by hallucinatory experience.)
Degree and duration of interests in topics, activities, or objects.
(Does the child flit ceaselessly from one topic to another?)
Spontaneous interruptions of attention.
(Is speech suddenly arrested, the point lost?)

Activity level

Gross activity.
(In particular, whether 'over-active' or 'hyperkinetic'.)

Intellectual function

Rough assessment of reading level, spelling, arithmetic, writing, general knowledge.
Write name and address, draw a man, copy triangle, diamond, cross and circle.
*Ideally, **testing by a clinical or educational psychologist** should be arranged, including assessment of basic intellectual ability, educational attainments, and specific learning problems.*

OTHER SOURCES OF INFORMATION

Obtain a school report or, for younger children, an account from nursery school or play group. Any other agencies that are involved with the child or the family should be contacted.

THE AETIOLOGICAL FORMULATION

Predisposing factors

Children's vulnerability to psychiatric disorders is increased by several factors. **Genetic influences** can be *direct*, as in the parent–child transmission of manic-depressive illness, or *indirect*, as when a child's **temperamental characteristics** lead to parental rejection which in turn leads to disorder. The *goodness of fit* between a child's characteristics and the environment seems to be especially important. For instance, difficult children who are brought up in stable, warm families are at lower risk of behavioural disorders than difficult children who are brought up in unstable, discordant families. Children with **mental retardation** or **specific developmental disorders** such as reading retardation are at increased risk of psychiatric disturbance.

The child's early **attachment relationships** to the parents can also be important. Brief disruptions of this relationship during infancy do not usually carry serious long-term consequences. Indeed, so long as alternative care is adequate, many children can survive even severe disruptions of attachment (such as parental death) without psychological damage. However, separations that are followed by chronic lack of care, or were preceded by severe family disruption, can lead to **insecure attachment**, which may in turn predispose the infant to problems later in childhood. Thus, children whose parents have divorced have higher rates of psychiatric disturbance than children who were separated from a parent by death. Other causes of insecure attachments include parental mental illness, personality problems in the parent, and being brought up in a poor-quality children's home.

Precipitants and maintaining factors

Psychiatric disorders in children are commonly precipitated by adversity, especially factors within the family such as marital difficulties. **Parental mental illness** is also strongly associated with problems in children, mainly because it leads to impaired quality of parental care. For example, depressed mothers are less able to respond to the child's needs and provide less consistent discipline. Emotional or sexual **abuse** may also be important.

Factors outside the family, such as difficulties at school or bullying, can also lead to psychiatric problems. Sometimes **physical injury** can trigger an emotional or behavioural disorder. For instance, severe head injuries may have a direct effect on brain function.

MULTI-AXIAL DIAGNOSIS

Different components of the child's problems are recorded separately using a **multi-axial framework**:

1. **Psychiatric syndromes.**
2. **Specific developmental disorders.**
3. **Intellectual level.**
4. **Medical conditions.**
5. **Psychosocial adversity.**

The use of this framework makes it much easier to devise a precise formulation of the child's difficulties. Thus, a child with conduct disorder (axis 1), specific reading disorder (axis 2), and epilepsy (axis 4), from a home in which the parents often fight (axis 5), would receive a coding on four areas.

PSYCHIATRIC SYNDROMES

Like psychopathology in adulthood, emotional and behavioural problems in children may be grouped into a number of distinct syndromes. It is important to note, however, that especially in younger children there is a great deal of overlap between these conditions. Thus, for example, depressed children commonly have other emotional symptoms such as anxiety. Similarly, children with hyperkinetic disorder often have conduct problems. There are, in addition, age differences in symptomatology. For instance, young children commonly respond to adversity with symptoms such as regression, whereas adolescents are more likely to become depressed.

Emotional disorders

Most emotional disorders of childhood are exaggerations of normal developmental trends rather than phenomena that are qualitatively abnormal in themselves. Their onset is usually during the developmentally appropriate age period. For example, it is normal for pre-school children to show a degree of anxiety over separation from people to whom they are attached. When this anxiety becomes severe, or persists beyond the usual age period, **separation anxiety disorder** is diagnosed. Similarly, when stranger anxiety (which is also normal in toddlers) persists beyond the pre-school years and/or is associated with impairment, the diagnosis of **social anxiety disorder** is justified. In adolescence specific fearfulness becomes less common, but when it does occur it usually takes the form of **school refusal**, or adult type neurotic disorders such as **social phobia** or **agoraphobia**.

Anxiety disorders are amongst the most common psychiatric problems in childhood, occurring in about 3 per cent of ten-year-olds. *Genetic factors* are of some importance, with children who are constitutionally 'slow to warm up' and inhibited being at greatest risk. The parents are often anxious and communicate their anxiety by behaviours such as over-protectiveness. Some cases of anxiety are precipitated by stress. This is especially so for specific fears.

Treatment consists of the *reduction of stress, behavioural treatment* of specific symptoms (for example, graded exposure to the feared situation), and general treatments for anxiety such as *relaxation*. Anxiolytics may occasionally be helpful for severe cases, but should never be prescribed for long periods. The prognosis of anxiety disorder is usually good, but about one-third will have another episode. Adult-type neurotic disorders arising in adolescence (such as agoraphobia) have a worse prognosis.

Affective disorders

Depressive disorders can and do occur in pre-pubertal children, though they are uncommon (prevalence of less than 1 per cent). By mid-adolescence the prevalence rises to about 2 per cent in boys and 4 per cent in girls. The main clinical features are similar to those found in adult depression (see Chapter 13), but depressed pre-pubertal children have more somatic complaints and anxiety than their adolescent or adult counterparts. Mania is extremely uncommon in pre-pubertal children, but about 10 per cent of adults with manic-depressive disorders have had their first episode in adolescence. Infants who have been severely deprived or abused sometimes show a state of withdrawal and retarded development (**anaclitic depression**).

Children and adolescents with depressive disorders tend to have parents who are depressed, but these links are probably more a reflection of environmental factors (such as parenting problems) than of genes. Depression in young people is commonly precipitated by adversity. Treatment consists of reducing this adversity, individual psychological interventions such as cognitive-behaviour therapy (which can be administered to children of ten years and older), and/or family therapy. Anti-depressants may be useful for severe adolescent depressions with endogenous features, but should be used with caution because of the dangers of overdose. Most depressed children will recover in a few months, but many will relapse within a year or two.

Suicide is very rare before puberty but does happen. **Self-poisoning** is much more common, but is usually an impulsive act that draws attention to an unsatisfactory situation rather than the result of depressive disorder.

Somatization

Unexplained physical symptoms, such as abdominal pain and headaches, are present in a substantial proportion of children attending medical services. Emotional disorders are found in excess in such children, but most of them are not otherwise psychiatrically disturbed. They tend to come from families in which there are health problems and high academic expectations. In many cases the child is in some kind of *predicament* in which other avenues have been blocked. For instance, the child may feel unable to perform academically according to the family expectations. Pre-existing physical problems in the child or in a relative may determine the kind of symptomatology that is shown. Treatment involves close liaison between the psychiatrist and the paediatrician, changing the family focus from physical to psychological issues, and an emphasis on leading as normal a life as possible (such as returning to school).

Conduct disorders

Conduct disorders are characterized by *repetitive anti-social behaviour that lasts for at least six months*. In young children the clinical picture is dominated by *markedly* oppositional behaviour such as defiance, hostility, and disruptiveness that is clearly outside the normal range. In older age groups behaviours such as stealing, truancy, fighting, lying, and running away are seen. In the most severe cases there may be fire-setting or cruelty to animals or other children. Conduct disorder is usually associated with poor peer relationships, but sometimes occurs in children who are generally well integrated into their peer group.

Conduct disorders occur in about five per cent of ten-year-olds living in towns, with lower rates in rural areas. They are twice as common in boys as in girls. Conduct disorder is *not* the same thing as delinquency (law breaking), which is much more common and shows a greater male preponderance. There is a strong link between conduct disorder and family factors, especially discordant intrafamilial relationships and personality disorder in one of the parents. Parents are often inconsistent in applying rules and are frequently very critical and rejecting of the child. The role of genetic factors is unclear, though temperamentally 'difficult' babies seem to be at greater risk of behavioural problems later in life. About one-third of children with conduct disorder have reading difficulties.

The kind of treatment that is offered will depend very much on the presenting problem and on the commitment of the parents. Behavioural techniques may be effective, especially in younger children. Parents will often benefit from simple advice on how to deal with their child's behaviour. Medication is of little value. Since children with conduct disorder commonly cause substantial disruption in the community, it is important to work closely with other agencies such as the school and the courts. Children who are severely disturbed may benefit from placement in special schools or other residential settings. The outcome of conduct disorder varies a good deal. Children with few symptoms and good peer relationships usually do well. Children with an early onset, poor peer relationships, and a large number of different kinds of symptoms are at risk of personality disorder and criminality. Almost all adults with dissocial personality disorder (see p. 63) have had conduct disorder as children.

Hyperkinetic disorders

Hyperkinetic disorders are characterized by the early onset of *over-active behaviour* and *marked inattention*. To diagnose the disorder these two problems should be evident in more than one situation (for example, home, clinic, classroom) and persist over time. The diagnosis is very difficult to make in children under the age of five as there is wide normal variation in activity levels in this age group. Several other abnormalities are associated with the disorder, including impulsiveness, conduct disturbance, and learning difficulties of one kind or another.

Prevalence estimates vary widely, from 0.1 per cent in the UK to 5 per cent in North America. This wide variation is probably the result of differences in diagnostic practice. Boys are four times more likely to have the disorder than girls. Brain dysfunction resulting from genetic processes or early brain damage is important in aetiology. Additives in the diet have also been implicated but attempts to prove this have not generally been successful. Hyperkinesis may occasionally be the result of early social deprivation.

The first step in treatment is to counsel the parents on the probable importance of biological factors. Behaviour modification programmes that aim to encourage the child to concentrate for increasingly lengthy periods can be effective, especially when they are carried out at school as well as at home. Many parents will have tried diets of one kind or another, and if these are not too restrictive and the parents feel they have helped then it is sensible to continue them. Stimulant medication, such as methylphenidate, can be very effective in severe cases, though side-effects such as depression and reduced appetite may occur. Hyperkinetic disorders are associated with an increased risk of conduct disorder in adolescence.

Pervasive developmental disorders (PDD)

This group of disorders is characterized by:

1. An onset before the age of three years.
2. Grossly abnormal social interactions (such as social withdrawal and lack of responses to other people).
3. Impairments in communication (such as lack of social usage and, in severe cases, absence of useful speech).
4. A restricted, repetitive repertoire of interests (such as pre-occupation with unusual activities).

The best known is **childhood autism (Kanner's syndrome)**. This has a prevalence of about 4 per 10,000 and is four times more common in boys than in girls. Two-thirds of children with autism have mental retardation. Autism is sometimes associated with medical conditions such as congenital rubella or the fragile-X chromosome anomaly (for description see p. 253), but in the majority of cases no diagnosable physical disorder can be found. Twin studies of such cases suggest that genetic factors are important. The prognosis of autism is very poor, with most cases unable to live independently in adulthood. Mild varieties of autism (**Asperger's syndrome**), in which there is no mental retardation or language disorder, have a better prognosis. Autism should be differentiated from the **disintegrative disorders**, in which there is loss of acquired skills. There is no specific treatment for autism, though children and their families can be greatly assisted by provision of appropriate educational facilities and other forms of practical help.

Adult-like psychotic disorders

Schizophrenia is very uncommon among pre-pubertal children, but there is a rapid increase in prevalence during adolescence. Diagnosis can be very difficult because the onset is often insidious and occurs in adolescents who were pre-morbidly withdrawn and odd. Differentiation from manic-depression can also be a problem. Psychotic adolescents usually require in-patient assessment and treatment.

Enuresis and encopresis

By the age of five years about 10 per cent of children will still be wet at night and about 3 per cent will be wet by day. **Enuresis**, *inappropriate emptying of the bladder in the absence of organic disease in a child over the age of five years,* may be nocturnal, diurnal, or both. The most common cause is an inherited delay in maturation of the nervous pathways that control micturition. However, referrals to child psychiatrists commonly have increased rates of behavioural problems, especially in girls and in association with daytime wetting. Enuresis can also be maintained by inconsistent or negative approaches to toilet training.

The first step in management is a careful history and physical examination. Symptoms like pain or dribbling are indications for further investigation, but usually urine microscopy and culture are the only investigations that are required. Children aged five or six years can be reassured that at least one of their classmates has the same problem and that improvement should occur over the next few months. In older children, behavioural measures such as rewards for dry nights, 'bladder training' (which involves encouraging children with daytime enuresis to pass urine at lengthening intervals), and enuresis alarms (which set off a buzzer when the child wets the bed at night) are indicated. Tricyclic anti-depressants can be useful when it is important that the child is dry for a few nights, such as when he goes off to camp, but should not be used routinely. Vasopressin may be effective in resistant cases.

By four years only 3 per cent of children show signs of faecal incontinence once per week or more, and by ten to eleven years this figure has reduced to less than 1 per cent. Most of these children are probably showing soiling secondary to constipation, and only a minority have **encopresis**, *the passage of normal stools in inappropriate places*. Encopresis is three times more common in boys than in girls, and has several causes including coercive and rigid patterns of potty training, emotional disorders, conduct disorders (in which soiling may be used for aggressive purposes), and life stress. Constipation, and occasionally anal fissures, are important precipitating and maintaining factors.

Assessment should include a full physical examination (including rectal), and careful charting of the circumstances and frequency of encopresis.

Treatment should start with the child being reassured that he is not the only sufferer from the problem. Parents should be advised not to punish the child for soiling but rather to encourage appropriate toilet habits, such as sitting on the toilet after every meal. This process, known as *shaping*, should be charted and a reward system should be devised (usually a star chart). It may also be necessary to treat associated psychiatric disorders. Bulking agents and oral laxatives should be prescribed.

Anorexia nervosa

Most cases of anorexia nervosa have an onset between fourteen and nineteen years. The clinical picture is similar to that found in adult cases, as is treatment, except that there is a greater emphasis on family work. The prognosis of pre-pubertal anorexia seems to be particularly poor.

School attendance problems

Although not a psychiatric syndrome as such, poor school attendance is a common problem and therefore requires some attention in its own right. The most common form is **truancy**, which may be defined as *not going to school while concealing the absence from parents*. Truancy is often a symptom of conduct disorder, and is therefore associated with factors like large family size, inconsistent parenting, and reading problems. It should be distinguished from **school refusal**, which may be defined as *remaining at home upset at the prospect of attending school*. School refusal is usually a symptom of emotional disorder, especially separation anxiety, and is frequently accompanied by depression. Complaints of illness are often used to secure staying at home. **School withdrawal** occurs when *children stay off school with the parents' consent*. Management of poor school attendance depends on the cause, but in all cases an effort should be made to return the child rapidly to school. Close liaison with the school and the educational welfare service is important.

SPECIFIC DEVELOPMENTAL DISORDERS

These disorders have an onset in infancy or childhood and involve impairment or delay in a *specific* psychological function such as speech, language, or reading. The course tends to be steady, without the remissions and relapses that occur in the psychiatric syndromes. The impairments often lessen as the child grows older, though some varieties, such as specific reading disorder, show strong continuity into adult life. From a psychiatric point of view, the most important specific developmental disorders are language disorders and reading disorders, both of which have a strong association with behavioural and emotional difficulties.

Specific developmental disorders of language may be sensory or expressive in nature. Both varieties present with slowness in speaking. There should be concern about children who show no interest in sounds by six months, or who fail to develop repetitive babble by a year, or who do not understand simple commands by eighteen months. Developmental language disorders should be distinguished from mental retardation, the most common cause of speech delay, by the fact that the delay is out of keeping with the general level of cognitive functioning. Other causes of delayed speech include deafness, autism, and elective mutism (which is characterized by an inability to speak outside the home but normal speech in the home).

In developmental language disorders there is commonly a family history of similar or related disorders, and it is likely that many cases have a genetic basis. However, in some cases environmental factors, such as deprivation or lack of stimulation, may be important. Such children are often helped by advice to parents on the ways to further communication, like having a special time to play with the child. Speech therapy and educational assessment are also helpful.

Specific reading disorder (SRD) is a *specific* and significant impairment of reading skills. It should be distinguished from *general reading backwardness*, in which reading problems are part of a general delay. SRD is three times more common in boys than in girls, and occurs in about 5 per cent of children. It is commonly accompanied by perceptual deficits, such as difficulty telling left from right. Social factors, such as large family size and lack of books in the home, seem to be important, but in some varieties there is probably a genetic component. There are increased rates of behavioural problems. Treatment is mainly educational, but some children are also helped by the treatment of associated psychiatric problems. Many children with SRD continue to show reading problems in adulthood.

PSYCHOSOCIAL ADVERSITY

As described earlier, **family influences** are very important in the genesis of psychiatric disorders in childhood. Family factors that carry a particularly high risk are chronic marital discord, inconsistent or harsh parenting, and lack of stimulation. Parental mental illness is also a factor, though the risk seems to stem more from the associated parenting and personality problems than from the illness per se. **Social adversities**, such as overcrowding or poverty, are also important.

Several forms of **abuse** are associated with psychiatric problems in children. Some parents can be so persistently hostile and rejecting towards the child that this constitutes *emotional abuse*. *Sexual abuse* can involve direct sexual assault, sexual intercourse, or the child being persuaded to stimulate the adult sexually. It can come to light when it is reported directly by the child. Alternatively, the child may present with physical symptoms (such as genital or anal pain), or with behavioural problems. Any kind of behavioural or emotional disorder can be present, but overtly sexualized behaviour in young children, or unexplained suicidal attempts or running away in adolescents, should raise suspicion of sexual abuse. In *Munchausen's syndrome by proxy* (see p. 238) symptoms or signs of illness in children are fabricated or induced by the parents.

GENERAL TREATMENT MEASURES

Discussion, clarification, diagnosis, reassurance

Most problems of child behaviour do not come to doctors and even fewer are referred to specialists. In the ordinary practice of medicine the chance to ventilate parental concern, seek guidance and clarification in problems of upbringing, or even face up to the ordeal of specialist referral will at times, of themselves, provide a basis for orientating to a problem or provide reassurance.

Psychotherapies

There are various strategies for exploring the situation that has arisen, for providing support, for achieving some understanding and resolving problems in relationships, and for reducing stress. Allowing a child to talk, explain his feelings, confess, relieve guilt may be helpful. Young children need a comfortable place to play, to enact their distress to the therapist. For adolescents groups of various sorts are used. Family therapy entails working with the whole 'living group' to illustrate and clarify the sorts of interpersonal reactions and tensions that exist and to work out better ways of functioning as a family.

Behaviour therapies

These are variously used to alter behaviour by eliminating unwanted and encouraging wanted behaviours – whether in encopresis, in conduct disorders, or in anorexia nervosa.

Drug treatment

Drugs are used sparingly and thoughtfully in child psychiatry, respecting our ignorance of their effects upon the immature brain, upon the developing child, and with regard to the problems of realizing some of their side-effects.

Day-hospital attendance

Day-hospital attendance is useful to allow detailed observation, provide for longer duration treatments, allow certain systematic therapies to be given (play therapy, for example), and provide relief to strained relationships.

In-patient admission

In-patient admission to a paediatric ward or to a specialist child psychiatry unit extends these possibilities.

Reception into care

Reception into care may be needed for children whose problem behaviour brings them into severe conflict at home or in trouble with the authorities. The law relating to children and families has been revised in the *Children Act 1989*. The main principles of the Act are that the welfare of children must be paramount, that parents have certain responsibilities, and that local authorities have a duty to promote the welfare of children in need. The act empowers the local authority to remove the child into care if they are likely to suffer significant harm.

FURTHER READING

Graham, P. (1986) *Child Psychiatry: A Developmental Approach.* Oxford: Oxford University Press.
Rutter, M. (1975) *Helping Troubled Children.* Harmondsworth: Penguin.

18 / SEXUAL AND REPRODUCTIVE DISORDERS

This chapter will be concerned with human sexual development throughout the life cycle. We will therefore start with gender identity disorders, since these start in the pre-school child, and pass on to consider homosexuality since it appears that events in childhood and adolescence are of some aetiological importance.

The second part of the chapter considers the common sexual problems of adult life, with emphasis on their aetiology and assessment. The section on paraphilias is short, since these seldom request medical treatment.

The third part of the chapter considers disorders related to reproduction, once more arranged in sequence from menstrual disorders, through pregnancy to the puerperium, and ending with disorders relating to the menopause.

DISORDERS OF EARLY DEVELOPMENT

Gender identity disorders (F64)

A person's *gender identity* refers to their awareness of being male or female, and *gender role* refers to the public expression of such an identity in clothing and behaviour. The aetiology of gender identity disorders is not fully understood. Most of those with such disorders are anatomically, hormonally, and genetically indistinguishable from other members of their biological gender. It has been suggested that prenatal endocrine influences on the developing brain may be important, and it can be shown that if androgens are given to a pregnant rhesus monkey her female infant will behave as a male. However, hormonal abnormalities have not been demonstrated in humans.

Patterns of early rearing are likely to be important: the *'assigned sex for rearing'* refers to being called 'John', dressed as a boy and given a toy aeroplane; or called 'Jane', dressed as a girl and given a cuddly doll. However, once more, the parents of transsexual patients usually deny that they brought the child up in an unusual way. The available evidence suggests that the gender-related behaviours acquired in the pre-school child are critically important in determining later satisfaction with gender role: any deviant patterns learned before going to school tend to be reinforced rather than disturbed by experience at the infant's school.

Minor degrees of *gender dysphoria* are relatively common at school, with effeminate boys stigmatized as 'pansies', and masculine girls ambivalently regarded as 'tomboys'. It seems clear that a developing child needs a satisfactory role-model with whom they can identify if an appropriate gender identity is to be developed.

Transsexualism

This rare disorder is characterized by the person's persistent sense of discomfort and inappropriateness about their anatomic sex together with a wish to be rid of their genitals and to live as a member of the opposite sex. These feelings take their origin in childhood. The patient wishes to be a member of the other sex and dresses in clothes of the desired sex without sexual arousal, but with a feeling of relief. The patients greatly dislike their genitalia, and request surgical removal of them. The idea of 'really' being a member of the other sex is an example of an *over-valued idea.* Males outnumber females by about three to one: the prevalence in England is 1 in 34,000 men and 1 in 108,000 women.

MEDICAL RELEVANCE

Such patients present to doctors requesting hormone treatment or sex-change operations. They should be referred to a specialist clinic. Sometimes previously normal patients can acquire all the features of the syndrome during a psychotic illness, most usually a schizophrenia. There is a strong association with depressive illness, and suicidal ideas and self-mutilation are common.

Homosexuality

It is a mistake to suppose that people are either homosexual or heterosexual, since many people are capable of either form of sexual activity. Figures from the USA suggest that approximately one-third of males have homosexual experience leading to orgasm at some time in their lives, most usually during adolescence, to be compared with about 6 per cent of women. Only about 3 per cent of men and 2 per cent of women have an exclusively homosexual experience.

Homosexual behaviour becomes much more common in conditions where the other sex is not available, such as prison; and it is common in those few societies where it is not stigmatized.

AETIOLOGY

Genetic factors are of some importance, since the MZ concordance for homosexuality is higher than the DZ concordance. Endocrine influences during pregnancy may determine gender behaviour in childhood, as mentioned above. The importance of *parental role-models* has also been stressed: homosexual patients coming for treatment typically report disturbed relationships with the same-sex parent. A boy who has been unable to identify with a weak or absent father, and whose nascent sexuality has been influenced by an over-protective mother, may be expected to have difficulties in acquiring sexual feelings about women. At about puberty a developing child must bring three things together: their gender identity, the developing capacity for sexual responsiveness, and the ability to develop close interpersonal relationships. Thus effeminate boys are likely to develop a homosexual orientation at puberty, and those who are unconfident about their masculinity may be unattractive to the opposite sex, so that early attempts at striking up relationships are painful. The same boys may be more than usually attractive to males seeking 'unmasculine partners', so that the adolescent enters the rather less competitive homosexual world.

Similar arguments apply to the acquisition of female homosexual behaviour, although here additional factors might be fear or disgust at the sexual behaviour of men ('heterophobia'), deliberate avoidance of men as part of a feminist stance, and poor performance in heterosexual situations.

MEDICAL RELEVANCE

The most important aspect of male homosexuality that involves doctors is the high prevalence of sexually transmitted diseases. Up to 16 per cent of patients with sexually transmitted diseases attending clinics in London have been found to be homosexual, but much lower rates are found elsewhere in the UK. Anal, oral, and genital lesions occur.

Until recent scares about AIDS, the enormous number of partners made recurrent infections likely. (Female homosexuals do not present the same problem of frequent short-lived relationships as homosexual men and their forms of sexual behaviour do not put them at such high risk; they therefore do not present with more sexually transmitted diseases.)

Although anxiety and depression have been reported frequently among homosexual men, there appears to be a truly increased prevalence only for those without a stable relationship. This inability to form lasting relationships may be indicative of interpersonal problems which go well beyond the patient's sexual orientation.

SEXUAL DISORDERS OF ADULT LIFE

The commonest forms of sexual disorders are those in which normal sexual activity is desired but not being achieved. **Primary sexual problems** are those which have been present since the onset of sexual activity, **secondary sexual problems** develop after a period of adequate sexual function.

Epidemiology

Few reliable statistics are available. One area with an established sexual problems clinic serving a defined area reports an annual consultation rate of 64 per 100,000 at risk; but data from surveys suggest that the prevalence of sexual problems is very much higher than this.

Sexual intercourse

Intercourse can be divided into three phases: *desire, arousal*, and *orgasm*, all under different innervation. Sexual interest is mainly under limbic control, arousal mainly under the control of parasympathetic (cholinergic and peptidergic) systems, while orgasm is mainly under sympathetic (adrenergic) control. The various sexual problems which arise can most easily be classified under these three headings.

Both men and women can experience disorders of sexual desire. Problems with arousal lead in the male to erectile difficulties and in the female to lack of lubrication and general sexual unresponsiveness. Difficulties in the orgasmic phase cause premature or retarded ejaculation in the male and orgasmic dysfunction in the female.

Male sexual problems

LACK OF INTEREST (F52.0)

This can occur as a primary complaint, often accompanied by general anxiety about sexual intercourse both between one individual and another and also at different times of life. Although psychological factors such as inhibitions from the past or relationship problems in the present are often important, organic factors may also be present. An increase in prolactin secretion which may be due to a cerebral tumour will cause loss of libido in both males and females. The ratio of testosterone to oestrogen in both sexes affects desire, higher testosterone levels stimulating it.

ERECTILE FAILURE (F52.2)

This may be primary or secondary.

Primary erectile difficulties arise because of inhibitions about sex or difficulties experienced in early sexual encounters. There may rarely be a basic organic defect.

Secondary erectile problems may arise after occasional failures due to alcohol, fatigue, etc., and this may lead to anxiety about the ability to perform, causing further failure and thus creating a vicious circle.

Organic factors may also be important and it has been estimated that up to 85 per cent of men with erectile difficulties have some physical problems, although even where these are present anxiety about performance is likely to make things worse. *Diabetes* and *multiple sclerosis* sometimes present with erectile failure, and problems are likely to increase with age. There are definite physiological ageing changes affecting the strength of the erection and the ease with which it is obtained, and further impairment may result from *atherosclerotic narrowing* of penile arteries. Where there has been serious illness, for example a coronary, the patient may also be anxious about the adverse effects of the exertion needed in intercourse.

PREMATURE EJACULATION (F52.4)

This is common, affecting up to 6 per cent of all males at some time in their sexual lives. It often arises after initial sexual experiences in situations where intercourse has to be hurried, for example the back of a car or in the parental home, and is then perpetuated by the anxiety that it will recur. Occasionally it can occur after a period of normal control, perhaps after a traumatic experience of some kind.

RETARDED EJACULATION

This is very much less common. It often occurs after medication, especially with tricyclic anti-depressants, but it may also occur in inhibited males who can usually masturbate normally to ejaculation.

RETROGRADE EJACULATION

This is ejaculation of semen upwards into the bladder instead of externally, and commonly follows prostatectomy, both transurethral and intra-abdominal.

PAINFUL EJACULATION

This is a rare complaint possibly due to infection and painful muscle spasm.

Female sexual problems

LACK OF DRIVE (F52.0)

In the female this is often due to inhibitions passed on from parents and society in general or from unfortunate past experiences such as rape or incest. It may also be caused by increased prolactin levels in the blood, and by a diminished testosterone/oestrogen ratio as in the male. Many women experience different levels of desire at different phases of the menstrual cycle, and many lose interest in sex after childbirth for a time, probably due to a combination of factors. These may include changing hormonal patterns, dyspareunia after episiotomy, changes in the general relationship, and fear of further pregnancy.

LACK OF AROUSAL (F52.2)
(GENERAL SEXUAL UNRESPONSIVENESS)

Arousal in the woman, as in the man, causes vasodilatation of the blood supply to the genital area. In the male this results in the cavernous sinuses of the penis filling with blood, and in the woman produces a cuff of dilated blood vessels encircling the lower part of the vagina. Some of the fluid from these vessels goes as a transudate into the vagina, producing the lubrication. A woman may not particularly desire sex but if adequately stimulated by a sensitive partner may be able to respond, lubricate, and reach orgasm. Inability to respond may be due to inhibitions from learned attitudes or past experiences or to adverse conditions in the present, including difficulties in the relationship. Any kind of anxiety connected with the situation, for example intercourse in the parental home or anxiety about the baby, may affect her ability to relax and respond. Inadequate stimulation from an inexperienced lover is often a cause of early difficulties. Lack of arousal will in all these situations cause dyspareunia (see below) because of lack of lubrication, and this can easily produce a vicious circle leading to avoidance of all sexual encounters. This commonly occurs after childbirth.

Arousal in the female may also be affected, as in the male, by drugs and neurological and vascular disease, and in post-menopausal women lubrication may be diminished because of lowered oestrogen levels.

DYSPAREUNIA (F52.6)

Pain on intercourse from any cause will inhibit arousal and may be caused by *emotional factors, vaginal infections, pelvic inflammatory disease, endometriosis, episiotomy*, and *operations affecting the cervix*, which may prevent the elevation of the uterus out of the pelvis which occurs in normal intercourse, leading to buffeting of the cervix by the penis.

ORGASMIC DYSFUNCTION (F52.3)

About 10 per cent of women never experience orgasm from any form of stimulation. About one-third of the rest reach orgasm in most acts of intercourse and most of the rest will respond to clitoral stimulation only. A small group respond to breast stimulation or even fantasy alone.

A few women lack the normal bulbo-cavernosus reflex (stimulation of the glans clitoris causing reflex spasm of the perineal muscles) and may be physiologically unable to reach orgasm. Many of the 10 per cent, however, may never have been adequately stimulated by their partners and have been too inhibited to masturbate themselves. Some women fear the momentary loss of control experienced during orgasm and are unable to 'relax and let it happen'.

VAGINISMUS (F52.5)

This is a spasm of the part of the pelvic musculature surrounding the lower part of the vagina making penetration difficult or impossible. It may be primary or secondary. Primary vaginismus may rarely be due to a small or even absent vagina or a very strong hymen, but is almost always psychological due to phobic anxiety to penetration. These women may respond normally to arousal and be orgasmic with clitoral stimulation but cannot let anything, even their own finger or a vaginal tampon, into the vagina. Secondary vaginismus may arise after painful vaginal lesions of all kinds.

Aetiological factors in sexual dysfunctions

PREDISPOSING

Psychological – inhibited upbringing in relation to sexual matters, inadequate sexual education, and traumatic early sexual experience such as incest or sexual assault.

Physical – these are rare causes of primary sexual problems, but anatomical problems such as hypospadias or Peronier's disease, or hormonal problems, may present in this way. Physically disabled people may have sexual problems, which can usually be overcome with a sympathetic partner.

PRECIPITATING

The first attempts at sexual intercourse form the precipitating factor in primary problems. Childbirth, infidelity, or other relationship problems commonly precipitate secondary problems. The onset of physical or depressive illness may also do so, as can a sexual problem developing in the partner.

Physical illness may precipitate sexual problems directly – as with diabetes – or as secondary complications. Following myocardial infarction, impotence and ejaculatory difficulties are common; loss of interest may result from depression or from the unfounded fear that sexual activity will cause further infarction.

Other physical illnesses that may cause sexual dysfunction are: renal dialysis, abdominal surgery leading to ostomies, mastectomy, neurological conditions that cause spinal cord damage, or peripheral neuropathy.

Hysterectomy usually leads to an improvement in sexual functioning because of relief of menorrhagia, but if this symptom has been used as a convenient excuse not to have intercourse a more overt problem may present after the operation. Vaginal shrinkage following the operation may cause pain and ensuing sexual dysfunction.

Both psychological and physical factors may occur together. About half of diabetic males develop impotence, especially the older men. But in many erections occur early in the morning and with masturbation so the mechanism cannot be entirely physical.

MAINTAINING FACTORS

These are often important. Anxiety occurring with sexual arousal leads to vaginismus and impotence, which often cause pain and shame. This can threaten the relationship so one or both partners may be afraid to attempt further sexual activity. If they do try they are anxious in anticipation, which exacerbates the difficulty, further failure ensues, and the problem is perpetuated. Poor communication between partners about sex, inadequate information about it, and conflicts in the general relationship all maintain sexual problems.

Assessment of sexual dysfunction

Although sexual dysfunction may require specialist treatment every doctor should be able to recognize and assess briefly such problems.

1. The sexual problem may be *presented directly* by the patient or the partner. Often it presents indirectly to the gynaecology, family planning, or infertility clinics. Depression, anxiety, or general problems in the relationship may also be presented when the patient is ashamed or embarrassed to describe the sexual problem directly.

2. The *exact nature of the problem and its duration should be assessed*. Is it the patient who experiences the difficulty or is it the partner? Is it primary or secondary? Which phase of sexual activity is affected? Can masturbation or sex with another partner occur satisfactorily? (If it can, organic causes need not be considered!) During such questioning the doctor will become aware of the patient's attitude to and knowledge about sex. A history indicative of *psychiatric or physical illness* in either partner must be sought as this could be responsible for a change in the sexual relationship. Similarly a drug history is required.

3. The patient must be *physically examined* to investigate the possibility of physical causes for the problem. It is especially important to examine the secondary sexual characteristics and the cardiovascular system, and to do a neurological examination of the lower limbs. Impotence may be the first sign of diabetes, so examine the urine and be prepared to examine the Valsalva response (see *Table 18.1*).

4. *The partner must be seen* so that a history of the problem and the partner's attitude to it may be assessed. When the two partners are seen together the doctor observes their ability to discuss sex, whether one partner blames the other, and their attitude towards treatment. It is essential to see each partner alone on at least one occasion so that the doctor can explore the possibility that one partner has had an extramarital affair. The upbringing and previous sexual experience of each partner are also evaluated individually. The couple's general relationship with one another should be assessed as well as their sexual relationship.

5. The expectations of, and preparedness to engage in, treatment must be assessed before it is commenced.

Treatment of sexual disorders

GENERAL MEASURES

Clarification of the problem and a full discussion of the sexual relationship will help the couple to discuss their difficulty more freely and this alone may lead to resolution of the problem. Improvement of the general relationship may be required before any improvement in the sexual relationship could be expected. However, this is not a medical problem.

Education and advice – a great deal can be done to help these patients by sex education, relieving anxiety, and helping to overcome inhibitions by giving them permission to enjoy their sexuality. Increasing communication between the couple is also important. All trained professionals can give simple counselling on these lines and this may be all that is needed for the couple to sort out their own problems. Where more help is required

Table 18.1 *The history and examination of the patient with secondary sexual problems*

history

sexually functional with another partner or by masturbation?		suggests psychogenic causes
is patient depressed?	*(males)*	erectile problems
	(either sex)	loss of libido
is patient anxious?	*(males)*	erectile problems
	(females)	delayed orgasm
recent illness or surgery?	myocardial infarct, ileostomy, colostomy, mastectomy	avoidance of sexual activity
problems with current sexual relationship?		lack of interest or enjoyment, erectile problems
what drugs is patient taking?		
• oral contraceptives		
• corticosteroids		decreased arousal
• parasympatholytics	propanthiline, phenothiazines, tricyclic anti-depressants	impaired erection
• sympatholytics	methyldopa, guanethidine, trazodone, thioridazine	impaired ejaculation

males

does history suggest autonomic neuropathy?	postural hypotension, bladder dysfunction	erectile problems
is there pain in buttocks on effort?	(refer to surgeon)	Leriche syndrome

females

does history suggest vaginal infection?		dyspareunia

on examination

general	look for hypertension, cardiovascular disease, diabetes	
loss of secondary sexual characteristics		hypogonadism, hypopituitism
autonomic neuropathy, Valsalva response	no rate change	diabetes
neurological signs in legs (include cremasteric reflexes, perianal sensory loss)		spinal causes, cauda equina lesion

specialist treatment needs to be directed towards increasing the positive stimuli to make the reverberating circuit fire off to orgasm where this is possible.

If there are fears of pregnancy, then *contraceptive advice* is needed. Sometimes fear of infertility interferes with normal sexual function and such fears must be dealt with before more specific treatment is attempted.

Reassurance that physical illness will not be exacerbated by sexual intercourse may allow the couple to resume their previous satisfactory relationship. Specific advice may be appropriate – for example, taking a beta-blocker before intercourse for the angina patient. Any underlying psychiatric or physical illness must be treated. Although anti-depressants can cause impotence, their appropriate use to treat depressive illness may lead to greatly improved sexual functioning.

Physical treatment – administration of testosterone has been shown to be useful where there is definite impairment of gonadal function. It has also been shown to increase libido even where testosterone levels are normal but will not then improve function. Penile prosthetic surgery has been used in cases of neuropathy. Injection of vasoactive drugs such as papaverine directly into the corpus cavernosum of the penis causes pharmacologically induced erections. Patients can inject themselves at home but require careful instruction in the technique because of the risk of drug-induced priapism. Mechanical aids to erection, consisting of a vacuum pump with a penile constrictor ring, are preferred by some patients. These methods can be used to overcome the performance anxiety and loss of confidence associated with psychological impotence, but are more commonly used when organic factors are present, as in diabetes mellitus.

SPECIFIC PSYCHOLOGICAL TREATMENT

Specialist treatment is usually the province of sexual dysfunction clinics but may be performed by any suitably trained professional. After individual and joint assessment, the couple are seen together for a number of sessions with the understanding that between each session they will be required to do certain exercises together.

The treatment is based on a behavioural model. It is assumed that sexual arousal leads to anxiety and the new response of relaxation must be learned instead. Since the anxiety is usually greatest with penetration, the treatment programme begins with *an absolute ban on attempts at full intercourse* for the first few weeks. This means that instead of experiencing frustrating failed attempts the couple can enjoy mutual pleasurable stimulation. Initially this is solely non-genital stimulation; later genital stimulation is introduced provided that increasing sexual arousal can be achieved while both partners remain relaxed. This must be practised over several weeks and discussed fully both with the therapist and with each other before steps toward full intercourse are taken. Specific techniques are used for premature ejaculation, vaginismus, and orgasmic failure (see Further Reading, p. 294).

As well as the behavioural techniques, counselling and education are usually required. Commonly resentment or embarrassment has developed between the partners and this must be faced and dealt with during sessions. If the problem has been labelled as that of one partner alone, both must recognize their role in the development and treatment of it. Suitable literature is available to guide the couple through sex therapy and to increase their understanding of normal sexual functioning.

Psychotherapy may be appropriate, either in the form of marital therapy if the couple's general relationship requires help, or individual psychotherapy if one partner is found to have problems of their own which will be helped with this form of treatment (see p. 111).

OUTCOME

Treatment of patients attending sexual dysfunction clinics leads to a satisfactory outcome in approximately two-thirds of cases. The outcome is best with vaginismus and premature ejaculation (often primary problems). The outcome of treatment depends on the quality of the couple's general relationship and motivation for treatment.

Paraphilias

In these disorders sexual arousal is repeatedly obtained from non-human objects, or with humans but involving suffering or humiliation or non-consenting partners.

FETISHISM

In fetishism a piece of clothing or part of the body, such as hair or feet, is used as a means of obtaining sexual arousal and orgasm. It is essentially a male perversion and there are many grades from using the fetish (often an item of female clothing) as an adjunct to normal sexual intercourse to using it as a sole means of gaining arousal.

PAEDOPHILIA

Paedophilia is the act or fantasy of engaging in sexual activity with young children as a repeatedly preferred method of achieving sexual arousal. Paedophilic acts usually take the form of immature sex play, with coitus or violence only occurring rarely. Paedophilia often involves a child previously known to the man and may be incest.

Aetiology – in adolescents paedophilia may be an exaggerated form of immature sexual activity. Among older men marital and social difficulties or social isolation are common and alcohol may be involved in releasing the behaviour.

Medical involvement may be required to assess the man or aid the child and their family. The former may be a request from a court.

SADOMASOCHISM

Sadomasochism is sexual gratification involving fantasy or acts of cruelty either to the person (masochism) or to another (sadism). The phenomenon may remain entirely confined to fantasy or may accompany coitus either as a general humiliation or as a highly specific ritual. Sadism is generally performed by men on females, other males, or animals.

TRANSVESTISM

Transvestism occurs in both sexes and involves the persistent wearing of clothes of the opposite sex. This is initially for sexual excitement and the person becomes intensely frustrated if cross-dressing is prevented. There are different forms with some men wearing female clothing in secret, others doing so overtly. If the purpose remains one of sexual arousal this is a kind of fetish; if the behaviour becomes continuous it may lead to a state resembling transsexualism. Both heterosexual and homosexual men and women cross-dress. It should probably be thought of as a minor form of gender dysphoria allied to deviant sexual practices.

Anxiety, depression, or marital problems may present to the doctor often with the spouse, rather than the patient, coming to the doctor. These are treated in the usual way, but if the cross-dresser is resistant to change the future of the marital relationship may be in doubt. Clarifying this issue with both partners will then need to be a first step in treatment.

EXHIBITIONISM

Exhibitionism is the repetitive act of exposing the genitals to an unsuspecting stranger for the purpose of achieving sexual arousal. The desire to shock the innocent party is strong. The man may masturbate but experience intense guilt later.

Depression is an important cause in the elderly, and the behaviour is occasionally accompanied by schizophrenia, organic brain damage, or mental handicap. Exhibitionism may be a short-lived episode in an otherwise normal person but persistent offenders tend to come from troubled family backgrounds, are immature, and under-achieve as adults.

The medical task is to detect treatable psychiatric illness if it is present, to try and prevent stigmatization of the occasional offender, and refer for *behaviour therapy* those who are well motivated to stop the behaviour. The anti-androgen, *cyproterone acetate,* is occasionally used for short periods in conjunction with other treatments.

In relation to court reports the doctor must remember that the majority of convicted exposers do not repeat the crime; it is the repeated offender who seems to be neither easily treatable nor deterred.

VOYEURISM

Voyeurism is sexual gratification through looking at people (usually strangers) who are naked, undressing, or engaging in sexual activity. The observer does not attempt to engage the person whom he has watched in sexual activity but masturbates afterwards.

REPRODUCTIVE DISORDERS

Premenstrual tension

EPIDEMIOLOGY

Estimates of prevalence range from one-third to three-quarters of all women of reproductive age, depending on the severity and duration of the symptoms included within
the definition and their timing in relation to the menstrual cycle. The frequency is such
that it is probably inappropriate to regard this condition as pathological, but the extreme
distress experienced by some women results in medical consultation.

CLINICAL FEATURES

The commonest physical complaints include breast tenderness and feelings of abdominal
distension, and mental symptoms include depressed mood, anxiety, and irritability. These
occur for up to ten days prior to a menstrual period and end one to two days afterwards.

DIAGNOSTIC CRITERIA

The physical symptoms are characteristic. All symptoms are limited to a maximum of
eleven to twelve days of each cycle. The 'biological' symptoms of depression do not
occur. The condition should be differentiated from the affective disorders, in which
symptoms may be exacerbated premenstrually but are more persistent throughout the
cycle. If a daily symptom diary is kept, this may reveal that the complaints are persistent
or intermittent throughout the cycle, indicating the possibility of the somatic presentation of an affective disorder.

AETIOLOGY

Despite the evident link between the timing of these symptoms and the menstrual cycle,
various aetiological theories concerning imbalance of ovarian or pituitary hormones
have not been substantiated. Symptoms of premenstrual tension disappear in about
two-thirds of women after hysterectomy (with intact ovaries), indicating that hormonal
factors are perhaps not of critical importance.

TREATMENT

Sympathetic explanation and reassurance are probably the most important aspects of
treatment. Psychosocial stress should be considered and psychological techniques such
as cognitive therapy and relaxation training may be helpful. Progesterone, bromocriptine, anxiolytics, vitamin B_6, anti-depressants, and diuretics have all been advocated.
There is little evidence that any of these has more than a placebo effect, and possible
teratogenic effects should be considered.

Disorders of pregnancy

EPIDEMIOLOGY

During the first trimester approximately 10 per cent of women experience a new episode of minor affective disorder. During the second trimester this rate falls and is probably similar to the frequency in the general population. There is evidence of an increase in affective disorders in the third trimester.

CLINICAL FEATURES

Any mental illness can have its onset during pregnancy, or may occur as a continuation of a pre-existing disorder. There does not appear to be any increased risk for illnesses characterized by psychotic symptoms, and the vast majority are affective disorders with a mixture of depressive and anxiety symptoms. However, thought content is likely to be focused on the pregnancy and its implications for the future, including the related social and psychological consequences.

AETIOLOGY

Affective disorders which have their onset during pregnancy are associated particularly with the experience of negative life events, such as bereavement, and chronic difficulties, particularly the lack of a confiding relationship. Other factors include a previous history of mental illness, marital conflict, and ambivalence about continuation with the pregnancy.

Onset during the first trimester is associated particularly with a previous history of termination of pregnancy and worries concerning the normality of the foetus.

INVESTIGATIONS

These will usually be limited to a search for evidence of particular aetiological factors which may play a part and the assessment should include interviews with the partner and possibly other informants. Particular attention should be paid to past history and pre-morbid personality, previous termination of pregnancy, recent life events and current difficulties, the marital relationship, and available sources of support.

TREATMENT

Supportive psychotherapy and counselling may be valuable to women for whom there is evidence of particular psychological difficulties, especially those who have failed to adjust to previous termination. *Joint marital therapy* may be indicated where there is evidence of particular difficulties in the relationship which may be highlighted by the pregnancy. Women who have material social difficulties and inadequate social support will need help, which should be available from local social services departments. It is particularly important to follow up patients into the puerperium, to assess the development of bonding between mother and child, and ensure a satisfactory level of child care.

COURSE AND PROGNOSIS

The outcome of affective disorders during pregnancy remains uncertain. Studies based on married women of higher socio-economic status suggest that most recover during the first three months of the puerperium; those based on less socially stable populations with lower socio-economic status indicate a more chronic course, with continuation during the puerperium and possibly for longer. It has been suggested that there are particular risks for subsequent child care and bonding between mother and child which may have long-term implications for child development.

Termination of pregnancy

In England and Wales approximately 100,000 women have terminations of pregnancy each year. Before the Abortion Act (1967) psychiatrists were frequently involved in assessing women prior to termination which was often carried out on grounds of suicidal risk due to depressive illness. Since the introduction of this Act recommendations for termination are usually made by the general practitioner and gynaecologist. Psychiatrists are involved mainly when there is a past history of serious mental illness or a particular need to assess the patient's likely response to termination.

Adverse psychological responses to abortion are rare. Although depression and anxiety are common during unwanted pregnancies these usually resolve within a few weeks after termination. However, there is some increase in the risk of post-natal depression in women with a history of termination, when past feelings of guilt may be re-evoked. By contrast, studies of women refused abortion show they are more likely to suffer depression later on, have an increased risk of suicide, have difficulty in adjusting to their unwanted children, and have children who are at greater risk of delinquency and difficulties at school.

Disorders of the puerperium (F53.0)

There is a well-recognized increase in the prevalence of mental illness following childbirth. Research has led to the classification of these disorders into three main groups which are considered separately below, but there is still much uncertainty about the extent to which these are different conditions and also their relationship to disorders occurring at other times.

'MATERNITY BLUES'

Epidemiology

Between 50 per cent and 80 per cent of all women develop the 'maternity blues' during the first week following delivery, and this has been a consistent finding in different countries, cultures, and ethnic groups. It is, therefore, doubtful whether this condition should be considered pathological, but it undoubtedly causes significant distress and requires medical recognition. No consistent relationship has been found to social class, parity, hospital as compared with home delivery, or obstetric complications.

Clinical features

Symptoms tend to develop in a predictable sequence starting on the *first post-partum day* with feelings of exhaustion, anorexia, and complaints of poor concentration. Mild perplexity and disorientation may occur. Weeping occurs in approximately 50 per cent of all women on the first day. However, about 80 per cent of all women also experience elation on the first day and this appears to be a normal response to childbirth, and in a minority (8 per cent) this persists or increases in the subsequent three days and is accompanied by garrulousness, over-activity, and excitability.

Symptoms which have their peak onset on the *third to fifth days* include depressed mood, restlessness, and irritability. Labile mood with swings from depression to elation on the same day is characteristic of this condition.

Weeping tends to be precipitated by minor events and in a substantial minority of cases depressive thought content includes low self-esteem, feelings of guilt, and pessimism concerning the future. Irritability and anger tend to be directed particularly towards the partner or to hospital staff and may lead to self-discharge from hospital.

Diagnostic criteria

'Maternity blues' invariably have their onset within the first week of parturition. The mood changes are characteristically brief and fluctuate rapidly, usually persisting for only a few hours at a time and at most for one to two days. For the majority there is sudden onset and sudden recovery, with duration usually lasting between one and three days, and never more than two weeks.

Differential diagnosis

The disorder must be differentiated from **post-natal depression**, which starts later, is more prolonged, and includes more persistent affective changes; and from **puerperal psychosis**, which has its onset at around the same time as 'maternity blues' and may have similar prodromal symptoms but then progresses with the development of psychotic features. **Acute toxic states** are suggested by evidence of clouding of consciousness or disorientation but are now uncommon where good obstetric care is available. Approximately 40 per cent of mothers experience either **lack of affection** or negative feelings towards their baby in the first few weeks or months of the puerperium but this is not necessarily related to 'maternity blues'. (It is associated with amniotomy and painful labour.) Mothers are usually extremely distressed by their lack of feelings, and may experience feelings of guilt. They may derive considerable benefit from reassurance that this is a common experience which rarely persists and is not indicative of either mental illness or inadequacy as a mother.

Aetiology

A biological contribution to the aetiology is strongly suggested by the relatively specific timing of onset and duration, the labile mood, and the lack of a clear relationship to psychosocial or cultural factors. Whilst there is a strong suspicion that the profound hormonal changes occurring at this time are implicated, most studies so far have failed to show any association between the presence or severity of 'maternity blues' and hormonal status.

In the first post-partum week there is a precipitate decrease in the circulating concentrations of oestrogens and progesterone. There are several sites in the CNS, including monoamine neurones and receptors, which are sensitive to these hormones.

There is a tendency for episodes (particularly more severe episodes) to be associated with a past history of depressive illness, including post-natal depression and affective symptoms in the third trimester of pregnancy. The latter tends to be associated with poor social adjustment and family and marital difficulties, fear of labour, and anxious and depressed mood during pregnancy. However, there is no evidence that life events other than childbirth contribute to onset and little evidence that there is any increase in risk of mental disorders generally.

Treatment

It is important to recognize the nature of the condition so that the patient and her family can be reassured about the likely course and outcome. Considerable tact and understanding are required by medical and nursing staff in their approach to the patient. Monitoring of the mental state should continue to ensure that complete recovery takes place, and that no other mental disorder is developing.

Course and prognosis

By definition recovery invariably takes place within two weeks without specific treatment and if this does not occur the diagnosis should be reviewed.

POST-NATAL DEPRESSION

Epidemiology

Between 10 per cent and 20 per cent of women develop a depressive illness during the first three months following childbirth and the incidence is, therefore, increased compared with the general population.

Clinical features

Generally symptoms develop after the patient has been discharged from hospital two weeks or more after parturition. The patient feels despondent, is tearful, and is distressed by feelings of inadequacy and inability to cope, particularly with the baby. There may be feelings of guilt, usually limited to self-reproach about not caring for the baby. The mood is often labile and depression tends to be worse in the evening. Commonly there is marked irritability, anorexia, fatigue, and feelings of exhaustion. Sleep disturbance is usually limited to initial insomnia. Almost always the patient exhibits excessive concern regarding the health of the baby and often shows hypochondriacal preoccupation with her own somatic symptoms.

Diagnostic criteria

The disorder is characterized by mixed symptoms of depression and anxiety which have their onset in the puerperium and persist for a minimum of two weeks.

Differential diagnosis

It must be differentiated both from the 'maternity blues' and from puerperal psychosis, and also from other non-psychotic disorders which have their onset before or during the puerperium.

Aetiology

There is no evidence that biological factors play any major part in the cause of post-natal depression, despite some claims to the contrary. There is an increased frequency in primiparae over the age of thirty. There is also an association with a history of a disturbed relationship between the mother and her own parents during her childhood. As with non-puerperal depressed women, there is evidence that adverse life events interact with social and personality vulnerability factors to induce depressive illness in the post-natal period.

Some studies have suggested that there is a relationship between anxiety during pregnancy and post-natal depression. For some women childbirth presents a maturational crisis, imposing a new psychological and physical burden and increased demands from others for dependency.

Investigations

No specific investigations are required, apart from establishing the time of onset of the disorder in relation to the puerperium and a careful assessment of the psychological and social significance to the patient of childbirth.

Treatment

Tricyclic anti-depressants are occasionally required, based on the usual indications. Claims for the effectiveness of specific treatment with **progesterone** on its own or in combination with monoamine oxidase inhibitors have been made but are at present unsubstantiated. For the most part treatment should focus on **supportive therapy** of the patient and her family by the primary care team, who should be particularly aware of difficulties that may occur in the process of bonding. With training, health visitors can provide **counselling** which results in early recovery by most patients.

Course and prognosis

The majority of patients recover within six to twelve months, but if untreated one-half of patients have failed to improve one year after childbirth. Chronic affective disorders starting after childbirth are not uncommon, tend to include poor libido and hypochondriasis, and may remain unidentified for many years.

PUERPERAL PSYCHOSIS

Epidemiology

Between one and two women per thousand deliveries develop a new episode of illness characterized by psychotic symptoms. The majority of these have their onset within the first two weeks of parturition. There is an increased risk particularly for primiparous women (double that for multiparous women) and possibly after caesarean section. No definite relationship has been found with other obstetric factors, with social class, or with marital status.

Clinical features

Symptoms generally have their onset between three and ten days after childbirth although a small proportion start in the subsequent two weeks. Usually they develop rapidly over the course of a few days. Any of the syndromes of the functional psychoses may occur but there is a particular tendency to find mixed states, with both **affective and schizophreniform** symptoms, and marked fluctuations in the type and severity of symptoms during the course of the disorder. **Depressive symptoms** predominate in over half these episodes and **manic symptoms** in about a third. Often these are mixed with **'first rank' symptoms of schizophrenia. Perplexity** occurs in the majority and a substantial minority are **disorientated** at some stage.

Diagnostic criteria

Any mental illness which includes psychotic symptoms and has its onset within four weeks after parturition is included in this category. It should be differentiated from episodes of illness having a previous onset but continuing into the puerperium and from acute toxic states (delirium).

Aetiology

After an episode of puerperal psychosis there is an increased risk of psychoses at times other than the puerperium, and there is also an increased risk of psychotic illness generally (although not of puerperal illness) in first-degree relatives. Thus there appears to be some general genetic and constitutional predisposition. There is no evidence of an excess of negative life events or difficulties during pregnancy. It is generally believed that these disorders are precipitated by the rapid and extreme changes in the hormonal state following parturition, but confirmation has proved elusive. Comparisons of psychotic puerperal women with non-psychotic puerperal women have shown the former to have higher levels of **thyroxin** and **prolactin** (and possibly oestrogen) and lower levels of **luteinizing hormone** and **progesterone**, but the significance of these findings is uncertain.

Investigations

Careful monitoring of the physical and mental state is required to rule out the possibility of an acute toxic state. Details of the patient's social circumstances and the available sources of support will be important in planning her treatment.

Treatment

It is usually necessary to admit the patient to a psychiatric unit and wherever possible this should be with her baby to a specialized mother and baby unit. Patients with a predominantly depressive syndrome in the puerperium tend to respond less well to anti-depressant drugs than those with depressive illnesses at other times. **Electroconvulsive treatment** is particularly effective and therefore tends to be used earlier than in other depressive illnesses. Those with predominantly manic or depressive illnesses are usually started on a **major tranquillizer** (chlorpromazine or haloperidol are suitable) and if there is no definite improvement within four weeks then ECT is started. Despite claims for the value of treatment with oestrogen and/or progesterone there is little evidence to support their efficacy. Expert nursing, including attention to nutrition and fluid balance, is important and should also include the mother's supervised **access to the baby**. As her mental state improves she should take increasing responsibility for the baby's care. Her ability to do this will require careful assessment which will determine the amount and nature of supervision needed once they are discharged from hospital.

Course and prognosis

With treatment virtually all patients improve or recover within three months. Of those patients who have further pregnancies about 30 per cent have a recurrence of puerperal psychoses. If the patient has a bipolar illness the risk in subsequent pregnancy is as high as 50 per cent. However, the risk of recurrence is by no means limited to the puerperium and about 40 per cent of all women who suffer a puerperal psychosis will have another episode of psychotic illness at some time.

INFANTICIDE

Depression in the puerperium carries a small but definite risk that the mother will kill her child. If this occurs within twelve months of the birth and there is evidence that 'the balance of her mind was disturbed' at the time, this act is described as **'infanticide'** and dealt with in British law as manslaughter rather than murder. Approximately half the women who kill their children in the puerperium also commit **suicide**.

The therapeutic use of drugs during pregnancy and the puerperium

1. Drugs taken by women of child-bearing age may have a teratogenic effect if they become pregnant.
2. Drugs taken at the end of pregnancy may result in withdrawal symptoms in the baby following delivery.
3. Drugs taken during lactation may result in toxicity in the breast-fed child.

In view of these possible effects it is desirable to avoid the use of any medication for the treatment of mental illness during pregnancy, and – if the mother wishes to breast-feed her child – during the puerperium. However, if there is a strong clinical indication for medication, this must be balanced against the risks.

TRICYCLIC ANTI-DEPRESSANTS

There is probably no evidence of a teratogenic effect when tricyclic anti-depressants are taken in therapeutic doses. Withdrawal effects occur in neonates and if possible it is preferable to stop these drugs a few days before delivery is expected. Tricyclics are excreted in the milk only in very small quantities and, therefore, **breastfeeding is not contra-indicated** when the mother is being treated with these drugs. However, the more sedating anti-depressants are best avoided as they can lead to respiratory depression and drowsiness.

BENZODIAZEPINES

There have been reports of congenital malformations, particularly cleft-lip and palate, in children born to women taking these drugs during pregnancy. Although the risk is probably small, the potential value of taking these drugs is unlikely to warrant their continuation during pregnancy and they should be avoided. Diazepam has been used for the treatment of pre-eclamptic toxaemia. This may result in toxicity in the neonate causing the *'floppy infant' syndrome*, as well as withdrawal symptoms due to prior physical addiction and both require specialized neonatal care. These drugs are excreted in milk and their **use should be resisted during lactation**.

PHENOTHIAZINES AND BUTYROPHENONES

There is little evidence that these drugs have a teratogenic effect and it appears that toxic effects in the neonate are rare. When taken by the lactating mother these drugs are absorbed by the baby in very small quantities and there is no evidence that this has a detrimental effect. Although best avoided during pregnancy and the puerperium, these drugs **may be used if there is a strong clinical indication**.

LITHIUM

It is well established that **lithium has a teratogenic effect**. It should, therefore, be stopped prior to a planned pregnancy, and contraception should be practised at other times. If essential it may be taken during the third trimester, but special precautions must be taken to control the serum level of the drug, which must be stopped before delivery. Lithium **passes into breast milk** and this can result in toxicity, but there is little evidence of any long-term effect.

Sterilization and hysterectomy

Recent prospective studies indicate that these procedures rarely contribute to the aetiology of mental illness. Sexual enjoyment is often enhanced by sterilization and regrets are uncommon. In a small proportion of cases there are prolonged difficulties in adjustment, including symptoms of anxiety and depression, and these are virtually limited to women in whom there is a past history of similar symptoms. Sometimes these procedures are embarked on as an unrealistic way of trying to deal with other problems, particularly in the marriage or in sexual adjustment. Therefore, a past history of mental illness or current interpersonal or social difficulties indicates a particular need for cautious assessment before surgery.

The menopause

There is no evidence that serious mental illness of any kind is commoner in women around the time of the menopause than at other times. The term 'involutional melancholia' was used in the past to describe severe depressive illness which was thought to be specifically linked to the menopause. The term is now obsolete, because this form of the disorder is related to the effects of age on symptoms of depressive illness, rather than to the menopause.

EPIDEMIOLOGY AND CLINICAL FEATURES OF MENOPAUSAL SYMPTOMS

Symptoms commonly complained of by menopausal and post-menopausal women fall into two main groups. Complaints of *hot flushes and excessive sweating* are commonest one or two years after the cessation of periods, when they are experienced by up to 90 per cent of all women and then gradually dwindle in frequency over the next few years. These are caused by vaso-motor changes, are closely related to reduced ovarian activity, and respond to treatment with oestrogen.

In the year following the end of menstruation approximately one-third of women complain of symptoms including *irritability, anxiety, fatigue, and headaches* and this is approximately 10 per cent greater than the frequency in pre-menopausal and post-menopausal women. These symptoms do not differ in quality from affective symptoms occurring in women at other times, or in men.

AETIOLOGY

There is no evidence that the affective symptoms are related to reduced oestrogen production: they are primarily psychological in origin. To some extent they appear to be determined by the *meaning of the experience* of the menopause. The end of potentially reproductive life is mourned by many women and regarded as a sign of ageing. However, it is welcomed by others, particularly in those cultures where contraception is not practised.

It is also a time when many other changes commonly occur in a woman's life, including the loss of children who leave home and the death of parents. These changes require considerable adjustment and it is not surprising if symptoms of minor affective disorder are commoner at this stage of life, particularly in those individuals who generally have difficulty in making appropriate adjustments to change.

Careful assessment of the nature and duration of symptoms will help to determine the possible value of medication. Each patient will require an individual appraisal of their current social circumstances and their psychological response to recent events.

TREATMENT

Symptoms of affective disorder occurring at the menopause do not respond to oestrogen any better than to placebos. Both tricyclic anti-depressants and benzodiazepines have been found to relieve some symptoms better than placebos, but their use should be restricted to the usual indications for these drugs. Psychosocial problems should be considered. Most patients will benefit from supportive psychotherapy.

FURTHER READING

Bancroft, J.H.J. (1983) *Human Sexuality and its Problems.* Edinburgh: Churchill Livingstone.

Brockington, I.F. and Kumar, R. (1982) *Motherhood and Mental Illness.* London: Academic Press.

Gath, D. and Cooper, P. (1982) Psychiatric aspects of hysterectomy and female sterilisation. In K. Granville-Grossman (ed.) *Recent Advances in Psychiatry* vol. 4. Edinburgh: Churchill Livingstone.

Gath, D., Osborn, M., Bungay, G. *et al.* (1987) Psychiatric disorder and gynaecological symptoms in middle aged women: a community survey. *British Medical Journal* 294: 213–18.

Greene, J.G. (1984) *The Social and Psychological Origins of the Climacteric Syndrome.* Aldershot: Gower.

Hawton, K. (1982) Sexual problems in the general hospital. In F. Creed and J. Pfeffer (eds) *Medicine and Psychiatry.* London: Pitman.

19 / DISORDERS OF OLD AGE

There has been a progressive increase in life expectancy this century throughout the Western world. This has meant that more and more people survive into old age and the proportion of the population of the United Kingdom aged over sixty-five years has risen from 5 per cent to 15 per cent. Similar changes in the age structure of populations throughout the rest of the world are occurring at an even more dramatic rate so that an understanding of the special characteristics of illnesses and the way that they present in old age is very important. Women survive into late life more often than men and in the years beyond the age of seventy-five men are outnumbered by three to one. From 1985–2041, population projections forecast that the proportion of those over the age of sixty will increase from 21 per cent to 26 per cent while the rise in the over eighty-fives will be from 6 per cent to 11 per cent (700,000 to 1,700,000).

Illnesses of all sorts and disabilities that arise from them are more common among the elderly than in other age groups. Old people are thus more likely to consult both general practitioners and hospital clinics. It is important to appreciate that most of these old people are not suffering from psychiatric disorders. Nor should the word 'senile' be used to indicate great age: most old people are not demented. It is unfortunate that although the noun 'senium' refers to the last part of the normal life cycle, the adjective 'senile' means demented in normal colloquial English!

However, it is also important to appreciate that changes in normal psychological functions are a necessary accompaniment of ageing. Old people are not involved in as wide a range of activities as young people, and this can be explained only partly by externally imposed factors such as retirement with a consequently reduced income, upper age-limits for some activities, or failing health. Drive and ambition are usually reduced, and there is a tendency to become less involved with new ventures.

Impulses and emotions are usually better controlled so that intemperate outbursts are uncommon. Specific skills and information acquired over a lifetime of experience are usually well preserved, but the acquisition of new skills or the response to new situations is not so good as it used to be. These normal changes of ageing bring with them a need for more time to cope with new tasks or situations, and there are limits to the amount of change that the individual can tolerate.

It should be remembered that the retired population tend to live alone. Those who stay on in the family home may find it difficult to maintain, and it may also lack modern amenities; while those who move into 'sheltered accommodation' often find it cramped and don't enjoy the feeling that they are in a 'ghetto' with other old people. When these adverse social circumstances are combined with failing physical health it is easy to see how psychiatric illness may be released. The same factors militate against quick recovery once disorder has occurred.

AETIOLOGY

Whilst retirement is often portrayed as tranquil and undemanding – rather like an extended holiday – it is in fact beset with stresses. Losses occur as a direct result of retirement: loss of income, loss of an imposed timetable, and loss of the territory of work and the challenges, company, and status that were an integral part of the Monday-to-Friday battle. In their stead come new challenges: husbands and wives thrown upon one another's company for longer periods than they have been accustomed to, and survival on a limited budget that cannot be supplemented by increased effort. Work has come to be viewed as a scarce commodity not to be shared with the old. Time tends to be unstructured other than by the alternation of night and day, the sequence of the seasons, and the *Radio Times*. Children and grandchildren may marry; grandchildren and great-grandchildren may arrive. Even these happy events carry mixed messages. Inevitably, time brings further losses: bereavements, destruction of favourite haunts by redevelopment, and, most significantly, loss of that sense of physical well-being that has hitherto been taken for granted. In its place come reduced mobility, impairments of the senses of sight, hearing, taste, and smell, and often pains associated with physical disease.

The most consistent characteristic of psychiatric disorders in old age is their association with physical illness and disability. This seems to apply across the whole range of psychiatric illness, including affective disorders and paranoid states as well as organic brain syndromes. Acute or subacute brain syndromes often complicate or act as presenting features of intercurrent physical illness, and dementing illnesses become progressively more common with increasing age.

Medical treatment prescribed for physical conditions may also produce psychiatric symptoms, and the intrusive attention from nurses and other carers which may become necessary is viewed as a further humiliation.

There are therefore many stresses in old age which are capable of provoking mental disorder, although by no means everyone exposed to such stresses does break down. Sometimes it is possible to uncover a history of illness in earlier life or a history of similar conditions in close relatives. Sometimes it seems relevant that the patient has known no model of successful ageing in their own family. Certainly long-standing personality traits and coping strategies developed in earlier life are very important in determining how an individual will respond to difficulties encountered in old age.

SYNDROMES COMMON IN OLD AGE

Organic brain syndromes

TERMINOLOGY

You are likely to encounter a bewildering variety of terms for describing much the same thing. The alternative terminologies reflect the inadequacies of simple classifications to cope with the complexities and variability of organic brain syndromes in old age, where aetiology is usually determined by many factors. It is particularly important to be aware that organic brain syndromes that have been present for many months may be reversible when all the contributory factors have been identified and corrected, and the brain has had time to readjust.

Acute and chronic *'brain failure'* are, quite simply, terms that are best avoided: the brain is a very much more complex organ than the liver or the heart, and cannot be said to 'fail' in the same way. Acute and subacute *'confusional states'* are widely used terms which can be used interchangeably with acute and subacute delirium: we prefer the latter terms, since 'confusion' is but one of the component parts of quite complex syndromes. Confusion has a number of uses varying from disorientation (in place, time, or person) to inappropriate behaviour (for example, getting into someone else's bed on the ward).

Acute and subacute delirium ('confusional states': F05)

CLINICAL FEATURES AND DIFFERENTIAL DIAGNOSIS (see p. 153)

These have been dealt with in pp. 153–6 and only features specifically of relevance to old-age psychiatry will be discussed here.

Delirium has to be distinguished from other organic brain syndromes on the one hand, and from affective illnesses like depression and hypomania on the other.

1. The distinction between a delirium and a **dementia** may present difficulties, since the presence of the latter makes symptoms of confusion and disorientation more likely when intercurrent illness strikes. A history from a reliable informant is the key to a successful diagnosis. Not infrequently an acute confusional state may overlie a dementia syndrome (see p. 155).

2. Patients with **depressive illness** may appear confused and disorientated if they have impairments of vision or hearing as well, or if physical illness limits their ability to move. **Pseudo-dementia** is the term given to a functional disorder presenting with features of dementia.

3. Rarer conditions which should be distinguished from delirium include **dominant hemisphere cerebrovascular accidents**, in which there is a jargon aphasia but in which non-verbal tests are performed normally, and **transient global amnesias** related to bilateral temporal lesions.

AETIOLOGY

It is usual for multiple pathologies to contribute to the development of both acute and subacute delirium in old age.

In the elderly the majority of cases of delirium are due to intercurrent physical illness, but another important cause is intoxication by (prescribed) drugs. Elderly people are often prescribed combinations of drugs for various illnesses, and their reduced hepatic and renal function may impair their ability to metabolize these drugs.In addition the brain may be much more sensitive to their effects so that blood levels that would be therapeutic in younger patients become toxic.

Problems arise because the symptoms of a delirium are often much more striking than the underlying physical illness. Indeed, the latter may be relatively silent: pneumonia without pyrexia, and myocardial infarction or perforated peptic ulcer without pain. Hypothermia – which is virtually confined to the elderly – may also present in this way.

In younger adults, the combination of reliable information from the special senses and an intact brain protect us from illusions, misinterpretations, and hallucinations. In the elderly neither of these can be taken for granted. Failing eyesight and deafness are common and may contribute to misinterpretations and illusions. Thus a poorly defined signal might be further distorted to produce an illusion. The random neural noise may itself come about in a number of ways. Anoxic or toxic effects on neurons may disturb neurotransmitter activity, either by impairing synthesis or by causing loss of re-uptake or inappropriate leakage. Such effects may be caused by events outside the brain, such as the effects of bacterial toxins or drugs. In addition, age-associated modifications to the blood–brain barrier make it more permeable to toxic substances, and structural changes to the brain itself make acute brain syndrome more likely to occur than in younger brains.

The other point to grasp is that many demented patients manage perfectly well in a protected environment which makes few demands of them, but they develop symptoms of acute confusion when they are stressed in some way. This is sometimes referred to as 'compensated' and 'decompensated' dementia. It is in this sense that stresses that produce symptoms of *depression* or *anxiety* can release a subacute brain delirium in a previously apparently healthy old person, and thus depressive illness and anxiety states are included in the differential diagnosis. However, it must be appreciated that *social and psychological stress* without clear evidence of an affective illness can also cause a dementia to decompensate and manifest itself to doctors as a subacute delirium: such stresses include anything that suddenly disrupts the environment: a spouse dying or being admitted to hospital, moving to a new house, being admitted to hospital for some other reason, or going on holiday.

Sometimes the cause seems to be loss of a familiar environment; sometimes it is too much stimulation from the environment. Thus a house with too much noise – perhaps dominated by the activities of teenage grandchildren – or a noisy ward with frightening machinery and frequent changes of staff may overload the patient with too much input.

COURSE

Most cases of delirium resolve with identification and treatment of the underlying cause, but there may be a lag of several days or weeks between the resolution of the physical problem and the return of normal psychological functioning. During the recovery period the patient should be encouraged to walk, talk, remember things, and exercise domestic and other skills. Rehabilitation including 'reality orientation' requires repeated practice and persistence to achieve one's full potential, and must take into account the patient's own baseline. However, sometimes even this can be bettered if the patient's eyesight can be improved with new spectacles, hearing improved by providing a hearing aid or syringing the ears, and discomfort from painful feet relieved by appropriate treatment. In the setting of an established dementia, rehabilitation will aim at producing a sufficient improvement to allow a supported life style outside hospital.

Dementia (chronic brain syndrome: F00–F02)

Dementia can be defined as an acquired impairment of higher mental functioning (intellect, memory, and personality) without impairment of consciousness.

Dementia is highly associated with age: 5 per cent of the population above the age of sixty-five, 25 per cent of those aged above seventy-five, and 60 per cent of those aged over eighty-five show some of the impairments described below. Dementia is rare under the age of sixty-five, and when it occurs it is called *'pre-senile dementia'* (see p. 161).

Only about one in seven of the old people suffering from dementia are housed in institutions (hospitals, nursing homes, or residential homes): yet all institutions caring for old people carry a disproportionately large number suffering from dementia – somewhere between 40 per cent and 60 per cent.

Multi-infarct dementia (F01.1: or arteriosclerotic dementia) tends to be commoner in men, and in the sixty-five to seventy-four age group than in those aged above seventy-five. On the other hand *Alzheimer's disease* (F00: senile dementia of Alzheimer type, or 'SDAT') tends to be seen more often in women, and is by far the most important dementia in those above the age of sixty-five.

AETIOLOGY (see p. 161)

A dementia can be produced by a number of pathological processes (see p. 167), but in old age it is not unusual for several processes to combine to produce it.

Remember the *potentially reversible causes* of dementias do occur in old age. **Hypothyroidism, vitamin B$_{12}$ deficiency**, and **anaemia** do not often produce dementia on their own, but they may each make a contribution to the causation, and certainly exacerbate the dementia produced by either Alzheimer's disease or multi-infarct dementia.

Chronic infections, constipation, impaired eyesight, reduced hearing, reduced mobility, depressions, and *an under-stimulating environment* are amongst the features that can contribute to a dementia. Finally, the effects of **drugs** deserve special mention and careful consideration in every case. They may have been prescribed in doses that are too high, they may be interacting with other drugs, or their side-effects (which may be more common in the elderly) may be contributing to the symptoms of the dementia.

DIAGNOSTIC CRITERIA (see p. 161)

There should be a history of progressive global deterioration of personality and intellect without associated impairment of level of consciousness, backed up by mental state findings indicating impairment of new learning. In making a diagnosis of dementia, each individual's performance should be judged relative to what might reasonably be expected of them, bearing in mind their past educational and occupational achievements.

DIFFERENTIAL DIAGNOSIS

1. **Distinction between Alzheimer's disease (F00: 'SDAT') and multi-infarct dementia (F01.1):** the latter is distinguished from SDAT by the history of sudden onset, step-wise deterioration, and the presence of arteriopathic and focal neuro-logical signs on physical examination.

2. **Other degenerative disorders:** Alzheimer's disease and multi-infarct dementia are relatively common, while *Huntington's chorea* (F02.2: see p. 163), *Pick's disease* (F02.0: see p. 162) and *Creuzfeld–Jacob disease* (F02.1: see p. 163) are seen only occasionally.

3. **Primary and secondary cerebral neoplasms** are suggested by evidence of raised intra-cranial pressure and confirmed by CT scan.

4. **Depressive pseudo-dementia** is described below (see p. 303).

5. **Normal ageing:** dementia must be distinguished from the effects of normal ageing described as benign *senescent forgetfulness* (now often called 'age-associated memory impairment'). In the latter condition patients forget part but not all of a task, retain insight into their disability, and respond well to cues. In dementia the patients may fill gaps by confabulation, and tend to mix up recent and past events.

COURSE

Alzheimer's disease can often follow a more benign course in the senium than in earlier life with a slow development of both symptoms and disabilities. This means that some patients with Alzheimer's disease die of intercurrent illness before developing the more severe symptoms: however, others will develop both parietal lobe dysfunction and fits. **Multi-infarct dementia** is characterized by episodes of sudden loss of function, any of which may release symptoms of an acute brain syndrome for a time. However, the extremes of disinhibited anger, aggressiveness, and sexual activity which can be encountered in pre-senile dementias are much less often seen in the older age groups.

Schizophrenia and allied states (F20: see p. 174)

CLINICAL FEATURES

Most patients who develop schizophrenia in early adult life will survive into old age. Some of these will have predominant defect symptoms (see p. 176), while others will have combinations of defect symptoms and florid symptoms – most usually persecutory delusions accompanied by appropriate hallucinations.

Some patients develop schizophrenia-like psychoses for the first time in old age, and because of their special features these illnesses have been called *persistent persecutory states of the elderly (F22.8)*. The principal abnormality consists of auditory hallucinations which are accompanied by delusions of persecution. Other patients develop persecutory psychoses with marked depressive features.

AETIOLOGY

Genetic factors are less important than in schizophrenias of earlier life.

Persistent persecutory states are commoner in women, and patients tend to have previous life styles and personalities characterized by emotional and sexual coldness. Social isolation, often exacerbated by failing vision, failing hearing, physical illness, or restricted mobility, facilitates both the hallucinatory phenomena and the persecutory ideas.

TREATMENT

Formation of a reasonable therapeutic alliance is an essential, although often very difficult, first step.

Hallucinations can usually be suppressed with neuroleptic drugs: but compliance is always a major problem, and symptoms return when the medication is stopped. If the patient can be persuaded to persist with medication they often return to their former lives as competent, rather distant individuals. Life expectancy is not reduced, and treatment as an out-patient is usually possible. Old patients treated with neuroleptics for prolonged periods are often troubled by apathy and reduced drive, as well as the well-recognized symptoms of Parkinsonism. However, anti-Parkinsonian treatment should be avoided if possible, and the patient maintained on the smallest dose of neuroleptic that is effective in controlling their hallucinations.

AFFECTIVE DISORDERS

Depressive episode (F32: see p. 195)

Symptoms of anxiety and depression are found in 10 per cent to 20 per cent of old people living at home, and even higher figures are found in those presenting for care to their general practitioner, to hospital out-patients, or to social services. Depressive illnesses are slightly less common than at earlier ages (although depressive symptoms may occur very commonly) and hypomania is comparatively rare.

Older patients are even more likely than younger patients to present with somatic symptoms when they are psychologically unwell (see Chapter 11). Those who will later be found to be suffering from a depressive illness will originally have sought help for complaints such as tiredness, weakness, palpitations, anorexia, constipation, breathlessness, and pains. It may be that physical pathology (for example, arthritis, a hemiparesis, or varicose veins) is indeed present and may account for some of these pains – but the symptomatology attributed to the physical disease is exaggerated by the mood disorder which itself may be hidden or denied.

Withdrawal from activities (*'Because I'm too old for them now and should give way to younger folk'*) and **reluctance to leave the house** (*'I'm not so good on my feet now, and if I fell I'd be such a trouble to everyone'*) may be presenting symptoms of a depressive illness, but the 'explanations' of the symptoms are easily accepted by relatives. Indeed, the 'understandability' of symptoms of depression and anxiety is a great hazard for the elderly, since detection and treatment are made less likely. There are therefore parallels with the depressive states secondary to malignant disease (see p. 136): in both cases, symptoms may respond to treatment, and they should therefore be regarded as morbid phenomena rather than as 'understandable' reactions to circumstance.

The risk of successful **suicide** increases with age and must always be borne in mind with depressed old people, especially if they live alone or are physically ill. Although some make suicidal threats for the effect that such threats have on others, it must be remembered that suicide becomes more common with advancing age. Thus any hint that an old patient is contemplating suicide must be taken seriously, and the doctor must ensure that adequate supervision is available and must provide active treatment. In practice, this will usually involve admission to hospital. Old people who have survived a suicide attempt should certainly be admitted to hospital – voluntarily if possible, but on a compulsory order if necessary.

Psychotic depression (F32.3: see p. 199)

In patients with psychotic depression, delusions of worthlessness, poverty, or nihilism occur at all ages, but delusions of infestation and cancer are also seen in the elderly. Psychomotor symptoms – either agitation or retardation – commonly accompany such delusions.

The differentiation of Parkinson's disease from psychotic depression can be difficult, since in both the patient may appear retarded: once more, correct assessment depends upon careful history-taking.

Pseudo-dementia

This refers to the situation when a depressed patient performs poorly on tests of short-term memory during the mental state examination, leading inexperienced clinicians to conclude that they are indeed demented. The differentiation of *depressive pseudo-dementia* from degenerative dementias should be made by careful history-taking. In the former condition there will be a short time scale of development with anxious and depressive symptoms predominating from the outset, and there may also be a history of earlier depressive episodes.

Even when the examination is confined to simple test material such as the Newcastle Scale, the patient manages to communicate severe depression and self-doubt with his answers:

> *I don't know. I don't know. Oh, don't be bothering with me . . . it's all beyond me now.*

In contrast, some demented patients produce inaccurate answers with confidence, sometimes amounting to confabulation.

Mania (F30: see p. 203)

This occurs in old people, but it is less common than in early adult life. Mixed states with both depressive and hypomanic features may bewilder both the patient and his relatives: the typical picture of earlier adult life is unusual. Irritability, downright combativeness, and even paranoid sensitivity are more common than elation and a sense of well-being. There is a real risk that excessive activity combined with lack of both sleep and food may put life at risk by precipitating serious cardiac or respiratory problems.

ALCOHOLISM AND DRUG DEPENDENCE (F10–F19: see p. 209–22)

Some of those dependent upon alcohol in early adult life manage to survive into old age; and many more are now surviving into old age dependent upon sleeping tablets and 'minor' tranquillizers. As such patients develop new pathology in their liver or brain they may lose their tolerance for alcohol or other drugs, and are therefore at higher risk for organic brain syndromes and other psychiatric disorders.

Some old people – mainly women – turn to drink or tranquillizers for the first time in old age. They have usually been prescribed such drugs for the symptomatic relief of symptoms of depression or anxiety, although in some dependence upon the drug has been released by the disinhibition of a dementing process. These patients typically come to medical attention through complications which include confusion, falls, and self-neglect; or the problem is reported by embarrassed relatives or home helps who have been prevailed upon to act as suppliers.

In theory treatment of those becoming dependent for the first time in old age should be straightforward, and should consist of withdrawal of the agent with appropriate treatment of the problem which has precipitated the dependence. However, in practice there are often real difficulties: partly because of the intractable nature of some of the associated social problems, but sometimes because of obstinacy on the part of the patient.

MENTAL RETARDATION (F70–F73: see pp. 249–58)

Those handicapped individuals who survive into old age are typically cared for by sisters or brothers after their parents' death. They may present as depressed or as 'confused' when the death or illness of a carer confronts them with their own limitations in coping ability.

INVESTIGATIONS IN OLD PEOPLE

Home assessments

There are many advantages in making assessments in the patient's home. Not only is this convenient for the patient, but it provides an opportunity for the doctor to see the patient functioning in the environment in which the problems have been identified. Information about current stresses and potential supports is readily available, as well as a great deal of useful information concerning the patient's personal life. If the patient is to be admitted to hospital, it is possible to make arrangements with relatives about how care will be resumed outside hospital when the time comes. However, some elderly patients may prefer to be seen at the hospital.

Physical examination

In addition to the usual physical examination including weighing the patient and testing the urine, it is important to remember to test eye-sight (with spectacles), hearing (with any hearing aid), to inspect teeth (and dentures), feet, balance, and coordination, and to carry out a rectal examination.

A full blood count, biochemical profile, and chest film should be carried out in every case, together with any further special investigations which are indicated by the special circumstances of the case. If they are available, CT scans should be carried out to investigate the possibility of intracranial pathology other than involutional changes.

TREATMENT OF THE ELDERLY PATIENT

It is of the first importance to build a trusting relationship between members of the multi-disciplinary team on the one hand, and the patient and their family on the other. Psychological treatments are usually exploratory or supportive. Dependence upon the therapist is unlikely to become intense, and can be sustained for relatively long periods whilst adjustment to new circumstances is achieved.

It is important that doses of psychotropic drugs are adjusted downwards, to take account of reduced body mass and reduced renal function in the elderly. High blood levels of drugs are easily attained, and may rise as the drug accumulates. The presence of other drugs, prescribed for other conditions, means that drug-interactions may complicate the undesired effects of any psychotropic drugs that are prescribed. It is therefore important to make sure that all drugs being prescribed are really necessary, and that none is being prescribed in doses that are too high.

The problems described above should not lead to failure to prescribe necessary drugs: mental illness in old age causes much preventable suffering, and is also associated with premature death by suicide.

Interview techniques with old people

When approaching an interview with an elderly patient it is important to *take account of their relative slowness*, their tendency to tire easily, and the greater likelihood that they will have difficulty with memory as well as problems with eye-sight, hearing, and mobility. Making sure that your face is at the same level as the patient, that your eyes and lips can be seen, and that you speak slowly and clearly take little trouble and is much appreciated – for it provides extra cues to supplement fading or unreliable hearing. However, do not assume that all elderly people are half-blind, half-deaf, and cognitively impaired!

Old people in particular have expectations about how a doctor will dress and behave: *a careful, polite approach is essential*. Repeated short interviews often achieve more than attempts to press on beyond the endurance of the patient. As in obstetric practice, two empty bladders are a good investment before you start.

Although you will encourage the patient to focus on their current problems as they give you the history, you should allow them to diverge from time to time to share a reminiscence with you – this shows an interest in them and their experiences, and will consolidate trust between you.

Since memory problems and confusion are common in elderly patients it is unwise to rely only on information from the patient, and you should always be sure to *talk to a relative as well*. It is not unusual for an elderly patient to be quite unaware of problems that others have noticed, and they may even deny that abnormalities reported by others have actually occurred.

Mental status examination in elderly patients

As with any other patient, this starts with *careful observation* and recording of the patient's appearance, behaviour, and spontaneous speech. If you are carrying out an assessment in the patient's home remember to include the situation in which the patient is living. Thus there may be evidence of long-standing self-neglect or failure to cope; or multiple locks and hostile messages may indicate a paranoid disorder.

There are occasions when this is all that can be achieved as more formal testing may be beyond the patient's ability. On these occasions be sure to obtain a history from a relative, and return to an assessment of the patient's cognitive state as soon as the patient's physical condition allows.

Examination of cognitive function is especially important as confusional states and dementing syndromes are common in the elderly. However, there are traps for the unwary. It is easy to elicit lack of awareness of current events and deficits in new learning in an old patient who is depressed, anxious, feeling physically unwell, in pain, or even just feeling uncomfortable in strange surroundings. You may conclude that the patient is demented or confused, when what is really wrong is that your test procedures were too fast, too long, too complex, or just badly presented. Short, simple tests that encourage the patient to do well with early items are better accepted and provide more worthwhile information. A number of question-and-answer tests have been developed that require the retrieval of knowledge acquired in the distant past and also require accurate recall of more recently acquired information. One such scale is Blessed and Roth's Newcastle Scale, which has the advantage that it has been validated against post-mortem findings: patients with high scores are found to have normal brains, while those with low scores and a history suggestive of dementia are found to have degenerative changes in their brains. The severity of these changes has been shown to correlate well with the lowness of their scores.

ADMINISTERING THE NEWCASTLE SCALE

You will find the abbreviated Newcastle Scale on the Card (also reproduced on the rear end-paper of this book). It is very easy to administer and score: jot down the actual responses with any comments of your own, and give one point for each correct answer. The 'recognition of persons' test is scored by asking the patient to identify other people in the room, or photographs of others which may be on the bedside table or mantelpiece.

INTERPRETATION OF THE SCORE

This is a rough and ready clinical test which should be looked upon as indicative of the state of cognitive impairment at the time of testing, rather than as diagnostic of a particular condition. Most old people without cognitive impairment will score within 1 or 2 points of the maximum possible. So, if you administer all 10 of the items, a score of 8 or less suggests cognitive impairment.

FURTHER READING

Arie, T. (ed.) (1992) *Recent Advances in Psychogeriatrics* (2). London: Churchill Livingstone.

Blessed, G., Roth, M. and Tomlinson, B. (1968) The association between quantitative measures of dementia and senile change in the grey matter. *British Journal of Psychiatry* 114: 797–811.

Blythe, R. (1981) *The View of Winter*. Harmondsworth: Penguin.

Jaccoby, R. and Oppenheimer, C. (1991) *Psychiatry in the Elderly*. Oxford: Oxford University Press.

Pitt, B. (1982) *Psychogeriatrics*. London: Churchill Livingstone.

Qureshi, R. and Hodgkinson, H. (1974) Evaluation of a ten item mental test in the institutionalised elderly. *Age and Ageing* 3: 152–7.

PART 4
PSYCHIATRY FOR THE HOUSEMAN AND LEGAL ASPECTS

20 / PSYCHIATRY FOR THE HOUSEMAN

During your time in the department of psychiatry as a student you will learn to take your time and do things thoroughly: however, during your pre-registration year you are going to have to learn some short cuts. The patients you will see in the accident room, and those that you admit to the wards, have a high incidence of affective illnesses, acute brain syndromes, and alcohol-related problems, and they also present difficult psychological management problems. You will become a far better doctor if you learn to recognize and treat these disorders.

After an opening section on interview techniques (the short cuts!) we will deal with breaking bad news to your patient's relatives; dealing with the psychological effects of surgery; dealing with dying patients and with those recently bereaved. A final section will deal with emergencies in the accident room, including violent patients and those who have deliberately poisoned themselves.

WHEN TO SUSPECT PSYCHIATRIC DISORDER

In Chapter 2 we drew your attention to the **verbal and non-verbal** cues which indicate possible psychiatric disorder (see p. 14); learn to notice these, and to give such patients the opportunity of telling you how they have been feeling as you take the history. Get into the habit of asking all patients:

> *How have you been feeling in your spirits?*
> *Have you been very worried about your health?*
> *How have you been sleeping?*

as you do the 'systems review' part of the interview: you will learn a great deal about your patients, and will often find yourself going on to the 'Short mental state for mood disorders', given below.

As you examine your patients, remember to observe their degree of **alertness**: if you have even mild doubts, carry out tests of **orientation** in order to detect acute brain syndrome. In elderly patients you will find the Newcastle Scale useful as an indicator of current cerebral impairment; for younger adults use conventional memory tests – both will be found on the Card.

Now you are sitting down, writing up your notes. Are the patient's symptoms quite typical of some recognized physical disease, or are they atypical, and peculiar in some way? If the latter, consider giving the short mental state examination relating to mood (see below).

Has the patient got any potentially alcohol-related disease (see p. 211)? If so, ask the 'CAGE' questions – also on the Card – and be prepared to go on to a drinking history (see p. 214).

A SHORT MENTAL STATE FOR MOOD DISORDERS (see 'The Card')

This should be given whenever you suspect a mood disorder. Many of the questions are perhaps those that you are used to asking anyway: but perhaps you are not used to allowing the replies to these questions to help you form a view about whether the patient is psychologically unwell. You will see that it consists of a set of rather general questions together with questions about anxiety and depression.

The **questions in emphasized type** should be asked of all patients, but it is only necessary to give the questions in parentheses if you have a positive reply to such questions.

Scoring and interpretation

The higher the score, the more likely is it that your patient has a mood disorder. The questions marked 'A' relate to anxiety, while those marked 'D' relate to depression. Ask yourself what relationship the disorder that you have elicited might bear to the somatic symptoms that have caused the patient to be admitted (see p. 136). Many patients who are anxious but not depressed will be found to have understandable anxiety symptoms that you can do a great deal to help. (For research purposes, diagnostic criteria for anxiety states and depressive illnesses are to be found on pp. 191 and 198.)

A short social history

Concentrate on the patient's present living conditions, rather than details of their past life.

Who is there at home?
Do you have any worries about them?
How do you get on together?

Anything happened to you recently that has upset you?
Any problems about the place you live in?
Any problems at work?
Any financial problems?

Seeing a relative

If you suspect a social or family problem, ask to see a relative. If you haven't time, or feel that the problem sounds too involved for you, ask the medical social worker for assistance.

Management

The management of the various disorders will be found on earlier pages. All require reassurance and explanation. If you haven't yet read the section on the management of somatization, maybe you ought to turn to p. 243 now.

BREAKING BAD NEWS TO RELATIVES

Telling a perfect stranger that their relative is dying is one of the most unpleasant tasks that will come your way. However, it will happen to you often during your pre-registration year. Perhaps because they are so uncomfortable about such interviews themselves, doctors often greatly increase the burdens that they impose on such relatives.

1. Start by introducing yourself, and asking whether you can 'have a word' with them. Take them to an interview room where you can have some privacy, and settle them down.

2. Open by saying something like *'I expect you've been very worried about him/her'*. **Pause** to give them time to reply. If they agree, ask *'How has it affected you – are you managing to sleep all right?'* Ask any further questions that might be indicated: this is your opportunity to learn something about the relative, and you will need this information later in the interview.

    You will also gain some idea about whether they have already feared the worst, or whether you are about to shock them badly.

3. Make a clear **transition statement,** like *'Well, the reason that I've asked to see you is that we have found out more about your [husband's] illness'*. This has the effect of focusing the relative's attention on what you are about to say.

    Now, explain exactly what has been found, without using any jargon. If there is a positive side to the news (for example, that a tumour is operable) *be sure to include it at this point*, but do not go into details of treatment yet.

4. Now, **pause** again. This gives the relative an opportunity of absorbing what you have said, and asking you any questions. Don't hurry this part, it is important.

5. You have almost certainly been asked about treatment; but if not, explain this now. Almost certainly, the treatment has a good and a bad side. Be very sure that you **start with the good side,** saying what can be expected from treatment. If there is a chance of a cure, tell them what it is: otherwise explain what the treatment is meant to achieve. For example, if a loop of gut is to be made to by-pass an inoperable carcinoma of the head of the pancreas, explain what will happen if the operation *isn't* done, and what can be expected if it is.

    Once the positive objective of any proposed treatment has been grasped, *go on to explain the bad side* of any treatment: the mortality of an intended operation, or the side effects of radiotherapy. In those few cases where there is no treatment to offer or discuss, you must emphasize that you undertake to keep the patient comfortable.

6. At this stage you will often be asked to predict how long the patient has to live. *Never give a precise time*: you cannot possibly know. If there is even a remote chance of cure, remember to say so. If you have an idea of the sort of range, err on the side of optimism: *hope keeps people alive; and despair kills them.*

7. Finally, the issue will arise about what the patient is to be told. You must never swear a relative to secrecy: they will know the patient much better than you do. It is very helpful if you tell the relatives what has been said to the patient so far. Ask the relative if they think the patient would want to be told. If they intend to tell the patient and you feel that the patient is too weak to receive such news immediately after surgery, *then it is your duty to tell the relatives this*. The decision about what to say to the patient is discussed further on p. 317.

8. Finish by offering to see them again if they think of further questions for you. Remember that the relative is very anxious: they will not absorb everything that you have told them first time round. Be prepared to repeat it on another occasion. If you are in any doubt, ask them to say it back to you.

If you are seriously concerned about the relative's health, suggest that they go to see their family doctor, and offer to ring the doctor up and explain the situation. The relative is not your patient.

THE EFFECTS OF MUTILATING SURGERY

There have been many studies of psychological problems and mental illness in patients who have undergone mutilating surgery, including mastectomy, hysterectomy, colostomy, and amputation. In each of these groups between 20 per cent and 40 per cent of patients are found to be suffering from mental illness, mainly affective disorders, and follow-up studies suggest that these disorders persist for at least one year. The changes observed are by no means limited to the effects of surgery as there are usually other major factors that influence the patients' mental state, including the effects of the disease – often malignancy – and the unwanted effects of any other treatment that the patient has already received.

The different ways in which relationships between physical and mental disorders may arise have been described in Chapter 11 and this section is concerned only with the psychological reactions to disease and its treatment.

Psychological reactions found after most mutilating procedures

1. **Uncertainty** regarding treatment procedures and their likely outcome and effect on the patient and her family give rise to **fear.**

2. **Helplessness** resulting from the sense of loss of control of one's own body and dependence on others.

3. **Guilt** and self-blame are often associated with the idea that the disease and its treatment are retribution for real or imagined imperfections.

4. **Sense of failure** is related to this and also to the idea that it may be too late to achieve past ambitions. (The above two phenomena may be part of a depressive illness.)

5. **Stigma** is anticipated due to disfigurement and its expected effect on others, for example, that they will be contaminated. The fear of being shunned may result in social isolation. . . .

6. **Isolation,** that is, the patient avoids others to save herself and others from embarrassment and consequently may lose the support of others at a time when it is most needed.

7. **Anger and resentment** at the loss of part of oneself and the disruption to normal function that may ensue is often exemplified by the question 'Why me?'

8. **Sexual problems** are common after mastectomy (in one-third of subjects) when there are feelings of loss of femininity and loss of self-esteem. After colostomy sexual relationships are often disrupted by fear of noise, smell, and rejection.

9. **Effects of associated treatments** for malignant disease include fatigue, nausea, vomiting, hair loss, amenorrhoea, and impotence due to cytotoxic drugs and/or radiotherapy.

10. **Maintenance of abnormal illness behaviour** after recovery from physical disease may result in long-term disability due to the gains that have been derived from illness (see p. 232).

The causes of adverse reaction

Although it may seem obvious that most patients subjected to mutilating surgery will suffer at least some of these psychological effects, the fact is that only a substantial minority develop overt mental illness; the majority appear to adjust well although they may take some time to do so. What factors determine who will show the most adverse reactions?

The strongest predictor for the development of an affective disorder is the presence of the psychological problems described above. Those with a *family history* of affective disorder, or a *past history*, are likely to be more vulnerable. Important aspects of the *pre-morbid personality* include the extent to which the subject has been able to adapt to previous stresses and to accept imperfections in herself: perfectionists tend to be more vulnerable.

Those who feel secure and have stable relationships are liable to maintain these and derive support, whereas those who tend to fear rejection will be more likely to isolate themselves and lack support.

A number of more immediate factors will also determine the nature of the response. Outward signs of disfigurement have a greater effect than when these are absent. The patient's knowledge of the likely outcome is also important: often uncertainty is more difficult to accept than a bad prognosis, although it is also important not to deny the patient some hope. Intercurrent problems, for example, with finance, work, and housing, or in relationships, will also add to the burden and increase the risk of a poor adjustment.

Management

RECOGNITION

The majority of mental illness occurring in patients following mutilating surgery is unrecognized by medical and nursing staff and most patients do not spontaneously bring their anxiety or depression to the attention of staff unless specifically asked. The management therefore requires awareness of the nature and frequency of these problems and their causes, and **active enquiry** by staff (preferably including routine screening) to identify those patients most in need of help.

It has been shown that staff in general wards reward those patients who 'keep smiling' (however inappropriately) by spending more time with them and view them more positively; patients who openly display negative feelings are more likely to be rejected by staff, and are placed in beds on the periphery of the ward or furthest from the nursing station.

RESPONSE

This should include the opportunity to *ventilate feelings* without rejection; if you also provide *clear and accurate information* it will help to reassure the patient. At all stages, but particularly early on, it is essential to ensure adequate *relief from pain*. Positive measures are essential to provide *counselling* regarding practical problems such as the management of a colostomy, the availability and use of prostheses, or the management of *sexual and work problems*. Where there is evidence of symptoms of an affective disorder this should be treated in the same way as a similar disorder arising in a person who is physically fit, except that serotonin re-uptake blockers such as fluoxetine or sertraline, or a noradrenaline re-uptake blocker such as lofepramine, appear to be better tolerated than tricyclics by patients on the general wards.

THE MANAGEMENT OF THE DYING

Many of the psychological problems and reactions that occur in those who have experienced malignant disease or mutilating surgery are also shared with the dying patient. The presence of these problems, and also of affective disorders, requires awareness by staff and active measures for management, in much the same way. Isolation in a hospital side-room surrounded by an aura of denial from staff and family is likely to increase fear and sadness and result in an undignified end.

Not all of those who are approaching death are aware of it but awareness is much greater than is generally supposed. Several surveys of patients who were dying suggest that *at least 75 per cent are fully or partly aware that they are dying*. However, most of these do not talk to hospital staff about it and only about half share this knowledge with their spouse. Patients sometimes express a wish 'to discuss their situation more fully', although not necessarily with a doctor. The following are some of the more important factors to be considered in the management of the dying.

1. **Relief from distressing physical symptoms** and the patient's clear knowledge that pain relief will be available *when necessary*, and not given on a four-hourly regime (see p. 150).

2. **A relationship with a doctor** who can be trusted to share the patient's values regarding the balance between trying to maintain life and reaching a comfortable and dignified end.

3. Provision of **counselling to relatives** who may have difficulty in accepting the patient's impending death and seek inappropriate and distressing treatments for the patient. They will also require help to face the patient, and to deal with their own grief, both before and after the patient's death.

4. Ensuring that the patient can **maintain close personal ties** with relatives and friends in order to share companionship and interests, and sometimes also the distressing experiences of grief. Explore the possibility that the patient might be discharged home, if the relatives say that they can manage, and the patient does not need hospital treatment.

5. **Symptomatic relief from extreme anguish** is necessary and available using tranquillizers or sedatives, and treatment with anti-depressants should be based on the usual indications. However, avoid unnecessary and excessive sedation which may add to the patient's distress by cutting him off from contact with others and may also prevent him from active participation in religious rites that he regards as important. Also remember that not all patients fear death: much depends for example on age, religious beliefs, and the extent to which the patient feels he has accomplished his aims.

6. There are many factors that affect the decision as to **what and how much to tell a dying patient**. These can be dealt with only briefly here. However, you should be aware that there is increasing public opinion in favour of doctors providing patients with the maximum information about themselves. This does not mean that every

dying patient should be informed that he is dying or that a direct reply should invariably be given to such questions as *'I will get better, won't I?'* Much experience and tact is needed to deal with such questions sensitively depending on the needs of the patient and your knowledge of him. Even for the experienced it is usually best to avoid giving an immediate direct reply, although this may come later. Do not avoid the issue when a patient raises it but encourage him to talk about his knowledge of his condition and its likely outcome and what he has already been told. Often this will reveal that he is already aware of the truth and is some way towards accepting it; or conversely that he is at present denying the truth and wants you to share in this. The ultimate responsibility for the decision concerning what the patient should be told will, of course, rest with the consultant and general practitioner.

BEREAVEMENT

Immediately following the death of a close relative a person goes through several stages of a normal grief reaction.

Initially the person is in a state of shock during which although he knows intellectually that the person has died, he has not yet come to terms with it. He is able to function quite well while arranging the funeral and sorting out affairs. Others may notice that the person 'is taking it so well', but the person himself feels numb and may experience depersonalization. Others will have episodes of crying even in this stage, and panic attacks may be experienced. This stage of numbness and shock usually lasts between five and seven days.

It is followed by a realization of the loss with a sharp increase in affective symptoms. This acute grief lasts for four to twelve weeks and resolves during the next three months. The phenomena during this phase are:

1. Intense **pining** for the lost person, and **preoccupation with thoughts of the deceased**, accompanied by weeping. There is a tendency to concentrate on aspects of the environment associated with the lost person. A clear visual mental picture of the deceased is often retained and there may be dreams of the deceased. Initially the thoughts may be distressing, later they can be comforting.

2. **Illusions** are common and everyday household noises are misinterpreted as the deceased coming in or moving about. Shadows in the dark or strangers may be fleetingly misinterpreted as the deceased. **Visual or auditory pseudo-hallucinations** occur in which the person sees or hears the deceased. A sense of the *presence of the dead person* is common, which may be comforting. In abnormal grief reactions the sense of presence may be accompanied by talking to the dead person and preparing meals, etc., for him (see 'Denial', p. 59).

3. **Depressive illness.** A triad of depressed mood, disturbed sleep, and weeping is seen in over 50 per cent of bereaved people. Other symptoms, such as anorexia, weight loss, tiredness, indecisiveness, anxiety, lack of interest and concentration, a

sense of futility, and guilty feelings also occur, so that many bereaved people will satisfy the diagnostic criteria for depressive illness (see p. 195).

4. **Somatic symptoms of anxiety** may predominate and severely distressed mourners may even express suicidal ideas because life seems hopeless without the deceased; they feel **guilty** about not having done more to prevent the death and may wish to join the dead person. The consultation rate for depressive or somatic symptoms of middle-aged widows increases three times in the six months following the bereavement. The somatic symptoms are sometimes similar to those experienced by the dead person.

5. The bereaved person may be **restless,** pacing the house and unable to settle. Withdrawal from social contacts occurs and consolation may be rejected. The bereaved person sometimes **searches** for the deceased, by making frequent visits to the cemetery and even calling out to him. She may constantly gaze at photographs of the dead person.

6. Feelings of **hostility** may be directed at other family members, God, or the doctor 'who let my [husband] die'.

All these phenomena should have largely subsided by six months after the death.

ATYPICAL GRIEF REACTIONS

These are commoner in women than men. They can be prolonged – an initial stage of numbness lasts more than two weeks and the whole grief reaction lasts over one year. It is also more severe, with *marked social withdrawal, inability to work, and suicidal acts.*

Persisting difficulty accepting the loss, *guilt* feelings, and *hostility* are severe. *Hypochondriacal symptoms* similar to those experienced by the deceased may occur.

Suicidal risk is raised two and a half times during the year following bereavement, with special risk at the *anniversary* of the death. Death from physical illness is also raised during the six months after bereavement, notably from cardiovascular disease.

Other forms of atypical grief include *delayed grief,* where the individual functions normally for a while, and then has a grief reaction; *denial of grief,* where the individual never appears to experience a grief reaction, but perhaps presents with otherwise inexplicable somatic symptoms much later. A psychotic form of denial was described on p. 59.

Atypical grief is more likely to occur when:

1. The death has been sudden and unexpected.
2. The person has been unable to view the body of the deceased, or to express appropriate grief at an early stage.
3. There was an ambivalent or hostile relationship with the deceased.
4. The loss involves a fully grown child.

5. The person experienced loss of their own parent as a child.

6. There are few relatives or other social supports.

ASSESSMENT AND MANAGEMENT

The aim of **assessment** is to decide whether the patient has a normal or atypical grief reaction. If it is the former, what stage has been reached and is the reaction proceeding? If the reaction is atypical, why is this so, at which stage has the reaction halted, and has the person developed a depressive illness? The presence of suicidal ideas must be assessed.

Management of those with an atypical grief reaction involves a special form of psychotherapy in which the person is guided through the remaining stages of grief. The patient brings photographs or belongings of the dead person and talks about the person. The patient is thus confronted with the reality of the loss and the emotional expression of grief is facilitated. *Anti-depressants* are prescribed if there is a depressive illness.

Grieving usually terminates naturally, but the patient may need encouragement to regain his former activities, or even start new ones, to combat loneliness and preoccupation with loss.

PSYCHIATRIC EMERGENCIES

This section is concerned with patients who present with violence or other disturbed behaviour and suicidal threats or acts. Although speedy action may be required, don't forget to use the usual format of history followed by examination to reach a diagnosis. In the accident and emergency department there is usually a relative or at least a policeman with the patient if they are unable to give you a proper history; the nurses can give you valuable information on the general wards. Psychiatric emergencies present more commonly in the accident and emergency department than in the general wards, where they may be preventable.

Assessment and management

Don't panic: remember that common things are common. In the general ward, a physically ill patient is most likely to have an acute brain syndrome; in the accident and emergency department, they are most likely to have a functional psychosis or an alcohol-related problem (including head injury!). If the patient is very disturbed, restless, noisy, and abusive you must first assess the risk of violence. It is preferable to approach the patient quietly, introduce yourself by name, and attempt to get the patient to talk to you. If you succeed in starting a conversation, ask the patient to sit down.

Any such approach must be made with **other staff in the background,** who will retire if the patient settles (tell them not to go too far away) but will come to your assistance if necessary.

As soon as calm prevails, you will need to consider the possible causes of disturbed behaviour, using the scheme shown in *Table 20.1.*

Table 20.1 *Emergency assessment of patients with disturbed or violent behaviour*

Has the patient clouding of consciousness?

Clouding	–	YES	–	acute brain syndrome – check for head injury; check pupils; careful physical examination to find cause; sedate with care . . .
Clouding	–	NO	–	*Does the patient appear psychotic?* (that is, show evidence of delusions or hallucinations)
Psychotic	–	YES	–	functional psychosis – check past history and attempt to identify features of schizophrenia or mania – consult psychiatrist. Avoid neuroleptics if possible. Sedate with diazepam and consider transfer to psychiatric ward
Psychotic	–	NO	–	*Does the patient have a mood disturbance?* elation; depression; anxiety; anger; despair *Is there evidence of intoxication?* alcohol; drugs

THE MANAGEMENT OF VIOLENT BEHAVIOUR

Since psychotic patients are usually frightened, try and be **non-threatening** in your approach: the presence of other staff nearby will often avert violence. You must **appear in control** (even if you don't feel it!). This is why it is best to have spoken, however briefly, to some other informant before you approach the patient.

The decision to sedate is crucial. You should **avoid sedation if you possibly can**, since it may make diagnosis of the cause of the patient's problems very much more difficult. However, if violence has already occurred or seems imminent despite your attempts to calm the situation, you may have no alternative. If it has to be done use **intramuscular chlorpromazine**, 50–100 mg depending on the patient's size; carry out the injection rapidly with plenty of male staff. The more staff you have, the less likely is it that anyone will get hurt. If you are fortunate enough to have four people assisting you, assign one to each limb of the patient. Be prepared to repeat the dose if necessary, after an appropriate interval.

If there is any question of epilepsy consider **haloperidol** or **paraldehyde** as alternatives. The former does not lower the convulsive threshold to the same extent that chlorpromazine does, and is the treatment of choice for acute brain syndrome. The latter is an unpleasant drug since it is both smelly and painful; but it is safe, will not suppress the symptoms of a psychotic illness, and is itself an anticonvulsant.

The advice of the duty psychiatrist is necessary at an early stage regarding both sedation and possible transfer to a psychiatric ward.

Dealing with angry patients

Angry patients demand attention in two situations:

1. One is the normal person who is **overwhelmed with an intolerable stress**, often a life-threatening disease. Crises of confidence between the renal dialysis patient and his medical attendants can present in this form, when in deep frustration the patient rips the drips from his arms and thrashes out at anyone who approaches.

2. The other kind of angry 'patient' is the **dissocial personality** (see p. 63) who not uncommonly presents to casualty threatening violence or suicide. He may just have had a row with his wife and may seek refuge in a hospital bed: he will often drop the talk of violence once his real need to find alternative accommodation is discussed.

In either case the important first step is to understand the situation, usually by gaining information from the ward staff or those who bring the patient to casualty. A dialogue regarding the real problem is likely to lead to a reduction in the patient's tension:

I can see that you're very angry. Would you like to tell me about it?

Listen carefully to what the patient has to say. If he complains about other members of staff, hear him out but do not take sides. If sedation is necessary, try to get the patient's prior agreement: always tell the patient what you are doing, and why.

SOME COMMON EMERGENCIES

You should be familiar with those conditions which might lead to a psychiatric emergency and see whether you can identify patients at risk beforehand:

Delirium (see p. 151)

The emergency will typically arise in the middle of the night, when the patient's hallucinatory experiences are most intense and disturbed behaviour ensues. Patients at risk are all those who have serious physical illness, but keep a special eye out for **drowsiness** and early signs of **clouding of consciousness** which are detectable during the day with careful examination. The nursing staff are likely to pick this up before you and they may be alerted to it by the patient's relatives, who notice that the patient is less alert at visiting time.

Take special note of the following:

1. The elderly patient on many drugs is especially at risk as are those who develop a chest infection.

2. The patient who has been a heavy drinker prior to admission (for example, for a hernia operation) may go into a withdrawal state, whose early signs of tremor, anxiety, and insomnia should be detected before delirium tremens develops.

3. The post-operative patient who is 'going off' represents a high risk. Take brisk action to correct electrolyte or acid-base disturbance, anaemia, or infection.

Treatment is of the delirium (see p. 156) but the patient who is up and pulling his drip out or trying to leave the hospital will require sedation as well as the special nursing care: **remember that *haloperidol* is the drug of choice.**

Functional psychoses

A relapse of schizophrenia or affective psychosis may occur while the patient is on a general ward as a result of the stress of the concurrent physical illness and its treatment. This is a good reason to ask about previous psychiatric as well as physical illness in your routine history-taking.

Any psychosis may present as disturbed behaviour especially if the patient experiences persecutory delusions. The mood disturbance of mania or depression should become clear if it is possible to engage the patient in conversation.

Treatment of the functional psychosis is along usual lines; but an early decision is needed, in consultation with the psychiatrist, regarding possible transfer to a psychiatric ward.

Panic attacks (see p. 190)

These can present as an emergency because the patient experiences sudden and intense fear (often of impending death) together with somatic symptoms of anxiety. The presence of medical personnel is often sufficiently reassuring to the patient.

Ask the patient what they are afraid is happenning. Ask them if they have ever felt like this before. Firmly tell the patient that what they are having is a panic attack, and that they are going to be all right quite soon. Reassure them about any irrational fears; if they have had them before remind them that they pass off naturally.

If this proves effective, advise the patient to tell themselves this if they have another attack in future – this is called 'self-talk'.

Rebreathing into a paper bag may help if hyperventilation is pronounced. A single dose of a benzodiazepine given orally or intravenously will bring the anxiety under control if other measures fail.

SUICIDE AND SELF-POISONING

The characteristics of those who successfully commit suicide and those who deliberately harm themselves without the intention of death may seem separate. The elderly man who takes himself to a lonely place with a lethal dose of barbiturates represents a different phenomenon from the young girl who impulsively takes a handful of tablets in front of her boyfriend in the context of a row. However, there is an area of overlap between these extremes.

Most of those who poison themselves have social problems, and many have psychiatric illnesses – usually affective illnesses. Most will have seen their doctors in the week preceding the episode, and may well have been given the tablets which have just been taken for an 'illness' that they do not even have.

Approximately 1 per cent of patients seen at hospital following an episode of self-poisoning eventually kill themselves, and this represents an increased risk of 100 times compared to the general population. Approximately half of successful suicides have previously deliberately harmed themselves.

The other problem is repetition. Such patients often cause great problems of management and they elicit resentment among those who try to help. Up to 20 per cent of self-poisoners seen at the hospital repeat the act within one year. The aims of assessment are therefore:

1. To identify those who are at greatest risk of suicide. The characteristics of these groups are given in *Table 20.2*.
2. To treat underlying disorders.

Evaluation of suicidal risk

Patients seen in casualty or admitted to the general wards who have taken an overdose or deliberately injured themselves may present acute problems of management.

When such a patient is seen in casualty there are two separate assessments to be made:

1. What is the severity of the physical damage resulting from the deliberate self-harm (or that is about to occur if the patient has ingested a drug whose adverse effects have not yet become apparent)?

Table 20.2 *Factors associated with increased suicidal risk*

Demographic and social
    Male
    Over forty-five years
    Separated, divorced, or widowed
    Social isolation
    Unemployment
    Recent bereavement

Medical
    Severe or chronic physical illness
    Depressive illness
    Alcoholism
    Anti-social personality disorder
    Previous episode of self-poisoning

2. What is the risk of further suicidal behaviour in this patient and what is the likelihood that he may successfully commit suicide? Risk factors are shown in *Table 20.3*.

INTERVIEWING

The **history from a relative** or other informant is especially important. If the patient is drowsy or in a coma, do this right away; otherwise after you have seen and examined the patient. This covers the same areas as the interview with the patient.

When **interviewing the patient** you need a quiet private place for the interview and to allocate a sensible amount of time for it. *Do not attempt to interview a patient drowsy after an overdose and expect to get a clear history.*

The patient is often an adolescent who is shy and reluctant to talk. She may be preoccupied with guilt about the episode of self-poisoning, still angry after a row (this anger can be displaced onto you!), or depressed and retarded. These will exercise your interview skills and may appear as apparent refusal to cooperate with you or refusal to see the psychiatrist. However, an assessment must be made and it is usually best to make this clear to the patient: be polite, but firm.

The **history** is taken in the usual way but the following are the points most directly related to assessment of suicidal risk:

1. **Detailed description of the episode of self-poisoning:**

   Objective:

   - Exactly what was taken, where and when, and was anyone else present? Were any precautions taken to avoid discovery?
   - Was there a **suicide note**? (If so, could you see it, please? The content may indicate increased or decreased risk.)
   - Was there any other act in anticipation of death?

Table 20.3 *Characteristics associated with repetition of self-poisoning*

Demographic and social
    Previous episode
    Not living with spouse
    Lower social class
    Unemployed
    Criminal record

Medical
    Alcohol and drug problems
    Previous psychiatric treatment
    Dissocial personality disorder
    Histrionic personality disorder
    Passive dependent personality

- Was action taken to alert potential helpers after taking the overdose?

Subjective:

- What was the patient's stated intent?
- What was the patient's **estimate of lethality** of the substances taken? (Even though you consider ten diazepam tablets relatively harmless the patient may have thought that dose would kill her: it is what the patient thinks that is important.)

2. Evidence of recent/current **psychiatric illness**, notably symptoms of depressive or psychotic illness.

3. Is there a **past history** of psychiatric illness or previous episodes of self-poisoning?

4. Is there any evidence of **alcohol or drug abuse**?

5. Recent **precipitating life event,** such as bereavement, redundancy, break-up of a close relationship. Are there job problems or unemployment, marital, family, or other interpersonal conflicts? Are there financial or other social difficulties?

6. Is there a **family history** of mental illness or self-poisoning? Does the patient **live alone**; if so, can he go and stay with someone for a while if necessary?

The **mental state examination** is performed in the usual way but evidence of depressed mood and continuing suicidal ideation is sought. Is the patient relieved or sorry to find himself still alive? The presence of psychotic phenomena and brief assessment of cognitive functioning are also important.

Now record your opinion about the whole episode. Why did the episode occur? What was the seriousness of suicidal intent? Who may continue to care for the patient?

> *Opinion: Self-poisoning with 10 'librium' tablets taken from mother's handbag following a row with boyfriend. Episode seems to have been demonstrative, and without real suicidal intent: told mother what she'd done almost at once; elder sister known to have taken 25 librium without ill effect. Discharge to care of mother.*

Does the patient need to be seen by a psychiatrist? Some hospitals have a policy that all self-poisoners are seen by a psychiatrist but this is gradually changing. Compare the above patient with this one:

> *Opinion: Self-poisoned with 50 aspirin, having hidden herself in garden shed. Increasing depression since death of husband last year, and pain from rheumatoid arthritis. Left note saying she could take no more, and disposing of her property. Discovered by son on chance visit to the house. Seems severely depressed with nihilistic ideas. She lives alone.*

It is necessary to make your assessment sufficiently detailed for a decision regarding discharge to be made if there is no continuing suicidal risk. Clearly, the last note should end with the words: 'Will psychiatrist please advise on further management?'

If in doubt, or if there is continued suicide risk, psychiatric illness, or the possibility that the patient may have to be compulsorily detained, it is essential to request advice from a more senior doctor on your own unit, or from a psychiatrist.

THE PATIENT WHO TRIES TO LEAVE BEFORE YOUR ASSESSMENT IS COMPLETE

If you have grounds for supposing that the patient may be a risk to themselves you may detain them with an Emergency Order. This requires agreement of the nearest relative or an approved social worker (see p. 331).

(See also *Table 21.1.*)

LONG-TERM MANAGEMENT

This will be determined by your senior colleagues, the social worker, and possibly the psychiatrist. The patient may be discharged to the care of the GP and local social services or other agency, in which case it is essential that you inform that person of the episode and the patient's discharge. This is best done by a phone call by either yourself, the ward sister, or the social worker, in addition to your letter.

The patient may be discharged with an appointment for the medical clinic. If this is to review social or psychological factors it is best done quickly (one or two weeks) or the patient may not attend.

Responsibility for the patient may be transferred to the psychiatrist. If this is transfer to a psychiatric ward it is usually straightforward. But if the patient is being discharged ensure that the appointment and any instructions regarding prescription are understood by the patient, psychiatrist, and GP before the patient leaves your ward. Do not prescribe potentially lethal drugs like tricyclic anti-depressants unless you have taken steps to reduce the risk of a repetition (see p. 201).

FURTHER READING

Blacher, R.S. (1987) *The Psychological Experience of Surgery.* New York: John Wiley.

Creed, F. and Pfeffer, J. (1982) *Medicine and Psychiatry: A Practical Approach.* London: Pitman Medical.

Hinton, J. (1967) *Dying.* Harmondsworth: Penguin.

Kubler-Ross, E. (1969) *On Death and Dying.* New York: Macmillan.

Parkes, C.M. (1986) *Bereavement.* 2nd edition. Harmondsworth: Penguin.

21 / LEGAL ASPECTS OF PSYCHIATRY

The law is now increasingly affecting the practice of medicine as a whole, but for many years there have been legal regulations about psychiatric work. The Mental Health Act (1983) controls the compulsory admission of patients to hospital, and there are legal principles which are vital in considering patients' fitness to appear in court, their responsibility for offences that they commit, their ability to make valid wills, and many other matters.

Most doctors will at some time in their working lives need to prepare a court report, perhaps in a case involving compensation for personal injuries, or to give evidence in court, most likely a coroner's court, or to deal with a disturbed patient who may require detention in hospital for treatment. Although forensic work is more frequent for those who take up psychiatry, some acquaintance with legal aspects of psychiatry is essential for all doctors who undertake clinical work.

FITNESS TO PLEAD

You cannot have a fair trial unless you are 'fit to plead', and for this you must:

1. Be aware of the charge against you – for example, that you are accused of burglary.
2. Know the difference between pleading guilty and not guilty.
3. Be able to follow the proceedings in court and challenge a juror (in practice, the solicitor or barrister for the defence does much of this).
4. Be able to advise lawyers about your defence, or to defend yourself.
5. Understand the verdict of the court – for example, 'Guilty and sentenced to six months in prison'.

However, let us suppose that you have been arrested and charged with burglary, but there is doubt as to whether you are fit to plead. A jury at a preliminary trial, at which evidence is given by two psychiatrists, one of whom is qualified under the Mental Health Act, decides if you are 'under disability'. If you are found fit to plead, a second trial takes place later, with a fresh jury, to determine whether you were guilty of the burglary. If, however, you are found to be 'under disability' (unfit to plead), usually a new jury will decide whether you really committed the burglary. They may acquit you, but if they are satisfied 'beyond reasonable doubt' that you did do it, the judge can order that you are detained in hospital for treatment, with or without a restriction order, or that you receive supervision community, or that you are absolutely discharged.

It is, however, good practice to delay the trial to allow treatment to take place first, with the aim of getting the defendant fit to plead. Permanent 'unfitness to plead' is usually due to severe mental handicap or to brain damage. If someone standing trial *refuses to speak* in court, there is a similar procedure to determine whether he or she is 'mute of malice' – which means keeping quiet to save your skin – or 'mute by visitation of God', which refers to muteness caused by mental illness. If muteness is caused by, for example, catatonic schizophrenia or psychotic depression, the individual is 'under disability', and is dealt with as if unfit to plead.

CRIMINAL RESPONSIBILITY

You cannot be convicted of most crimes in an English court unless two ancient Latin requirements are satisfied:

1. **Actus reus:** it must be proved that the offender did the illegal act (for example, stole some meat from a supermarket), and
2. **Mens rea:** it must be established that he did the act in a certain state of mind – with a guilty intent (for instance, that he took precautions to avoid being detected, and did not just absent-mindedly carry the meat out of the shop).

You may be exempted from criminal responsibility by:

1. **Mistake** – about the fact, or the situation; not about the law (for example, you buy stolen property in all innocence).
2. **Accident** – a child runs in front of your car and is seriously injured when you are driving with due care and attention, and within the speed limit.
3. **Duress** – with a gun in your back you are forced to open your employer's safe and hand over his money.
4. **Necessity** – killing in self-defence.
5. **Age** – you cannot be tried and punished for an offence, even if you have committed it, before you reach the age of ten. Between ten and fourteen you are *doli incapax*, and it has to be proved that you knew that what you did was wrong. By the age of twenty-one you become liable to the full rigours of the law.

6. **Drink and drugs** – to be acquitted you must be 'so drunk as to be incapable of forming an intent' (too drunk or drugged to be able to decide to offend). A habitual heavy drinker is usually expected to be able to forecast the deleterious effects of alcohol on himself, and should have decided to limit his drinking if he knows he may become violent after, say, eight pints of beer.

7. **Automatism** – post-epileptic automatism or confused behaviour in a hypogly-caemic state rarely provides a defence. (And if it succeeds, you are likely to be committed to a Special Hospital for a long time!)

8. **Insanity** – the **McNaughton Rules.** These state that a defendant must be 'labouring under such defect of reason due to disease of the mind, as not to know the nature and quality of the act, or, if he did know it, that he did not know he was doing wrong'. These are difficult conditions to satisfy. However, if you are so mad that you either do not know what you are doing, or do not know that it is wrong – then you will be found 'Not guilty by reason of insanity', and will be dealt with as 'under disability' with the same range of disposals as if you had been found 'unfit to plead'.

The **Homicide Act (1957)** allows a person to be convicted of manslaughter rather than murder if he 'is suffering from such abnormality of mind . . . as substantially impaired his mental responsibility' for the killing. (Abnormality of mind may include learning disability, mental illness, psychopathy, or head injury – although these conditions are described in legal rather than medical terms in the Act.)

Amnesia does not exempt you from criminal responsibility: forgetting the details of an offence, whether because of intoxication with alcohol, head injury, hysterical dissociation, or for other causes, is not a defence!

It is now government policy that, wherever possible, mentally disordered people should be 'diverted' from the criminal justice system and should instead receive care and treatment from the health and social services.

COURT REPORTS

These should be clear, free from jargon, and systematically set out using headings:

1. An **introduction** which states the evidence on which the report is based – the number of interviews you have had with the defendant, the documents that you have read, and the other professionals whom you have consulted.

2. A section giving the defendant's **background**, and stressing the psychiatric aspects. (In serious cases, a full **history** goes in here.)

3. A cautious comment on the **offence**, concentrating on the defendant's **mental state and circumstances** 'at the material time'.

4. A summary of his **mental state** at the time of your examination, with a clear indication of whether you consider him to be suffering from a psychiatric disorder.

5. A **conclusion**, which sums up what has gone before, and deals with questions of **criminal responsibility** and **fitness to plead** where these are relevant, and ends, if possible, with a **recommendation to the court** such as:

> *I therefore recommend that the Court considers dealing with the case by placing Mrs Smith on probation, with a condition of attending the City Hospital for treatment as an out-patient.*

APPEARING IN COURT

The doctor giving evidence in court should be formally dressed, should speak clearly and simply, avoiding or translating medical jargon, and should remember that he is trying to explain technicalities with which he is familiar to laypeople to whom they may be new. The English legal system is an *adversarial* one, so questions may be asked first by the side which has asked you to appear (for instance, the defence). This is known as the *examination in chief,* and is followed by *cross-examination* by the opposite side (for instance, the prosecution); and then *re-examination* by the original questioner.

The judge or magistrates may also question the witness. Remember that the truth will often lie somewhere between what is being put forward by the opposing sides, and that it is important not to be drawn by the questioning too far over to either the defence or the prosecution view, unless you whole-heartedly endorse that idea. Useful phrases are 'I cannot comment on that'; or 'I cannot go that far' – followed, if possible, by a restatement of your view.

THE MENTAL HEALTH ACT

Until the Mental Health Act (1959) almost all psychiatric in-patients were compulsorily detained. Since then the proportion has fallen progressively, so that now the vast majority are informal, with the same rights and freedoms as any other hospital patients. Only about 7 per cent are now compulsorily detained and there are restrictions on the powers of psychiatrists to treat them without their consent.

The Mental Health Act (1983) is like most Acts of Parliament in that it is a lengthy and forbidding document, and like other Acts its paragraphs are numbered. This leads to potentially confusing references to 'Section 37' or the 'Sectioning' for compulsory detention. It is preferable and more intelligible to refer to each section by name: to a 'Treatment Order' (rather than Section 3), to a 'Hospital Order' (rather than Section 37), and so on.

There are complex and varying conditions for the making and renewal of each detention order: an 'Assessment Order' (Section 2) and a 'Treatment Order' (Section 3) are used most often, and so examples of these will be given in what follows.

Assessment Order

An Assessment Order (Section 2) requires two medical recommendations, one from a qualified psychiatrist (approved under Section 12 of the Act) and one from another doctor, who may be the patient's general practitioner. The consent of the nearest relative – or an approved local authority social worker – is also needed (except for orders made by the courts or the Home Office). This kind of admission is used when a patient:

1. Is suffering from a mental disorder (the type need not be specified).
2. Is unwilling to be admitted to hospital.
3. But needs to be admitted *either for his own health* **or** *safety or for the protection of others*.

The wording 'health *or* safety' is important, since it means that if the patient has an illness that is a threat to health they may be detained. This allows the doctor a certain amount of latitude – compulsory powers are not confined to suicidal patients, or those whose clinical state is a threat to others.

The admission is for assessment, but this can be followed by treatment. It lasts up to twenty-eight days, and the patient may appeal within the first fourteen days to a *Mental Health Review Tribunal*. This is a small informal court with three members: a legally qualified president, an independent psychiatrist (in practice this means from another health district), and a lay person. The tribunal has the power to discharge the patient from the order, so that he could then decide to leave or to remain as a voluntary patient.

Treatment Order

If the patient needs to be kept in for longer than twenty-eight days a 'Treatment Order' (Section 3) can then be made, detaining them for up to six months. Because this order deprives the patient of liberty for much longer, there are more stringent requirements:

1. The patient's mental disorder must be specified as either *mental illness, severe mental impairment, mental impairment*, **or** *psychopathy*, and details of the disorder must also be given.
2. It must be *of a nature or degree which make it appropriate for him to receive treatment in a hospital*, and
3. Treatment cannot be provided unless he is detained.
4. In the case of the milder disorders (mental impairment and psychopathy) treatment must be likely to 'alleviate or prevent a deterioration of his condition'.

Tables 21.1 and 21.2 deal with commonly used compulsory admissions, with longer-term admissions (you must be sure to be well acquainted with these), and with orders involving courts.

The Mental Health Act Commission

The Mental Health Act Commission has about ninety members, including psychiatrists, psychologists, nurses, social workers, lawyers, and lay people. These are appointed by the Secretary of State for Health and Social Services for up to four years, and they have generally supervisory responsibilities for detained patients, including:

Table 21.1 *Compulsory emergency admission under the Mental Health Act (1983)*

Section number	description	signatures needed	patient in	maximum detention
4	Emergency Order	any doctor, nearest relative, or social worker	not specified	72 hours
5(2)	Admission Order	doctor-in-charge	hospital	72 hours
5(4)	Holding Order	qualified nurse	hospital	6 hours
136	admission by police	police constable	public place	72 hours

Table 21.2 *Longer-term admission under the Mental Health Act (1983)*

Section number	description	signatures needed	patient in	maximum detention
2	Assessment Order	two doctors (one approved); nearest relative or approved social worker	unspecified	28 days
3	Treatment Order	two doctors (one approved); nearest relative or approved social worker	unspecified	6 months renewable
37	Hospital Order	two doctors, magistrates or Crown Court	unspecified – but often in prison	6 months renewable
41	Restriction Order	Crown Court judge	unspecified	indefinite

1. Reviewing the **use of powers of detention**.
2. Interviewing and visiting detained patients and **investigating their complaints**.
3. Supervising **consent procedures**. (Detained patients can only be treated against their will in a serious emergency, of if an independent psychiatrist appointed by the Commission agrees.)
4. Preparing **Codes of Practice** on admission procedures and on the medical treatment of mentally disordered patients.

TESTAMENTARY CAPACITY

Any doctor may be asked to assess testamentary capacity, meaning the ability to make a valid will. A patient's general practitioner is much more likely to be asked to do this than a psychiatrist. If a patient is seriously ill, or even dying, he may decide to make a will, and may ask the doctor attending him to witness it. If the doctor does this he is said to have 'attested the will', and should have considered the patient to be of *sound disposing mind*. If the will is subsequently contested, he may have to answer questions in court about the patient's mental state.

Anyone over the age of eighteen who is not 'of unsound mind' can make a will. Mild dementia would be unlikely to affect a simple will, although it might invalidate a complex one. However, someone who is confused, forgetful, or even deluded may be able to draw up a will with legal assistance.

Having a *'sound disposing mind'* involves:

1. Knowing what property you own.
2. Knowing who has claims on it: you should know the names of your nearest relatives.
3. Being able to form a judgement on the relative strengths of these claims, without undue distortion due to mental abnormality.

FURTHER READING

Code of Practice (to 1983 Mental Health Act) (1990). London: HMSO.
Faulk, M. (1988) *Basic Forensic Psychiatry*. Oxford: Blackwell Scientific.
The Mental Health Act (1983) (1983). London: HMSO.
Review of Health and Social Services for Mentally Disordered Offenders and Others Requiring Similar Services. Final Summary Report. Chairman: Dr John Reed (1990). London: HMSO.

GLOSSARY

Acute dystonia consists of muscle spasms, often painful and alarming in appearance, which may have their onset within the first week of starting a neuroleptic drug. They may include spasms of the tongue, neck, back, and extrinsic ocular muscles (oculogyric crisis). They respond rapidly to anti-cholinergic anti-Parkinsonian drugs.

Agitation is a state of increased motility which accompanies tension and is seen in some depressed patients. It may take the form of poorly organized but purposeful activities such as cleaning, in which the patient starts the same activity frequently, becomes distracted, starts an alternative activity, and so on. There may be repetitive hand wringing leading to excoriation of skin, or head rubbing resulting in hair loss. Behaviour may be importunate. For example, a patient may knock at a door, start to ask a question, break off and walk away, only to repeat this behaviour each time the door is closed. The inexperienced commonly fail to recognize that such behaviour may be caused by agitation and use meaningless terms such as 'attention-seeking' or 'hysterical' to describe the patient. The degree of agitation is not directly related to the severity of subjective anxiety, and a retarded patient may also describe inner feelings of great tension.

Akathisia is a state of increased motility accompanied by a subjective feeling of restlessness and is an extra-pyramidal effect of neuroleptic drugs.

Akinesis is a reduction in motor activity particularly affecting muscles of facial expression, and accessory movements such as arm swinging when walking. It is a feature of Parkinsonism and is commonly drug-induced. Thus there is a particular risk of failing to differentiate this treatment side-effect from depressive retardation and of consequent inappropriate treatment.

Ambivalence. Refers to vacillation of motivation. Also used to mean vacillation between complying and refusing when asked to do something.

Approximate answers or 'answering past the point'. Replies to questions which are almost (but not) correct and imply a knowledge of the correct answer, for example: 'How many legs has a sheep?' 'Five.'

Automatism. A simple or complex motor act, often inappropriate to the circumstances (for example, undressing in a supermarket), carried out while apparently unaware of the environment and without conscious motivation. Associated with organic cerebral disorders, particularly epilepsy, and with dissociative disorder.

Blunting of affect is a disorder that may be seen in schizophrenia, particularly in those with a chronic disorder. The usual modulation of mood is lost, and the patient lacks warmth, but does not convey the lowering of affect seen in severely depressed patients.

Catatonic symptoms. A collective term for a variety of motor behaviours, including ambivalence, negativism, posturing, and waxy flexibility.

Compulsions are closely related to obsessions, but are repetitive acts rather than thoughts. They may be simple actions, such as repeated checking, for example to see whether a door is locked before going to bed, or there may be complex rituals involving sequences of actions, each of which the subject feels compelled to repeat for a 'magical' number of times. For example, a patient may feel compelled to wash his hands seven times to avoid contamination, then he thinks this must be repeated in case he touched the sink, which might have been contaminated, and so on. Sometimes, as with obsessions, there is an attempt to resist compulsive actions. However, some patients practise compulsive acts in order to relieve the distress caused by an obsessional thought. For example, compulsive hand washing may be welcomed and practised to avoid the obsessional idea of contamination. The patient knows the actions are his own and based on his own will, even though they distress him and he may struggle to avoid them. In this respect they differ from passivity phenomena, from which they must be distinguished.

Depersonalization is an unpleasant perception of change in mental functions or body image. The patient may no longer experience usual feelings towards others. Parts of his body may look unfamiliar, although correctly identified as his own. The experience may be accompanied by **derealization**, in which the external world seems altered and unfamiliar: the experience is unpleasant. Both can occur as isolated symptoms – especially due to fatigue – but they commonly accompany affective illnesses, or any other mental illness higher in the hierarchy.

Depressive delusions. Delusions of guilt, self-blame, poverty, infestation, and infection are associated with depression and reflect the low self-esteem and hopelessness for the future which are characteristic of that mood. Of course such ideas occur commonly in depressed patients without necessarily being delusional in quality. Nihilistic delusions are extreme variants in which the patient believes that he is losing his physical or mental functions due to disease, or that he is already dead. For example, a depressed patient insisted that his head was shrinking, that his forehead was growing smaller so that he no longer had a place to wear his glasses, and that this state would soon be incompatible with life.

Dissociative amnesia is differentiated from other memory defects by the characteristic loss of personal information, both recent and long term. For example, the patient is unable to remember his name and address or whether he has family, and fails to recognize close relatives. By contrast, he appears to have no difficulty in recognizing, naming, and using equally familiar objects, such as food and drink. Such profound and selective memory loss does not occur in other disorders.

Fugue. A disturbance of behaviour characterized by wandering, without conscious motivation, in a state of altered or diminished consciousness; subsequently there may be amnesia for the event. Associated with organic (including epileptic) and dissociative states.

Grandiose delusions include beliefs that the patient has special powers, is chosen by God, or has been sent to save the world. For example, following laminectomy a greengrocer believed he was in hospital because he was a famous neurosurgeon, was there to operate on the other patients, and that the staff were there to assist him. He strutted about the ward issuing imperious commands and held his hands as though 'scrubbed up'. Such beliefs are particularly likely to occur in manic patients, but are also found in schizophrenics and those with organic cerebral disorders.

Incongruous affect is a display of affect which is inappropriate to the patient's subjective mood state. For example, a patient may smile to himself briefly when describing a recent bereavement. Never assume that this is inappropriate, based on your own expectation of what the patient's mood should be. Ask the patient why he smiles. He may say he feels sad and does not know why he smiles, in which case this is probably an example of incongruous affect. However, he may say he was remembering an amusing incident at the funeral or thinking of the legacy he expects to receive. Inappropriate affect is a characteristic of schizophrenia.

Labile mood is when fluctuations occur in response to circumstances, but show rapid and excessive variation with loss of control. It is strongly suggestive of organic brain disease and may be a feature of dementia, but can also occur in histrionic personalities and in some manic-depressive illnesses.

Mannerisms. All people have certain mannerisms, which are habitual and meaningless movements, such as stroking the face or hair or clearing the throat, which tend to increase when they are tense. They imitate purposeful movements and can be brought under voluntary control.

Mutism is total absence of speech. It may occur as a feature of stupor in depressive illness, schizophrenia, or organic brain disease. Occasionally it may be a hysterical symptom. **Elective mutism** is seen mainly in disturbed children and is characterized by mutism which occurs in some settings but not in others. For example, the child may speak normally at home, but is mute at school.

Negativism. The response to a request which is the opposite to that which is required. Sometimes also used to mean failure to carry out a task.

Obsessions are repetitive thoughts which the subject feels are forced into his conscious mind against his wishes, that is, he feels compelled to have them. The nature of these thoughts is unpleasant and, therefore, he tries to resist having them. Both the thoughts and the attempt at resistance are associated with anxiety. An essential feature is that the patient knows these are his own thoughts, that is they originate in his own mind, even though their content is contrary to his own wishes. For example, the patient may find the idea forced into his thinking that his hands are contaminated by faeces, that he has failed to wash his hands properly, and that he may poison others for whom he is preparing food. It is also important to note that the idea is not a delusion: the patient is not convinced that his hands are contaminated, but fears that they might be and is unable to put this fear from his mind, although he may know intellectually that it is 'foolish'.

Over-activity becomes a problem when the actions are either inappropriate or not completed. Manic patients may display considerable energy, start many activities, but fail to complete them. **Loss of inhibition** may also lead them to inappropriate activities, such as spending sprees or sexual excesses.

Passivity. Delusions of passivity are included in the phenomena that characterize schizophrenia, which appear to be based on a breakdown of 'ego-boundaries', that is, the normal awareness of the boundaries between ourselves and other people in the world outside ourselves. Included are beliefs that one's body is under the control of other people or forces, that other people control one's thoughts, are able to place thoughts into or remove them from one's mind, can read each thought as it goes through one's mind, or that the thoughts in one's mind do not belong to oneself. These beliefs are extremely concrete, that is, that a thought can actually be taken out of one person's mind and placed in another mind. The subject may feel physically controlled, like a marionette. It is easy to identify such beliefs incorrectly by asking inaccurate questions.

Perplexity. A mood state of bewilderment, with uncertainty about the nature of immediate experience of the environment. The subject usually appears puzzled.

Phobias are fears of specific objects or situations which are not generally regarded as dangerous, such as spiders, mice, heights, or crowded or enclosed places. The phobic person will tend to avoid the feared situations, but will not always do so. It is crucial to the definition of a phobia that the subject is aware that the fear is irrational, because the object of fear is not dangerous. Thus it must be differentiated from a delusion. For example, an agoraphobic patient may be house-bound, but will know that there is nothing harmful outside the house. A patient with persecutory delusions may also fear to go out, but this is because he believes there is danger, for example a gunman waiting to kill him, and that it is, therefore, a sensible precaution to remain in the house.

Posturing. Used to refer to abnormal body posture. Manneristic posture is a stilted exaggeration of normal posture. Stereotyped posture is non-adaptive, rigidly maintained, and often uncomfortable.

Pressure of speech describes the rapid outpouring of ideas which is characteristic of mania. This is accompanied by an increase in the quantity of speech and often in the volume. It may be difficult to interrupt, to ask questions, or to direct a conversation successfully with a patient who shows this disorder. The continuity of thinking is often, but not necessarily, also affected.

Reference. Ideas (or delusions) of reference involve beliefs that events in the environment have special meaning for the subject and refer particularly to him. For example, the news reader on television mentions an epidemic of fever, and the patient knows that this is a message specially intended for him rather than others and that it is a warning to guard himself against infection; the patient hears laughter from a nearby room and is sure that people are laughing at him: a stranger on a bus is overheard saying 'He's gay' and the patient knows he is referring to him. Ideas of reference occur in a wide range of disorders, including depression, mania, and schizophrenia, and have little diagnostic specificity.

Retardation of movement involves delay in initiating movement, slowness in subsequent performance of the movement, and also a reduction in the total quantity of movement. It is usually accompanied by retardation of speech (see next entry) and is most commonly seen in depressive illness.

Retardation of speech is often associated with retardation of movement. It is characterized by delay in the initiation of speech, for example in response to a simple question, as well as by a slow rate of speech production. The volume of speech may be so low as to make it difficult to hear what is said. The quantity of speech may be greatly reduced. Retardation is usually symptomatic of depressive illness. Depressed patients who show retardation of speech do not usually experience slowness of thinking, but often describe their thoughts as being in a state of turmoil. The examination of the mental state of a retarded patient calls for great tolerance and patience on the part of the interviewer.

Secondary delusions. This refers to delusions which are secondary to some other abnormality, such as a hallucination. If you hear voices of spies planning to kill you, you may develop the belief that such plans exist! Other examples of secondary delusions would be those that can be understood in terms of abnormal emotion, or those which can be attributed to coarse brain disease, such as a cerebral tumour.

Stereotypies. Utterances or movements which are monotonously repeated, non-goal-directed, executed in a uniform way, and have no obvious significance for the subject, for example rocking to and fro on a chair, or endlessly repeating the same oath, or the same barking noises.

Stupor is characterized by total immobility, except for following movements of the eyes, and mutism. (Confirm by moving the patient's head yourself and seeing whether he moves his eyes to continue to fixate points in the visual field.) It can occur in depressive illness, in which it appears to be an extreme form of retardation. However, it can also be found as a catatonic feature of schizophrenia or due to organic cerebral disorders.

Tardive dyskinesia is a syndrome which may include many different rhythmic or jerking movements and tremors: these may be multiple, affecting most of the body, and are then disfiguring and extremely distressing. Most commonly they have their onset several months after the start of neuroleptic drugs. They are liable to become worse initially when the drug is stopped, and there is at present no reliable treatment.

Thought block is experienced by the patient as an interruption in the flow of thinking, so that thoughts are totally absent for a period of a few seconds. It is common in anxious people – for example, students during vivas. In psychotic illness the patient may suddenly go silent, for example in mid-sentence, look blankly, and then continue on the same or a different theme. It is important to ask the patient what he noticed during this interlude, and what he was thinking about. Often it emerges that he was distracted by other thoughts, sounds, and so on, rather than experiencing total absence of thoughts, in which case thought block did not occur. This phenomenon must also be differentiated from petit mal epilepsy. Thought block occurs in some schizophrenics and is often associated with secondary delusions of interference.

Thought broadcasting. The delusion that one's private thoughts are being made known to others, perhaps throughout the world.

Thought echo. The experience of thoughts being repeated or echoed with very little interval between the original and the echo.

Tics are sudden, involuntary twitchings of muscle groups often mimicking expressive movements and particularly involving the face, for example frowning or 'screwing up' the eyes. They occur commonly in children at times of tension and may persist into or emerge during adult life.

Torpor. A state of pathological drowsiness with a tendency to fall into a dreamless sleep.

Tremor at rest is a common feature of anxiety. Static tremor may also occur in Parkinsonism. All tremors, both static and intentioned (due to cerebellar disorders), are exacerbated by anxiety, and tremor in an anxious patient may, therefore, be due to an organic cerebral state in addition to the anxiety.

Twilight state. Conscious awareness is narrowed down to a few ideas and attitudes which dominate the subject's mind.

Volition is the state of energy and drive which directs our purposeful activity. Loss of volition is, therefore, a state of inertia in which a person fails to carry out necessary or usually enjoyable activities although the ability to carry them out is in other respects preserved. It is often difficult to assess during an interview.

Waxy flexibility. On moving parts of the patient's body into a new posture the examiner notes a plastic resistance, and the posture may subsequently be maintained.

INDEX

THE PSYCHIATRIC HISTORY

History of present condition

Duration, chronological development of symptoms, associated disability, systems review, treatment received.

Family history

Parents, siblings, listed in order: age, age and year of death, occupation, physical and mental health, relationships.

Personal history

Childhood experience: stability, separations.

School: duration and types, higher education, qualifications.

Sexual development: menarche, information, menopause.

Marriage(s): age, separations and other problems, sexual and other relationship; spouse, age, occupation, health.

Children: list names, age, health, problems.

Occupation: number of jobs, longest, problems, present employment.

Present social circumstances: housing, members of household, relationships, financial difficulties, friends.

(Forensic: trouble with police, charges, convictions, in chronological order.)

Past medical history: physical and psychiatric.

Pre-morbid personality

Interests, mood, friendships, alcohol, drugs.

THE MENTAL STATE

Appearance and behaviour

Description, level of consciousness; reaction to interviewer; motor activity, speed, quantity, posture, involuntary movements.

Speech

Speed, quantity, continuity.

Mood

Subjective account; observed mood – level, fluctuation, appropriateness; autonomic activity.

Thought content

Suicidal ideas, preoccupations, ruminations, abnormal beliefs.

Perception

Illusions, hallucinations, depersonalization.

Orientation

Time: hour, day, date. Place. Person.

Attention and concentration

Days of week backwards; months of year backwards; sevens from 100 (threes from 20).

Registration and short-term memory

Digit span.

Stanford-Binet sentence:

Dull intellect – 'Yesterday we went for a ride in our car along the road that crosses the bridge.'

Dull–average – 'The aeroplane made a careful landing in the space which had been prepared for it.'

Average – The red-headed woodpeckers made a terrible fuss as they tried to drive the young away from the nest.'

Superior – 'At the end of the week the newspapers published a complete account of the experiences of the great explorer.'

Name, address and flower: immediate, 2 minutes, 5 minutes.

Recent memory

Experiences in last few days: e.g. duration in hospital, television, news.

Remote memory

Past personal events, e.g. school, marriage. Six towns, five fruits, prime ministers.

Intelligence

Calculation; difference and similarity between a fence and wall; direction of wind; reading and writing.

Abstraction

Proverbs.

Insight and judgement

Ill? Nature, cause, treatment.

Interviewer's reaction to patient

THE CARD

This card contains screening tests for **alcohol problems and mood disorders**, and a reminder of the points to be covered in an assessment of **suicidal risk.**

It also contains the abbreviated **Newcastle scale** for assessing cerebral impairment in an elderly person, and a reminder of the points to be covered when assessing the **psychiatric history and mental state.**

You will find these tests useful on the general wards and in the accident room.

ISBN 0-415-10611-7 (hbk)
ISBN 0-415-10612-5 (pbk)

ASSESSMENT OF SUICIDAL RISK

1. **Recent self-poisoning (or injury)**
   Objective. What drugs were taken? How much? When? Where? Who else was there? Who did patient inform about it? Arrangements to avoid being found?
   Subjective. Patient's statement about purpose; knowledge concerning drugs taken; attitude to being alive now?

2. **Illnesses associated with increased risk**
   Does history and mental state examination suggest evidence of:
   depressive illness
   alcoholism, other addictions
   schizophrenia
   dementia
   epilepsy
   antisocial personality
   chronic, painful physical disease?
   What does patient say about suicidal thoughts and intentions **now**?

3. **Demographic and social data**
   Age, sex, social class, occupation, marital status.
   Social isolation.
   Unemployment.
   Bereavement.

REMEMBER: the best predictor of suicide is an episode of self-poisoning.

THE ABBREVIATED NEWCASTLE SCALE

	Score
1. Age (nearest year)	0/1
2. Time (nearest hour)	0/1
3. Address for recall at end of test – this should be repeated by the patient to ensure it has been heard correctly; you may repeat it until patient has it right: 42 West Street	
4. Year	0/1
5. Name of institution	0/1
6. Recognition of persons (if none available, omit question and score test out of 9)	0/1
7. Date of birth (day and month sufficient)	0/1
8. Years of Second World War	0/1
9. Name of monarch	0/1
10. Count backwards from 20 to 1	0/1

Score of 8 or less out of 10 (or 7 or less out of 9) suggests impairment.

TWO SHORT MOOD SCALES

A. Anxiety

1. Have you felt keyed-up, and on edge?
2. Have you been worrying a lot?
3. Have you been irritable?
4. Have you had difficulty relaxing?

(If 'YES' to any ONE of above, go on to:)

5. Have you been sleeping poorly?
6. Have you had headaches or neckaches or tightness in head?
7. Dizzy; trembly; sweating; diarrhoea; frequency; tingling, etc. (autonomic anxiety)?
8. Been worried about health?
9. Difficulty falling asleep?

D. Depression

1. Low energy?
2. Loss of interest?
3. Lost confidence in yourself?
4. Felt hopeless?

(If 'YES' to any ONE of above, go on to:)

5. Unable to concentrate?
6. Lost weight? (due to poor appetite)
7. Early waking?
8. Felt slowed up?
9. Felt worse in mornings?

1 point for each positive answer.
Add A-score; add D-score. Anxiety states usually score at least 4 on A; depressives at least 4 on D.

THE CAGE

C Have you ever felt you ought to CUT down on your drinking?

A Have people ANNOYED you by criticizing your drinking?

G Have you ever felt bad or GUILTY about your drinking?

E Have you ever had a drink first thing in the morning to steady your nerves or get rid of a hangover (EYE OPENER)?

If you get positive replies to any **TWO** of these questions, it is worth taking a proper 'drinking history'.